DOCUMENTATION
FOR PHYSICAL THERAPIST PRACTICE

A Clinical Decision Making Approach

JACQUELINE A. OSBORNE, PT, DPT, GCS, CEEAA

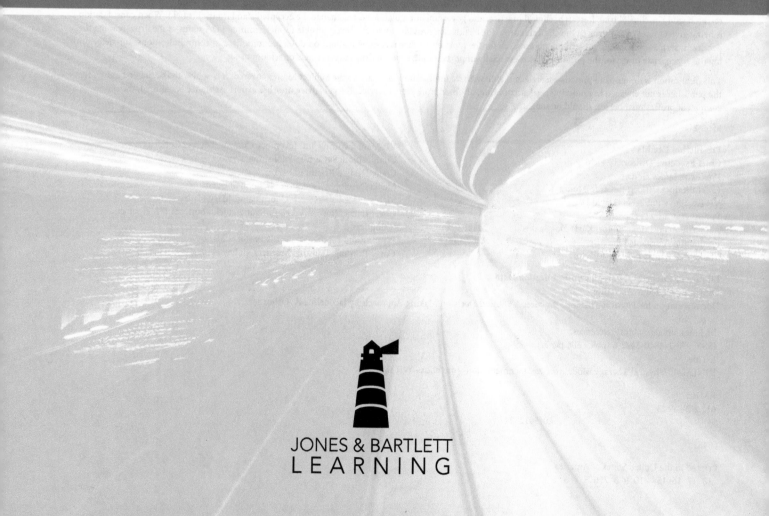

JONES & BARTLETT
LEARNING

World Headquarters
Jones & Bartlett Learning
5 Wall Street
Burlington, MA 01803
978-443-5000
info@jblearning.com
www.jblearning.com

Jones & Bartlett Learning books and products are available through most bookstores and online booksellers. To contact Jones & Bartlett Learning directly, call 800-832-0034, fax 978-443-8000, or visit our website, www.jblearning.com.

Substantial discounts on bulk quantities of Jones & Bartlett Learning publications are available to corporations, professional associations, and other qualified organizations. For details and specific discount information, contact the special sales department at Jones & Bartlett Learning via the above contact information or send an email to specialsales@jblearning.com.

8563-8

Production Credits
Chief Executive Officer: Ty Field
President: James Homer
Chief Product Officer: Eduardo Moura
VP, Executive Publisher: David D. Cella
Publisher: Cathy L. Esperti
Associate Acquisitions Editor: Kayla Dos Santos
Production Assistant: Talia Adry
Marketing Manager: Grace Richards

VP, Manufacturing and Inventory Control: Therese Connell
Composition: S4Carlisle Publishing Services
Cover Design: Kristin E. Parker
Media Development Editor: Shannon Sheehan
Rights & Media Research Coordinator: Mary Flatley
Cover Image: (top) © VikaSuh/Shutterstock, (bottom) © Melpomene/Shutterstock
Printing and Binding: Edwards Brothers Malloy
Cover Printing: Edwards Brothers Malloy

Library of Congress Cataloging-in-Publication Data
Osborne, Jacqueline A., author.
Documentation for Physical Therapist Practice: A Clinical Decision Making Approach/by Jacqueline A. Osborne.
    p. ; cm.
Includes bibliographical references.
ISBN 978-1-2840-3422-6 (pbk. : alk. paper)
I. Title.
[DNLM: 1. Physical Therapy Modalities. 2. Documentation—methods. WB 460]
RM705
615.8'2—dc23
                          2015012324

6048

Printed in the United States of America
18 17 16 15   10 9 8 7 6 5 4 3

Contents

SECTION II   Physical Therapy Documentation Content   47

SECTION III   **Critical Issues in Physical Therapy
Documentation**   **153**

Preface

I am a physical therapist with a passion for the physical therapy care of older adults. I am an educator in a post-professional residency program facilitating clinical expertise in my residents. I am a mentor who provides feedback to clinicians regarding clinical reasoning and decision-making at all levels of clinical care including documentation. I am also a clinician who documents. I have a great respect for what my documentation represents primarily because early in my career I was subpoenaed to be an expert witness in a court of law for an individual whose motives regarding her physical therapy care were questioned. As her physical therapist, my documentation was also questioned in an effort to gain insight into her claims of continued dysfunction and pain. When I learned that my presence was requested in a court of law and that I would be engaging in a conversation about my job, I could not think. Who was this patient again? Who was the third-party payer? Did I follow all the rules and regulations? Did I perform a thorough enough initial examination? Did I complete the re-examination on time? Were my interventions clearly described? Did I show that the care I delivered was necessary? Did I write what I was supposed to write?

It turns out, I did write what I was supposed to write. There were no issues identified that could implicate the care that I delivered to my patient or my license in anyway. But how was I to make sure that I write what I am supposed to write every single time I document? It seemed so daunting to try to create the content of my notes based on who I thought might read them. How was I to know that I would be defending my documentation to a lawyer in front of a judge more than a year after I wrote it? Thankfully, I didn't have to remember the patient or the clinical situation because as I reviewed the health record in preparation for my day in court, I realized I had documented my clinical reasoning. In other words,

my thought processes and justification for every decision I made were clarified by my documentation from my chosen tests and measures to the interventions included in my plan of care. It was my clinical reasoning that added value to my documentation. It was my clinical reasoning that validated my actions as a physical therapist. It was my clinical reasoning that preserved my license. I realized then what an asset my documentation was to me in my clinical practice and I have treated it as such ever since.

Documentation is the vehicle that validates your delivery of physical therapy services. You document to relay what happens with your patient or client during a clinical encounter. You document to communicate with other health care providers regarding the care of your patient or client. You document for the patient or client and for the patient or client's family members. You document to get paid and you document to keep your license. However, successful documentation is more than simply keeping a record of the patient or client's comings and goings in the form of a physical therapy plan of care. It is the justification of your clinical reasoning to others. The American Physical Therapy Association supports infusing clinical reasoning into your documentation and has adopted the position that documentation with focus primarily on clinical reasoning and decision-making should occur in the provision of physical therapy services.[1]

It is a goal of this text to help you deem documentation as essential an element of your daily practice as manual techniques and exercise prescription and to help you recognize that documentation is not an ancillary responsibility but is in fact an integral component of your practice that permeates the care you provide as a clinician. The efficiency, consistency and utility of your documentation will reflect its purpose as a tool that will support rather than hinder your clinical practice. It is important to realize that the content of successful documentation does not depend on the consumer of the note, the purpose of the documentation, or the payer source. In other words, successful documentation includes any information that the consumer needs to make a well informed decision, whether that consumer is you, a colleague, an internal auditor, an external auditor or a third-party payer.

Many barriers exist that derail intentions of producing successful documentation. Time constraints in the clinical setting usually mean shortcuts in documentation so that more time can be spent in direct patient or client care. Documenting within an electronic health record may present even further challenges to timely, meaningful and successful documentation. Individual clinic policies further confuse the issue of what should actually be included in the health record. Nonetheless, your professional responsibility as a provider of physical therapy services is to persevere under the influence of these barriers and recognize that the consequences of poor documentation can be severe.

An additional goal of this text is to provide practical guidance in using the terminology and framework developed by the American Physical Therapy Association and the World Health Organization to create successful documentation across all practice settings in patients and clients with any health condition regardless of the payer source. The intention is to illustrate how the common and standard language of The Guide to Physical Therapist Practice and the International Classification of Functioning, Disability, and Health (ICF) model can be integrated with a physical therapist's clinical reasoning process and a physical therapist assistant's skill set to produce successful documentation.

This text has 12 chapters divided into three sections.

○ **Section I: Utilizing a Clinical Reasoning Framework for Documentation** includes Chapters 1 and 2. These chapters present the framework used to facilitate a common documentation language among physical therapists and physical therapist assistants using terminology from The Guide, the APTA's documents on Defensible Documentation, and the WHO's ICF model.

○ **Section II: Physical Therapy Documentation Content** includes Chapters 3 – 7. These chapters investigate the explicit details of the content that belongs in initial examination notes, daily notes including intervention flow sheets, home exercise programs, re-examination notes, and conclusion of the episode of care summaries.

○ **Section III: Critical Issues in Physical Therapy Documentation** includes Chapters 8 – 12. Chapter 8 describes the relevance of the principles of measurement such as reliability, validity, and responsiveness to documentation. Chapter 9 illustrates how to document alternative forms of communications to other health care providers in the health record such a phone conversations, interactions that occur outside the context of a patient or client visit, and creating letters of medical necessity. Chapter 10 compares and contrasts paper-based documentation systems and electronic systems. Additionally, the relevant features of using electronic health records in documentation as well as recognizing the advantages and disadvantages of using electronic health records for documentation are introduced. Chapter 11 relays information about the current state of health care reform and its impact on physical therapy documentation. Finally, Chapter 12 demonstrates why sound documentation is vital should any interaction between a clinician and a patient or client come into question by the legal system.

Key Features

○ **Electronic Health Records** content are featured in each chapter to relay which concepts developed in that chapter may have special considerations in an electronic documentation system. This content is also intended to facilitate the notion that successful documentation is not determined by the system in which this information is stored or by the source from which physical therapy services are reimbursed.

○ **Learning Objectives** at the start of each chapter help focus learners on key concepts.

○ **Keywords** listed at the beginning of each chapter and defined in an end-of-book glossary provide learners with the vocabulary for successful documentation.

○ **Case Study Questions** and **Discussion Questions** are intended as opportunities for both students and practicing clinicians to apply the information from the text. These questions are designed to get readers to think about the decision-making that goes into creating successful documentation and to facilitate the identification of errors and shortcomings in documentation.

Instructor Resources

○ Answers to End of Chapter Questions provide instructors with tips and tricks in assessing students' responses to the **Discussion Questions** and **Case Study Questions**.
○ Robust **Test Bank** with Chapter Quizzes, Midterm, and Final.
○ Lecture Slides in PPT Format to aid instructors in teaching the content in their course's **Image Bank** of key elements in the text.

Audience

This text is intended for an audience with a range of experience levels and includes complex scenarios that clinicians may face at any level of clinical training or practice. Suggestions for introducing these scenarios to students who may not yet have access to patients or clients include creating opportunities for a student to shadow or interview a practicing clinician. Students on clinical affiliations could engage in discussions with clinical instructors. Additionally, the content of this text could be delivered directly before or concurrent with clinical experiences so that learning can be maximized with application.

Medicare

Specific billing scenarios related to Medicare beneficiaries are not relayed in this text because interpretation of billing rules and regulations by Medicare Administrative Contractors, entities who process Medicare claims, are extremely varied. Billing practices vary by practice setting and by which individuals (physical therapists, physical therapist assistants, students) are involved in the clinical scenario. It is paramount that a clinician be aware of the billing codes that can and cannot be reported together in order to avoid fraudulent billing practices. However, because of the complex nature of the law, this is one area of documentation that students and entry level clinicians will need to glean support from their colleagues in the settings in which they practice, resources available from the APTA, or the payer's themselves.

Abbreviations

It is recommended that abbreviations are used judiciously in physical therapy documentation.[2] Therefore, a specific list of recommended abbreviations are not provided in this text. Chapter 12 however includes details regarding error prone abbreviations as well as abbreviations that have dual meanings that may lead to medical errors. Additionally, the need to establish specific policies and procedures for the use of abbreviations in any one clinical practice is also reinforced.

Summary

My sincere hope is that the content presented in this book will serve as a valuable resource to guide you in creating consistently successful documentation. Remember, successful documentation includes common details that are present in *every* note, regardless of the note's consumer. When writing the content of a health record the author need not write for an intended audience. Rather, the author should write so that any one note could be used by multiple consumers for multiple reasons.

Acknowledgments

This work would not have been possible without the initial ideas and prompting from my friend and colleague Marilyn Moffett, PT, DPT, GCS, PhD(c) who contributed to Chapter 10 on electronic health records, or the invaluable contributions of Raine Osborne, PT, DPT, OCS, FAAOMPT who authored Chapter 8 on the Principles of Measurement in Documentation and, Sheila K. Nicolson, Esquire, PT, DPT, MBA, MA who authored Chapter 12 on Legal Considerations in Documentation. Most importantly I could not have attempted or completed this project without the companionship and support of my husband, Raine Osborne, who loves me enough to engage in ridiculous, philosophical arguments.

Jacqueline A. Osborne

References

1. American Physical Therapy Association (APTA). *Physical Therapy Documentation Reform*. Alexandria, VA: American Physical Therapy Association; June, 2013.

2. APTA. *Defensible Documentation General Documentation Guidelines*. Alexandria, VA: American Physical Therapy Association; 2012.

About the Author

Jacqueline A. Osborne, PT, DPT, GCS, CEEAA is the Director of the Geriatric Residency Program at Brooks Rehabilitation, a non-profit rehabilitation system in Jacksonville, Florida. In addition to this role, she maintains a clinical practice at Brooks Rehabilitation and serves the American Physical Therapy Association (APTA), the American Board of Physical Therapy Specialties (ABPTS), the American Board of Physical Therapy Residency and Fellowship Education (ABPTRFE), the Florida Physical Therapy Association (FPTA), and the Florida Injury Prevention Advisory Council (FIPAC) as a member of a variety of workgroups and taskforces.

Dr. Osborne received a Bachelor of Science degree in Business Administration with a concentration in Operations Management from the University of Delaware in 2000 and a Doctor of Physical Therapy Degree from Beaver College (now Arcadia University) in Glenside, Pennsylvania in 2003. She obtained Board Certification in the area of Geriatric Physical Therapy from the American Board of Physical Therapy Specialties in 2007. She also obtained the credential of Certified Exercise Expert for Aging Adults (CEEAA) from the Section on Geriatrics (now the Academy of Geriatric Physical Therapy) of the American Physical Therapy Association in 2012.

Dr. Osborne has a passion of for the care of older adults. She is an advocate for this group in many ways. One way that she works on behalf of older adults on routine basis, however, is through her clinical documentation. There is little more valuable than obtaining needed resources known to benefit patients or clients because of successful documentation! With this text, she hopes to share an approach to documentation rooted in clinical decision-making that will continuously serve as an adjunct to clinicians to advocate for patients and clients in clinical practice.

Contributors

Marilyn Moffett, PT, DPT, GCS, CEEAA, PhD(c)
  Assistant Professor of Physical Therapy
  Wingate University, Wingate, NC

Sheila K. Nicholson, Esq., DPT, MBA, MA, PT
  Quintairos, Prieto, Wood & Boyer, P.A. – Partner
  Tampa, FL

Raine Osborne, PT, DPT, OCS, FAAOMPT
  Brooks/University of North Florida Orthopedic
  Residency Program Coordinator,
  Brooks Institute of Higher Learning, Brooks
  Rehabilitation, Jacksonville, FL

Reviewers

Linda Csiza, PT, DSc, NCS
Assistant Professor, Assistant Director of
Clinical Education
Physical Therapy Department
Texas Woman's University
Fort Worth, TX

Regina Enwefa, PhD, CCC-SLP, ND
Professor
Speech Language Pathology Department
Southern University
Baton Rouge, LA

Kent E. Irwin, PT, MS, GCS
Assistant Professor & Co-Director of Clinical
Education
Physical Therapy Program
Midwestern University
Downers Grove, IL

Janet Konecne, PT, DPT, OCS, CSCS
Assistant Professor, Director of Clinical
Education
Department of Physical Therapy
Western University of Health Sciences
Pomona, CA

Sarah E. Luna, PT, DPT, GCS
Assistant Professor
Physical Therapy Department
University of the Incarnate Word
San Antonio, TX

Valerie Dong Olson, PT, PhD
Program Director
Physical Therapy Department
Dominican College
Orangeburg, NY

Jacqueline Randa, DPT, OCS, PhD(c), PT
Assistant Professor
Physical Therapy Department
Touro University
Nevada Henderson, NV

Linda J, Tsoumas, PT, MS, EdD
Dean and Professor of Physical Therapy
Physical Therapy Department
MCPHS University
Worcester, MA

Christopher Wilson, PT, DPT, GCS
Clinical Assistant Professor
Program in Physical Therapy
Oakland University
Rochester, MI

Nancy Wofford, PT, DPT, OCS, Cert MDT
Assistant Professor
Physical Therapy Department
Armstrong State University
Savannah, GA

Utilizing a Clinical Reasoning Framework for Documentation

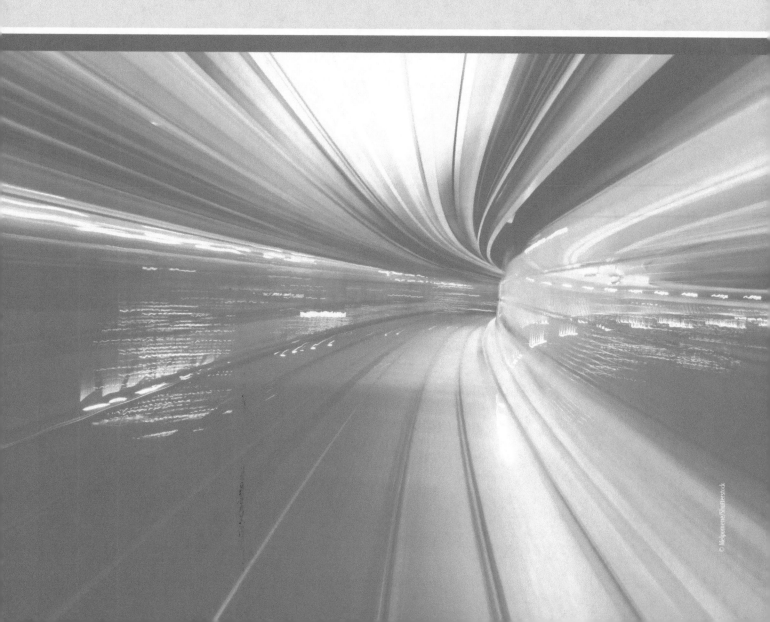

CHAPTER 1

Documentation: An Essential Element of Physical Therapist Practice

CHAPTER OBJECTIVES

1. Define "successful" documentation.
2. Define the purpose of documentation.
3. Recognize how clinical reasoning concepts can be applied to the development of successful documentation.
4. Recognize that a thorough clinical picture of a patient or client is generated through many entries

   into the health record starting with the initial examination and ending with the conclusion of the episode of care.
5. Recognize that proper documentation is imperative for the delivery of a comprehensive physical therapy plan of care regardless of the medium: paper-based or electronic.

KEY TERMS

Clinical decision making
Clinical reasoning
Electronic health record
Feedforward

Feedback
Reflection
Successful documentation

Introduction

Accepting documentation as an integral part of clinical practice is vital to the development of clinical expertise. This chapter is designed to relay the criteria that define **successful documentation**. Equally important is understanding who the users or consumers of your documentation are and the purposes for which your documentation might be used. This chapter also relays the importance of infusing your documentation with your clinical reasoning skills and self-reflecting on the documentation you create so that you consistently produce quality documentation that is meaningful to multiple users. In addition, this chapter introduces the idea that a complete clinical impression of a patient or client is developed through multiple interactions with the patient

or client by many healthcare providers. The quality of the account of each of these encounters will further enhance your clinical expertise and your ability to provide quality care to your patient or client. Lastly, this chapter develops the need to apply successful documentation regardless of the documentation medium: an electronic or a paper-based system.

Defining Successful Documentation

What is "good" documentation? If you were reviewing a physical therapist's or a physical therapist assistant's documentation, what characteristics would you look for?

What criteria would you use to judge the documentation as "good"? As a physical therapist or a physical therapist assistant reviewing a colleague's documentation, you might decide that it is "good" if the information you are looking for is included. Now consider that you are in charge of completing internal chart reviews for your company. Or, consider that you are a third-party payer reviewing documentation to determine reimbursement to the physical therapy provider for services rendered. Do your criteria change regarding what constitutes "good" documentation since the individual using the documentation changed? No. In fact, in all three scenarios the criteria are the same: "good" documentation contains the information that the consumer needs to make a sound decision. Consumers of physical therapy documentation are many and can be found listed in TABLE 1-1. Often there are multiple consumers of one clinical note, each of whom reviews it to make different decisions.

Critically reviewing documentation for content and actually creating "good" content requires two different skill sets. Conducting a documentation review to establish if documentation is in fact "good" is a feedback type of process, where you read and judge the content against some predetermined set of criteria to make a determination about outcomes. Refer to APPENDIX 1-A: American Physical Therapy Association (APTA) *Guidelines: Peer Review Training*.[1] In motor control, **feedback** is used to check the effectiveness of a response and allows for adaptation should the motor pattern generated be different from the actual planned movement.[2] Similarly, when you review a note, you are checking for specific details and making recommendations if you do not find what you are looking for. The criteria you utilize might be part of a formal internal quality assurance process or a more informal set of criteria that you impose as you attempt to extract the desired information. In contrast, creating "good" content is more of a feedforward process that requires you as the author to recognize what detail should be included in that content. A **feedforward** process in motor control allows an anticipatory response, one that is learned from the memory of past successful movements.[2] Hence, knowing the details that constitute "good" documentation will help to facilitate the formation of more "good" content.

If a feedforward framework is used to create documentation, then you will ensure that the content will not be based on the documentation's consumer. For example, a student should not modify his documentation based on the physical presence or absence of his clinical instructor. Likewise, a physical therapist or physical therapist assistant providing care to a Medicare beneficiary, an individual with private health insurance, or an individual who is paying cash should not document differently based on the different payer sources. Rather than tailor your physical therapy documentation to meet the needs of the documentation's consumer, simply include the details required to make well-informed decisions. This is the criterion that defines "successful" documentation. In other words, the term "successful" documentation indicates that which includes all of the information that the consumer wants.

The patient or client health record is a product that has many potential consumers. Therefore, it must possess the utility necessary to meet the needs of each end user. If the end user is a physical therapist assistant, then the documentation must include the interventions that meet the goals outlined in the plan of care as well as any information such as precautions or contraindications that allows

TABLE 1-1 Documentation Consumers

Consumer	Purpose for Documentation Review
Physical therapist, physical therapist assistant, physical therapist aide, or physical therapy student colleague	Gather information needed to provide comprehensive physical therapy care to a patient or client.
Physical therapist supervisor	Internal audit.
Member of the patient or client healthcare team (referring or attending physician, surgeon, nurse, occupational therapy professionals, speech language pathologist, case manager, etc.)	Review patient or client progress or status, make further healthcare decisions.
Patient or client; family members of patient or client	Record keeping.
External consultation service	External audits and clinical reviews.
Third-party payer	Determine reimbursement for services rendered.
Legal system	Verify claims against a physical therapist for services rendered.

the physical therapist assistant to deliver care safely. If the end user of your documentation is the patient or client's referring physician, then details that relay the patient or client's progress with physical therapy should be included. If the end user of your documentation is a third-party payer, then objective data that substantiates the need for skilled physical therapy care is warranted. Third-party payers use daily notes and progress notes for example, to determine continued medical necessity, progress through the plan of care, and remaining deficits including impairments in body functions and structures, activity limitations, and participation restrictions that impact the daily functioning of a patient or client. Consider the following scenario.

You are working with a teenager who had an anterior cruciate ligament (ACL) reconstruction 8 weeks ago. The frequency of your plan of care is three times per week and the patient or client's goal is to participate in soccer tryouts in 6 months. The patient or client has achieved full flexion and extension active range of motion at the knee and the current focus is re-strengthening the vastus medialis oblique muscle. Towards the end of the session, the patient or client's father asks for a copy of the clinical note you just completed so that his daughter can take it to the appointment with her surgeon, which is in 45 minutes. Your note reads as follows:

> Patient states knee is doing fine. No problems with home exercises.
>
> See flow sheet. Added resisted hip abduction in standing.
>
> Patient tolerated treatment well.
>
> Continue plan of care.

Does this note meet the criteria for successful documentation? Does it contain the information you would want as the patient or client's father or patient or client's surgeon regarding the physical therapy care the patient or client is receiving? You could argue that you would have written your note differently had you known that the patient or client was to follow up with the surgeon that afternoon. However, remember that the content of consistently successful documentation does not depend on the note's consumer. This same note could be reviewed by a team internal to your practice for quality assurance or by a third-party payer to determine reimbursement to your facility for services you provided. Furthermore, this note could be reviewed by a legal team who is working to resolve a billing dispute or to address an inquiry or complaint from a patient or client regarding the physical therapy services he or she received.

Regardless of the note's consumer, every entry into the patient or client's health record should relay the journey through the plan of care from the initial examination to the conclusion of the episode of care summary. In other words, your documentation should tell a story with the end goal of providing the support for why skilled physical therapy services were warranted. In general, high-quality creative writing practice includes knowing your audience and tailoring the content so that the author can connect with the reader to relay a message. Applying this framework however to the documentation in a patient or client's record, a more technical form of writing, may lead you to mistakenly omit content that is vital to the entire clinical picture. With each entry into the patient or client's health record, you are building a case for why your patient or client should receive skilled physical therapy care. Perhaps a more complete note, one you would be proud to copy and give to the patient or client's father for the follow-up visit with the surgeon, might read as follows:

> Patient reports a 3/10 pain at the medial right knee joint line when performing transitional movements like turning or when rolling over in bed.
>
> See flow sheet. 8 weeks status post ACL reconstruction; vastus lateralis oblique exercises dosed for motor control (4 sets of 30). Reviewed lower extremity positioning during transitional movements. Added resisted standing hip abduction bilaterally dosed for increasing strength (3 sets of 10; 1 RM).
>
> Knee Active ROM = 0 to 126 degrees.
>
> No extensor lag noted during straight leg raise performed after session. Decreased stance time on right when ambulating clinic distances after session.
>
> Add treadmill walking with focus at terminal stance, no limp.

This note includes specific information regarding the patient or client's status, what was done during the treatment session including education to address the patient or client's pain complaint, an outcome measure (range of motion), the patient or client's response to the intervention provided that session, and the plan for the following session. While not a formal reassessment of all of the outcomes measured for this patient or client, a clear, succinct, and informative update is relayed. Furthermore, it is apparent from this note why physical therapy services are still warranted for this patient or client and that the care provided met or exceeded the standard of physical therapy care.

Defining the Purpose of Documentation

If successful documentation includes all the details necessary to make informed decisions, what then is the *purpose* of successful documentation? Take a moment to reflect on this question. Would you say that the purpose of successful documentation is to serve as the log of services you provide to a patient or client at a given time? Would you say that the purpose of successful documentation is to serve as a mechanism for you to communicate with the other healthcare providers involved in the health care of your patient or client? Would you say that the purpose of successful documentation is to serve as a legal representation of the care you delivered to a patient or client for optimal reimbursement from a third-party payer? What if the patient or client pays out of his or her pocket for the physical therapy services that you provide? Does the purpose of successful documentation now change? In fact, the purpose of successful documentation is multifaceted; however you need not be concerned with the exact purpose if you are consistently precise about the content. Knowing which details signify the content of successful documentation regardless of the consumer involves recognizing how to transfer your thoughts, and therefore your clinical reasoning processes, from your brain to the patient or client's health record. If your reasoning is clear then communication between you, the patient or client, and the rest of the patient or client's healthcare team will also be clear. Likewise, anyone who accesses your note would be able to extract the content they seek to make a sound decision.

Clinical Reasoning and Self-Reflection in Documentation

Clinical decision making is a deliberate and dynamic process used by clinicians to synthesize data collected from an encounter with the patient or client.[3] It requires an ability to integrate knowledge and technical skill when making decisions about a patient or client's care.[4] **Clinical reasoning** is the framework that supports why you have made these decisions and ultimately, why you do what you do with each patient or client. It includes knowledge of evidence in practice, but also the cognitive process of reflection to achieve successful outcomes in patient or client care.[4] It stands to reason that as long as you have a firm, evidence-based rationale for why you chose a certain clinical test and measure, outcome measure, or intervention for a patient or client, then your actions based on this reasoning are justified. Furthermore, your execution of the patient or client's plan of care is guided by this rationale and exemplary care is offered. If your reasoning is reflected in your documentation, you or your employer will likely be reimbursed for the physical therapy services you provide, and potential inquiries by the legal system will not evolve into threats to your professional license.

Expert clinicians continuously challenge their knowledge base by constantly reflecting on the clinical decisions made in patient or client care. Characteristics shared by expert clinicians include clinical reasoning that is centered on the individual patient or client and that is further enhanced by a strong knowledge base, skills in differential diagnosis, and the ability to engage in self-reflection.[5] **Reflection** involves allowing future behavior to be guided by a systematic and critical analysis of past actions and their consequences.[6] Self–reflection is being able to self-direct this developmental process for proficiency in clinical practice. Wainwright and colleagues report that a specific skill set is required for effective self-reflection (TABLE 1-2). These skills include self-awareness, description, critical analysis, synthesis, and evaluation. Consider the following scenario.

> Your patient or client is a 71-year-old female who was referred to outpatient physical therapy for knee pain. You start the initial examination 15 minutes late because the patient or client got lost on the way to the clinic. She also required some assistance completing the Western Ontario and McMaster Universities Osteoarthritis Index (WOMAC), a self-report questionnaire. You decide to begin your examination using the items from the WOMAC as a guide. You ask her to stand and she does not. When you repeat your request, she stands and starts to walk across the room. You decide to allow her to continue so that you can

TABLE 1-2 Skills Needed for Reflection

Skill	Description
Self-Awareness	The ability to assess how the situation has affected the person and how the person has affected the situation
Description	The ability to recognize and recall salient events
Critical Analysis	The ability to examine, identify, and challenge assumptions, and imagine and explore alternatives
Synthesis	The ability to integrate new knowledge with existing knowledge to solve problems and make predictions
Evaluation	The ability to make judgments about the value of something

Reprinted from Novice and Experienced Physical Therapist Clinicians: A Comparison of How Reflection is Used to Inform the Clinical Decision-Making Process by Sunsan Wainwright, PHYS THER. 2010; 90:75-88. http://ptjournal.apta.org/content/90/1/75, with permission of the American Physical Therapy Association. © 2010 American Physical Therapy Association.

observe her gait pattern. You proceed with other tests and measures and end the session prescribing a home exercise program to improve her knee extension range of motion. She has a difficult time understanding your instructions for the exercise so you decide to try schedule her next appointment the following day so that you can get started on intervention right away.

After an interaction such as this, what is your impression of the patient or client's behavior? Completely answering this question requires reflection on the interaction. For example, you could assume that your patient or client has cognitive impairments based on the fact that she arrived 15 minutes late to the appointment, required assistance to fill out a self-report outcome measure, misunderstood your directions during the examination, and had difficulty executing an exercise you prescribed. However, making a judgment regarding cognitive status based on her behavior is an inappropriate assessment strategy. Since you did not assess her cognition, you cannot make this assertion. An alternative approach to formulating your impression based on your observations alone includes utilizing self-reflection to determine if alternative solutions exist that explain the behaviors you observed (TABLE 1-3).

Creating successful documentation is as important a skill as perfecting your hand placement for a manual technique or appropriately prescribing exercise. Therefore, reflecting on your documentation to extract content and examine the context can serve to improve your ability to successfully document. One does not become an Olympian without taking the time to train and practice. Likewise, you will not become a proficient documenter if you do not take time to review your work. Therefore, the concept of reflection can be applied to documentation to improve the content of the patient or client's health record so that you can rely on it as an adjunctive tool to your

TABLE 1-3 Results of Clinical Reflection

Consider that events may have occurred prior to the patient or client's arrival at the clinic that may have affected her behavior.
- Never had physical therapy before and is nervous about the encounter.
- Had a poor previous experience in physical therapy.
- First time in an unfamiliar location.
- Disturbing phone call with family member prior to entering the clinic.
- Presence of comorbid conditions not obvious from the external documentation you received.
- There was an error in the map and directions to the clinic that she received from the front office staff.

Consider that impairments exist in body structures and functions that you did not assess.
- Visual impairment kept patient or client from independently completing the self-report assessment tool.
- Hearing impairment kept patient or client from being able to follow verbal instructions.
- Cognitive impairments affected the patient or client's executive functions.

Consider that your communication style did not meet the patient or client's needs.
- You do not make eye contact or directly face your patient or client when speaking to her.
- Your voice volume was not adequate.
- Your verbal instructions were unclear.

clinical practice. In other words, the well-constructed health record serves not only as a tool you can use to accurately and precisely keep track of the plan of care you created for your patient or client, but also as a tool used by other consumers of your note. The APTA *Guidelines for Peer Review Training* (APPENDIX 1-A) indicate that

"... a physical therapist performing a peer review must have an understanding that documentation is a:

- Chronological record of the physical therapy provided.
- Legal medical document.

○ Means of communication with other healthcare providers.
○ Reflection of medical necessity.
○ Rationale for care.
○ Method to demonstrate outcomes.
○ Record of the effectiveness of intervention.
○ Means to support reimbursement."[1]

Consider inserting the word "self-review" for "peer review." It is important to apply the above definition of what documentation is to your documentation every time you create an entry into your patient or client's health record so that you are consistently precise about any given note's content. Recognizing what your documentation represents will help you to consistently identify relevant content.

Limited physical therapy research is available regarding the use of reflection to develop clinical expertise.[3,4,5,7–10] Furthermore, an area of study that has not been explored is the use of reflection to develop expertise in physical therapy documentation and linking this development to improved patient or client outcomes, higher reimbursement, decreased claims denials, and decreased litigation due to poor documentation. In the example above, engaging in a systematic reflective process regarding your interaction with your patient or client may reveal content that should be reflected in your documentation to support a longer episode of care, to support a referral to a different healthcare provider, or to support your rationale for the assessment and intervention choices you make. **TABLE 1-4** provides a list of questions to use when self-reflecting on the documentation you create.

TABLE 1-4   Questions for Self-Reflection on Documentation

○ What did you record regarding your patient or client's status?
○ Why did you choose to capture this information?
○ What gains did the patient or client make since the last session?
○ What are the patient or client's remaining deficits?
○ What did you do during your physical therapy session?
○ Why did you choose to perform these interventions?
○ What was the result of what you did with your patient or client during the session?
○ What did you accomplish with your patient or client?
○ What was the outcome of your session?
○ How did the patient or client respond to your interventions?
○ Why do you think these outcomes occurred?
○ What information did you use to formulate your clinical impression of the patient or client?
○ What is your plan for the next session?
○ Why did you choose this content for the next session?

Capturing the Whole Clinical Picture through Documentation

Consider that every aspect of your interaction with a patient or client generates a data point that you ultimately use when formulating your patient or client's plan of care. As you and your patient or client exchange initial greetings with each other, you immediately begin formulating what is likely the most appropriate communication level and style for that individual. The breadth and depth of data that you collect during your history and systems review support the development of a preliminary clinical impression of your patient or client's chief complaint. As you further examine your patient or client, you select tests and measures and outcome tools based on additional results from your examination. This process assists you in refining your clinical impression allowing you to develop an appropriate physical therapy diagnosis and prognosis, including the frequency and duration of the episode of care as well as an intervention plan. It is important to recognize that you develop judgments or opinions based on every interaction you have with your patient or client.

You have likely been taught to "document what you do." However, using this axiom as a guide for your documentation will fall short of helping you produce successful documentation. If you simply document what you do, you are omitting the patient or client's perception of their progress, the patient or client's response to your interventions, your clinical impression of your findings, and your plan for the next visit. In fact, documenting what you do is analogous to completing only the examination element of patient or client management, or only the objective portion of a daily physical therapy note. The APTA *Guide to Physical Therapist Practice* indicates that an examination occurs when a physical therapist "conducts a history, performs a systems review, and uses tests and measures to describe and/or quantify an individual's need for services."[11] During the examination, the physical therapist must also "determine if the individual would benefit from physical therapy, develop a plan of care, progress the plan of care based on the individual's response to intervention, and determine if a referral to or consultation with another provider is indicated."[11] The Guide also confirms that there are other essential components to patient or client management in addition to collecting data. Remember, the examination is but one of the five elements of patient or client

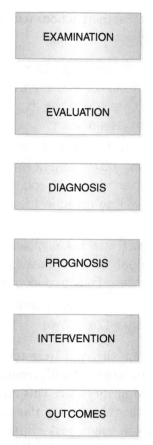

FIGURE 1-1 Elements of the Patient/Client Management Model.
Reprinted from the Interactive Guide to Physical Therapist Practice, online version; 2003, with permission of the American Physical Therapy Association. Available at http://guidetoptpractice.apta.org/content/1/SEC2.body. © 2003 American Physical Therapy Association.

management leading to optimal outcomes to physical therapy care (**FIGURE 1-1**).[11]

The online version of the APTA *Guide to Physical Therapist Practice* was developed to serve as an electronic resource to physical therapists and physical therapist assistants to help influence knowledge as research develops and examination and intervention strategies evolve.[11] The Guide was also developed as a resource to educate other healthcare professionals as well as the community about the physical therapy profession. Furthermore, the Guide lays a valuable foundation for successful documentation because it can be used to standardize terminology across practice settings to optimize communication within and about the profession.

The APTA's *Defensible Documentation for Patient/Client Management* also serves to promote consistently successful documentation. These guidelines exist to raise awareness among physical therapists and physical therapist assistants of documentation issues regarding legal, regulatory, and payer requirements as well as providing

tools including templates and tips for documenting medical necessity and evidence-based care.[12]

Along with documenting what you do, you may have also been taught that "if you didn't document it, you didn't do it." This axiom demonstrates the weight given to a patient or client's health record in that it serves as the legal representation of the services you actually provided. APTA's *Defensible Documentation* guidelines emphasize that appropriate documentation is crucial because it represents a physical therapist's and physical therapist assistant's responsibility to a patient or client and helps to ensure safety and quality in the delivery of services.[12] Ultimately when creating your documentation, it is important to become proficient at identifying the balance between too much documentation and not enough. Consider the following daily note.

> Mrs. A reports that she is noticing more and more mobility in her arm and is trying to use it more during her daily activities although she notes that she is still unable to reach the back of her head when washing her hair and is not able to reach across her body with her right arm to put on her seatbelt when in the driver's seat of the car. She reports a 6/10 pain by the end of the day in the lateral aspect of the right upper extremity to the elbow that is also interfering with her ability to get to sleep.
>
> See flow sheet for completed exercises. Added functional reaching tasks with emphasis on postural positioning of the cervical spine, glenohumeral joint, scapulothoracic joint and thoracic spine in standing, as well as an emphasis on motor control. When reaching overhead Mrs. A displayed limited right shoulder elevation to 110 degrees with approximately 5 cm of scapular elevation and 40 degrees of scapular upward rotation. Mrs. A demonstrated 30 degrees of a lateral trunk lean to the left with increased weight bearing through the left lower extremity and decreased weight bearing along with increased plantarflexion with the heel lifting off the ground on the right.
>
> Continue to improve motor control of the shoulder girdle and progress to a strengthening dose of the lower trapezius, middle trapezius, and rhomboid musculature as able.

What do you think about the level of detail in this note? Is there enough information to determine how to proceed with the next session? Is there enough detail to relay medical necessity and to show why physical therapy services are warranted? While the note appears to include the content necessary to appropriately and accurately support the services you provided, it also relays many other details that do not add value to the note. Now consider this note.

> Mrs. A reports improved mobility at the right shoulder; she continues to experience limitations reaching to don her seatbelt in her car and washing her hair. She reports a 6/10 pain in the lateral shoulder to elbow by the end of the day that limits her ability to fall asleep.
>
> See flow sheet. Added lateral functional reaching tasks with an emphasis on motor control.
>
> Mrs. A demonstrates poor scapular stability during lateral functional reaching tasks requiring moderate tactile cues for positioning.
>
> Isolate scapular depressors and adductors next session for improved static positioning and add functional reaching tasks as stability with straight plane movements improve.

What do you think about the level of detail in this note? This note appears to include relevant information in terms of relaying medical necessity and supporting the services you provided in a succinct and efficient way. Clinical circumstances regarding the safety of your patient or client may also warrant a certain level of detail in a daily note. Consider the following example of a daily note for your patient or client in the inpatient rehabilitation setting who is recovering from a fall that resulted in a concussion and a humeral fracture who also experiences tachycardia and shortness of breath during your session.

> Mr. B reports extreme fatigue.
>
> Appears to be short of breath; pulse rate fast but regular. Skin clammy.
>
> Unable to complete any exercise or functional training today due to fatigue.
>
> Continue plan of care as able.

Are there any details missing from the above note that would help to complete the clinical problem that this patient or client has experienced? You may have ultimately communicated with the rest of your patient or client's healthcare team and suspected that this individual was experiencing symptoms related to congestive heart failure; however if you did not record your patient or client's vital signs or communications you had on his behalf,

then it is assumed that these actions were not taken. Now consider this daily note.

> Mr. B reports increased fatigue and that when he woke this morning he did not feel rested. He reports that he felt unable to propel his wheelchair with his legs like you taught him yesterday.
>
> Baseline vital signs: BP rest = 145/89 mmHg; HR rest = 122 bpm; RR rest = 20 breaths per minute on room air; oxygen saturation = 98% on room air; skin appears clammy; no swelling noted in the lower extremities bilaterally.
>
> Exercise program was not completed today due to tachycardia and shortness of breath at rest. Consulted nursing staff to relay findings during session.
>
> Mr. B's therapies are on hold until results of further medical assessment are known.

This note relays that you were responsible for determining your patient or client's medical stability and that you practiced quality care. This note also includes the details that other members of this patient or client's healthcare team can use to make further clinical decisions regarding your patient or client's status and need for further assessment.

If your documentation were to come under review, from either a colleague following the care of your patient or client, a patient or client inquiring about his or her own plan of care, an internal audit conducted by your employer, or an external audit conducted by a third-party payer, you should be assured by the fact that your documentation is successful, meaning it relays to the consumer exactly the information needed. Consider that your documentation should be so succinctly complete that there is little need for clarification. Your colleague should not have to ask for a quick synopsis of the patient or client you initially examined prior to initiating care. Rather, a colleague should know that he or she can go to your initial examination documentation, as well as any follow-up notes or progress notes and identify exactly *why* that patient or client has sought physical therapy services, *what* he or she has been doing in physical therapy, *how* he or she has responded to date, *what* the plan is for that visit, and *where* he or she is in the journey through the current plan of care. Indeed it is beneficial to verbally confer or to conduct rounds with your colleagues regarding patient or client management. In fact, the purpose of conferencing on a patient or client's care is to relay the clinical reasoning and rationale used to support the organization of your plan of care. Opportunities may then exist for your colleagues to provide you with constructive feedback regarding this rationale to help you grow as a clinician. Unfortunately, however, what should be documented in writing regarding a patient or client's plan of care is often only shared verbally among colleagues. One shortcoming of this practice is that the treating physical therapist or physical therapist assistant is influenced by the verbal information being shared by other providers involved in the patient or client's care. The treating therapist or assistant then organizes thoughts and makes clinical decisions based on information that is not clearly represented in the health record. These clinical decisions are the product of the clinical reasoning process and should be captured in the health record. Consider the following scenario.

> You practice in a busy inpatient rehabilitation environment. You work with individuals who have suffered a neurological event such as a cerebrovascular accident or a cerebral aneurysm. You have already discussed and planned your schedule for the day with your occupational therapist, speech therapist, and therapy aide team members. A physical therapist from another team approaches you with a request to include one of her patients or clients on your schedule due to a conflict that she has to ensure that the patient or client receives her full amount of therapy allotted for the day. As you look at your schedule you see that you have a 30-minute window of time when you can provide care for this patient or client.

As the treating therapist or assistant you are now responsible for the safe delivery of care to the patient or client, which requires you to be aware of the plan of care including the patient or client's functional status, cognitive status, precautions or contraindications, comorbid conditions, and goals for therapy. In addition, you may want to know how the patient or client responded to the last physical therapy session. To gather this information you decide to review the patient or client's health record and find the following information from the initial examination:

> FIM transfers: moderate assistance × 1 via sliding board transfer
>
> FIM locomotion: 2 – maximum assistance (patient can perform 25% to 49% of task)

> Fugl-Meyer Assessment UE Motor Function Score: 10/66
>
> Fugl-Meyer Assessment LE Motor Function Score: 12/34
>
> Trunk Impairment Scale: 13/23
>
> Left neglect, left upper and lower extremity hemiparesis, aphasia; the patient is receiving IV fluids and has a PEG tube

The physical therapy daily note from the previous session reads:

> Required maximum assistance × 1 to stand in parallel bars for weight-bearing and pre-gait activities such as weight shifting.

After reviewing the health record you might decide that it would be beneficial to transfer the patient or client to the edge of the mat to work on sitting balance and to help her orient more to midline using visual and verbal cues. Based on the reported outcome measures and the goals established in the initial examination this appears to be an acceptable and beneficial way to spend 30 minutes of intervention with this patient or client. When you relay your ability to work with the patient or client, your colleague shares that the patient or client is very confused and became agitated when the team attempted to use the body weight support system for overground walking. During a session yesterday the patient or client was unable to consistently follow simple one-step commands and became agitated during a dependent transfer from her wheelchair to the bed. Your colleague adds that the patient or client has been difficult to work with since her admission 2 days ago and is not willing to participate in therapy.

Does your intervention plan for this patient or client change now that you are aware of additional information about her? If you were to listen only to a verbal account of the team's perception of the patient or client, you may formulate inaccurate opinions regarding the patient or client and make clinical decisions based on this information without fully assessing why the she became agitated. A more complete daily note from this patient or client's previous physical therapy session might include the following to reveal a more accurate clinical picture:

> Required maximum assistance × 1 to stand in parallel bars for weight-bearing and pre-gait activities such as weight shifting. Patient became agitated at attempt

to use body weight support system for pre-gait activities. Variable ability to follow one-step commands. Required a dependent transfer × 2 from wheelchair to bed at end of session.

Having access to this additional information during your review of the patient or client's health record might lead you to further investigate the change in the patient or client's transfer status from moderate assistance × 1 to dependent × 2. You might also decide to communicate with the patient or client's nurse regarding the patient or client's behavior at various points in the day. Perhaps further discussion would identify a need for a toileting schedule or a medication change, for example. You might also decide to conduct a brief cognitive screen to assess the patient or client's current ability to respond to your cues. Furthermore, you might decide to conduct her session in a more closed, private, and calm environment or take time to educate her further on the use of a body weight support system and how it can prepare her for walking. Essentially, the verbal information that was shared with you by your colleague may have generated further productive discussion regarding the care of the patient or client. Remember, that verbally conferencing about a patient or client should occur to complement your documentation and further develop your clinical reasoning that drives the choices you make in the delivery of physical therapy care to a patient or client.

Being responsible for a patient or client's care requires that you are an advocate for his or her health by documenting why the care he or she received was medically necessary. The APTA *Standards of Practice for Physical Therapy* state that

"The physical therapist of record is the therapist who assumes responsibility for patient/client management and is accountable for the coordination, continuation, and progression of the plan of care."[13]

Consider the following scenario.

You practice in an outpatient clinic and are filling in for a therapist who is out sick. There is a new patient or client on the schedule so you are to provide the initial examination for this individual to determine the physical therapy plan of care.

Even though another physical therapist will be working to carry out the plan of care you created for this patient

or client, you are considered the physical therapist of record unless your documentation explicitly indicates that you are transferring the care to another physical therapist. The *Standards of Practice for Physical Therapy* also state that

"The physical therapist of record is responsible for 'handoff' communication."[13]

Your documented plan of care might reflect this information as follows:

> John Doe will benefit from daily skilled physical therapy intervention to improve his ability to manage his wheelchair and to perform independently all of the activities required of him throughout a 6-hour school day including mobility, pressure relief, toileting, and lower extremity range of motion from a wheelchair level. The treating physical therapist will be different than the evaluating therapist, and therefore John Doe's physical therapy plan of care is being transferred to the treating therapist for any subsequent physical therapy management of this plan of care.

The detail in this note ensures that you are not only meeting the requirements of successful documentation by alerting the note's consumer of the actual circumstances surrounding this plan of care, but that you are also following the *Standards of Practice for Physical Therapy*.

Documentation in an Electronic Health Record

Documentation skills develop over time as experience mounts and self-reflection occurs regardless of the medium used to record it, written or electronic. You likely do not have the option of choosing your preferred documentation format, and therefore you must be comfortable successfully documenting in both formats. **Electronic health records** (EHRs) are not standardized and vary greatly across and within practice settings. However, what should not vary are the key elements utilized to create successful documentation (**TABLE 1-5**). Your clinical reasoning processes should not change when creating your documentation, but could however be influenced by some of the features of EHRs. For example, drop-down menus and pre-populated fields could halt your clinical reasoning process. Your ability to use a feedforward framework could also be compromised.

TABLE 1-5 Key Elements for Creating Successful Documentation

Transfer clinical reasoning processes from thoughts to medical record.
Use a feedforward framework.
Include details required to make well-informed decisions.
Provide support for why physical therapy services are needed.

For example, premade templates could guide your decisions and determine the flow of your encounter with a patient or client rather than be used as a means to quickly record collected data carefully selected for that individual. In addition, your ability to include all of the details you prefer to make well-informed decisions regarding the components of your plan of care may be constrained by the features of an electronic system such as character limits or areas that require selecting items from a list rather than an area available for free text. Alternatively, these elements of an EHR, such as drop-down menus, pre-populated fields, templates, and lists can serve to improve your documentation time, accuracy, and efficiency as long as you preserve your professional obligation to create meaningful and usable information. Overall, the ability to be a proactive documenter in an EHR rather than reactively entering data will afford you the ability to provide evidence that the physical therapy care you provided was medically necessary and of value to your patient or client.

Additional benefits of EHRs include facilitating communication within and among healthcare providers to ensure that a patient or client's health record is accessed and updated in real time for the most accurate information possible for sound clinical decision making. EHRs may also reduce medical errors and improve operational efficiency[14] thereby saving money. Recognize however, that the data input into an electronic system is only as good as its creator. For the contents of electronically written documentation to be usable by multiple consumers, the key elements of successful documentation must be at the foundation.

Summary

Creating successful documentation is a complex process that evolves over time and likely requires practice to ensure that all the necessary elements are included. For example, successful documentation involves the ability to accurately capture quality content including any elements that may be required from a regulatory standpoint in a time efficient manner. This text is designed to help you include the content that you need within every note to meet these objectives. As mentioned above, creating sound documentation is a skill that is just as important to your success as a physical therapist or physical therapist assistant as your manual skills or your ability to prescribe effective exercise for a given clinical scenario. To become refined, skills must be sharpened. Just as you create goals and collect outcome measures from which to gauge the success of your plan of care, so too should you have goals when striving to create successful documentation. These goals might include creating a process for critically reviewing your own documentation or the documentation of your peers with the intention of providing constructive feedback.

Capturing your clinical reasoning within the context of your documentation will ensure that the interaction you had with your patient or client was accurately represented. In other words, anyone who reads your note would know the details of the session and be able to make decisions based on this information. As you review a note that you created, remember to ask yourself why you included certain details of your note and determine if you omitted any details that you think may have been useful to include. Reflect on how you will change your documentation the next time you create a daily note or document the results of an initial encounter with your patient or client. Using a feedforward framework such as this to practice refining your documentation skills will help you identify gaps in your plan of care and ultimately help you to improve your expertise as a clinician. Another key element important for the creation of successful documentation is ensuring that the details required to make informed decisions are included. For example, you should be able to review your documentation and make decisions about various aspects of the plan of care including determining the prognosis, setting goals, and developing intervention strategies from the information you collated from each part of the examination. Furthermore, you should look at your documentation and be able to defend why your skilled services are necessary. If you are able to do this, then you have likely created successful documentation!

Discussion Questions

1. What is meant by the term *successful documentation*?
2. If you were to judge one's documentation as "good," what information would be included?
3. What is the purpose of documentation?
4. For whom should you document and why?
5. What is the difference between the concepts of feedforward and feedback? How can you use these concepts as frameworks for structuring clinical documentation?
6. Describe the skills helpful for engaging in critical reflection of documentation.
7. Take a few minutes to recall a clinical scenario where your patient or client had a successful outcome with physical therapy. Now retrieve your documentation for this patient or client. Based on what you reviewed in your documentation, reflect on the following:
   a. Why did your patient or client have a successful outcome with physical therapy?
   b. Does the history and systems review follow a logical sequence and structure?
   c. Can you determine why certain tests and measures and outcome measures were collected based on the information documented in the history and systems review?
   d. Is there a clear rationale obvious from the history, systems review, and physical examination that leads to the development of the clinical impression or diagnosis?
   e. Is there a clear rationale that leads to the prognosis?
   f. Is there a clear rationale that leads to the frequency and duration of the episode of care?
   g. Can you determine the rationale behind why each goal was written?
   h. Can you determine the rationale behind the inclusion of each intervention?
8. Take a few minutes to recall a clinical scenario where your patient or client had an unsuccessful or negative outcome with physical therapy. Now retrieve your documentation for this patient or client. Based on what you reviewed in your documentation, reflect on the following:
   a. Why did your patient or client have an unsuccessful or negative outcome with physical therapy?
   b. Does the history and systems review follow a logical sequence and structure?
   c. Can you determine why certain tests and measures and outcome measures were collected based on the information documented in the history and systems review?
   d. Is there a clear rationale obvious from the history, systems review, and physical examination that leads to the development of the clinical impression or diagnosis?

e. Is there a clear rationale that leads to the prognosis?
f. Is there a clear rationale that leads to the frequency and duration of the episode of care?
g. Can you determine the rationale behind why each goal was written?
h. Can you determine the rationale behind the inclusion of each intervention?
9. Choose a patient or client with whom you have recently had a follow-up physical therapy session. Reflect on the following questions:
   a. What did you record regarding your patient or client's status?
   b. Why did you choose to capture this information?
   c. What did you do during your physical therapy session?
   d. Why did you choose to perform these interventions?
   e. What was the result of what you did with your patient or client during the session?
   f. What did you accomplish with your patient or client?
   g. What was the outcome of your session?
   h. Why do you think these outcomes occurred?
   i. What information did you use to formulate your clinical impression of the patient or client?
   j. What is your plan for the next session?
   k. Why did you choose this content for the next session?
10. Gather your documentation from two of your patients or clients. Include all elements of patient or client management. Exchange documentation with two of your colleagues. Critically review the documentation and provide constructive feedback using the following guidelines:
    a. Does the history and systems review follow a logical sequence and structure?
    b. Can you determine why certain tests and measures and outcome measures were collected based on the information documented in the history and systems review?
    c. Is there a clear rationale obvious from the history, systems review, and physical examination that leads to the development of the clinical impression or diagnosis?
    d. Is there a clear rationale that leads to the prognosis?
    e. Is there a clear rationale that leads to the frequency and duration of the episode of care?
    f. Can you determine the rationale behind why each goal was written?
    g. Can you determine the rationale behind the inclusion of each intervention?
11. Ask your clinical instructor or one of your colleagues to access the health record for one of your patients

or clients and to develop an intervention plan after a 5-minute review of your documentation. Was he or she able to formulate a plan that was similar to your own? What information did he or she look for when creating this plan? Was there any information that he or she sought in developing this plan that could not be found? How can you use the information to improve your documentation?

12. Ask your colleague to review your documentation for one of your patients or clients, preferably a patient or client with whom he or she is not very familiar. Ask him or her to describe this patient or client to you based on what he or she read in your documentation. Is the description accurate? Does it match your description of this patient or client? Ask your colleague what information he or she used in the documentation to develop the clinical picture of your patient or client in his or her mind. How can you use this information to improve your documentation?

Case Study Questions

1. Assume that you work for a home health agency and are filling in for a therapist who is sick. You are to make a follow-up visit to an older adult who was discharged from the hospital 3 days ago after an open reduction internal fixation of an intertrochanteric fracture of the femur. You are reviewing the clinical note from the last visit and see that the patient or client's vital signs are within normal limits and that the patient or client reported a 6/10 pain at the lateral aspect of the right hip that is relieved with pain medication. You also see the following information:

   > Patient has no new complaints to report.
   >
   > Performed ankle pumps, resisted knee flexion and extension exercise, hip adduction squeezes. Gait not performed. Independent with transfers. Reviewed safe positioning for sleeping.
   >
   > Patient tolerated treatment well.
   >
   > Continue POC.

   a. Does this note meet the criteria for successful documentation? Why or why not?
   b. Does it contain the information you would want as the treating therapist?
   c. What would make this note more complete? Rewrite the note to reflect successful documentation.

2. You are working in a busy outpatient clinic. As you review your schedule for the day, you see that your 8:00AM patient or client is the new patient or client that you examined yesterday afternoon at the end of the day. Your plan was to finish documenting the plan of care for this new patient or client first thing in the morning; however when you arrived at work, you had to return a few e-mails and help organize a shipment of new equipment that arrived the evening before. You did not have time to complete your documentation prior to the patient or client's arrival for their first follow-up appointment.

   a. Should you initiate the first follow-up session without having completed the documentation from your initial encounter with the patient or client?
   b. What are the consequences, if any, of initiating this session? Of postponing the session?
   c. If you choose to treat your patient or client for the first follow-up session, how should you start this session? What information did you use to make this decision?
   d. What will you do to avoid this situation in the future? How will you implement this strategy?

3. Your patient or client is an 81-year-old male who suffered a myocardial infarction 8 days ago. He was admitted to the inpatient rehabilitation facility in which you work 3 days ago. You are the physical therapist who will be responsible for his physical therapy plan of care over the weekend. He has a 10-year history of diabetes and moderate-to-severe osteoarthritis at the left knee. His heart rate and blood pressure have been regulated with medication; however, he is having difficulty maintaining a steady blood oxygen saturation level on room air. You review the primary physical therapist's note from yesterday's session and find the following:

   > Patient reports that he gets short of breath when rolling in bed.
   >
   > Bed mobility activities performed (rolling and supine to sit) at bedside.
   >
   > Pt required minimum assistance × 1 with bed mobility activities.
   >
   > Continue to improve tolerance to functional activities.

   a. Does the information above meet the criteria for successful documentation? Why or why not?
   b. Develop one short-term and one long-term goal based on the information given in the above scenario. Provide a rationale for why you chose to

write your goals in this way. Are they functional, measurable, and objective?

c. Develop a 15-minute intervention session based on the information given in the above scenario. Provide a rationale for why you included this information in your intervention plan.

d. Was there any information that could have been included in the note above that may have helped you to better plan your intervention without having met the patient or client? Rewrite the note to reflect this detail.

4. Your patient or client is a 76-year-old female with severe osteoporosis. She was recently admitted to the skilled nursing facility where you work after a 3-week stay in an inpatient rehabilitation setting. She experienced spontaneous fractures of three ribs one of which punctured her lung 4 weeks ago. She has intermittent pain at her low back and hips that limits her ability to participate in tasks such as transfer and gait training.

At the end of your session, you recommend the use of an assistive device such as arm troughs on a walker to determine if this assistance improves her ability to transfer and ambulate short distances for increased independence with tasks such as getting to the bathroom. She responds to your suggestion that she does not want to use a walker and will not participate in physical therapy if you suggest she use one.

a. Imagine yourself in this situation. What is your immediate response to your patient or client's comment?

b. What is your impression of this patient or client's behavior? Use the skills required for self-reflection to generate an interpretation of the situation above.

c. Does your interpretation after critical self-reflection of this situation differ from your immediate response above?

d. How might you approach this patient at your next session?

References

1. American Physical Therapy Association (APTA). *Guidelines: Peer Review Training*. Alexandria, VA: American Physical Therapy Association; March 2005. Available at: www.apta.org/uploadedFiles/APTAorg/About_Us/Policies/BOD/Practice/PeerReviewTraining.pdf. Accessed on July 15, 2014.

2. Umphred DA. *Neurological Rehabilitation*. 4th ed. St. Louis: Mosby; 2001:141, 424

3. Wainwright SF, Shepard, KF, Harman LB, Stephens, J. Novice and experienced physical therapist clinicians: a comparison of how reflection is used to inform the clinical decision-making process. *Phys Ther*. 2010;90:75–88.

4. Atkinson HL, Nixon-Cave K. A tool for clinical reasoning using the international classification of functioning, disability, and health (ICF) framework and patient management model. *Phys Ther*. 2011;91:416–430.

5. Resnik L, Jensen GM. Using clinical outcomes to explore the theory of expert practice in physical therapy. *Phys Ther*. 2003;83:1090–1106.

6. Driessen E, van Tartwijk J, Dornan T. The self-critical doctor: helping students become more reflective. *BMJ*. 2008;336:827–830.

7. Hayward LM, Black LL, Mostrom E, Jensen GM, Ritzline PD, Perkins J. The first two years of practice: a longitudinal perspective on the learning and professional development of promising novice physical therapists. *Phys Ther*. 2013;93:369–383.

8. Black LL, Jensen GM, Mostrom E, Perkins J, Ritzline PD, Hayward L, Blackmer B. The first year of practice: an investigation of the professional learning and development of promising novice physical therapists. *Phys Ther*. 2010;90:1758–1773.

9. Greenfield B, Jensen GM. Understanding the lived experiences of patients: application of a phenomenological approach to ethics. *Phys Ther*. 2010;90:1185–1197.

10. Plack MM, Santaiser A. Reflective practice: a model for facilitating critical thinking skills within an integrative case study classroom experience. *J Phys Ther Edu*. 2004;18(1):4–12.

11. APTA. *Guide to Physical Therapist Practice* 3.0. Alexandria, VA: American Physical Therapy Association; 2014. Available at: guidetoptpractice.apta.org/. Accessed on July 15, 2014.

12. APTA. *Defensible Documentation*. Alexandria, VA: American Physical Therapy Association; last updated March 8, 2012. Available at: www.apta.org/Documentation/DefensibleDocumentation/. Accessed on July 15, 2014.

13. APTA. *Standards of Practice for Physical Therapy*. Alexandria, VA: American Physical Therapy Association; last updated October 1, 2013. Available at: www.apta.org/uploadedFiles/APTAorg/About_Us/Policies/Practice/StandardsPractice.pdf. Accessed on July 15, 2014.

14. APTA. *Support of Electronic Health Record in Physical Therapy*. Alexandria, VA: American Physical Therapy Association; last updated August 15, 2012. Available at: www.apta.org/uploadedFiles/APTAorg/About_Us/Policies/Practice/SupportEHR.pdf. Accessed on July 15, 2014.

Appendix 1-A

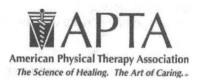

American Physical Therapy Association
The Science of Healing. The Art of Caring.

<u>GUIDELINES: PEER REVIEW TRAINING</u> BOD G03-05-15-40 [Amended BOD 03-04-17-41; BOD 03-01-14-50; BOD 03-99-15-48; Initial BOD 06-97-03-06] [Guideline]

I. Purpose

<u>Guidelines: Peer Review Training</u> provide direction to APTA chapters and sections, to physical therapy services, and to individual physical therapists who want to develop or pursue training in the peer review of the provision of physical therapy. These <u>Guidelines</u> are APTA-approved, nonbinding statements of advice intended to promote standardization both in the content of peer review training and in the performance of peer review. They also may be helpful as a tool for self-review. It is important to note, however, that these <u>Guidelines</u> do not provide the training itself.

Specifically, these <u>Guidelines</u>:
- Describe peer review.
- Delineate the underlying principles of peer review.
- Describe the content areas required for peer review training.
- Provide a framework for the training process.
- Provide a list of tools required both for peer review training and for the performance of peer review.

In addition to having the knowledge described in these <u>Guidelines</u>, a physical therapist providing external peer review services:
- Should be a licensed physical therapist, with no history of   license suspension or revocation.
- Should be a member of APTA.
- Should have current clinical expertise in the area of the review.
- Is recommended to have a minimum of 5 years of clinical experience.

II. Description of Peer Review

The purposes of peer review are to educate physical therapists to: (1) uphold professional standards, (2) be accountable to the public, and (3) be consistent in interactions with payers and managed care organizations. Peer review provides a framework to evaluate the quality, the medical necessity, and the appropriateness of the physical therapy provided. It can lead to identification of the need for corrective actions and can provide instructive feedback to practitioners.

Definitions

Claims review: Review of the billing record that may result in identification of issues that may require medical review.

Guidelines: APTA defines "guidelines" as a statement of advice.

Medical Review: Review of the medical record based on standards of practice in regard to medical necessity and appropriateness of care.

Peer: A person of the same profession who is like-licensed.

Peer review: A system by which peers with similar areas of expertise assess the quality of physical therapy provided, using accepted practice standards and guidelines.

    Internal: The process in which a physical therapist reviews the services provided by peers within a physical therapy service

    External: The process in which a physical therapists reviews physical therapy provided by a peer outside of the reviews physical therapy service a the request of a payer, a medical review organization, a professional organization, or a regulatory agency.

Utilization review: Utilization review is a system for reviewing the medial necessity, appropriateness, and reasonableness of services proposed or provided services to a patient or group of patients. This review is conducted on a prospective, concurrent, and/or retrospective basis to reduce the incidence of unnecessary and/or inappropriate provision of services. Utilization review is a process that has two primary purposes: to improve the quality of services (and patient outcomes) and to ensure the efficient expenditure of money.

Internal peer review and external peer review are based on the same principles and guiding documents (e.g., APTA's <u>Standards of Practice for Physical Therapy</u> and the Criteria, and the *Guide to Physical Therapist Practice*.) They differ, however, in the source of the request for the review, the party to whom the report is sent, and the final actions. Internal peer review may result in self-correction (by an individual physical therapist or physical therapy service), whereas external peer review may result in a reimbursement, provider status, licensure, accreditation, or credentialing decision. Internal peer review processes may include additional requirements that reflect the type of practice setting or the individual service's policies and procedures.

An internal peer review process may assist a physical therapy service with the following:

- Performing quality improvement review.
- Providing for continuing professional competence and growth.
- Assessing medical necessity, effectiveness of intervention, and patient/client outcomes.
- Identifying problems and possible corrective actions.
- Meeting the requirements of regulatory agencies.
- Preparing for credentialing (e.g., by managed care organizations) of an individual physical therapist or a physical therapy service.

An external peer review process may assist with the following:

- Determining (concurrently or retroactively) medical necessity and appropriateness of care for payers, managed care organizations, provider networks, and governmental agencies (e.g., agencies governing Medicaid and Medicare, state physical therapy licensing boards) that request a review of a physical therapist's performance or a physical therapy service's performance.
- Providing a quality assurance review.
- Determining fair and equitable levels of reimbursement.

III. <u>Training Content</u>

A. Principles of Peer Review

A physical therapist performing peer review must have a working knowledge of the following principles:

- A peer review process performed by a physical therapist assesses the physical therapy provided based on APTA's <u>Standards of Practice for Physical Therapy</u> and the Criteria; the *Guide to Physical Therapist Practice*; other core documents; and, when applicable, state laws and chapter documents.

Peer review of physical therapy services is provided only by physical therapists who possess an active license without current sanctions to practice physical therapy. This peer review shall be based on American Physical Therapy Association (APTA) <u>Standards of Practice for Physical Therapy</u> and other pertinent documents including state practice acts. APTA is opposed to any activities related to peer review that may adversely impact a physical therapist's plan of care or intervention without the involvement of a physical therapist peer reviewer. Adverse physical therapy patient/client management decisions made without the involvement of a physical therapist reviewer may constitute the unlawful practice of physical therapy. (<u>Peer Review of Physical Therapy Services</u>, House of Delegates Position).

- The peer review process is a quality improvement mechanism that applies to all physical therapists and to all patient management provided by physical therapists.
- The peer review process, both internal and external, is appropriate for use in a variety of physical therapy settings.
- APTA core documents, including the <u>Standards of Practice for Physical Therapy</u> and the Criteria and the <u>Guidelines: Physical Therapy Documentation of Patient/Client Management</u>, and the *Guide to Physical Therapist Practice* put forth minimal requirements for documentation and practice and apply to all physical therapy settings. The physical therapy service is encouraged to set optimal requirements to promote quality improvement in practice.

- The clinical expertise of the physical therapist providing the peer review should be commensurate with that of the physical therapist(s) whose services are being reviewed and have a minimum of 5 years of clinical experience.
- A physical therapist should apply the <u>Guidelines</u> and standards for peer review of the provision of physical therapy.
- Peer review must be performed with impartiality and objectivity.
- In the performance of peer review, as in other areas of practice, physical therapists are legally and ethically accountable for the services provided.

B. Documentation

A physical therapist performing peer review must have a working knowledge of physical therapy documentation as described by APTA's <u>Guidelines: Physical Therapy Documentation of Patient/Client Management</u>. Training should be based on the understanding that documentation is a:

- Chronological record of the physical therapy provided.
- Legal medical document.
- Means of communication with other health care providers.
- Reflection of medical necessity.
- Rationale for care.
- Method to demonstrate outcomes.
- Record of the effectiveness of intervention.
- Means to support reimbursement.

Documentation should reflect the critical thinking and sound professional judgment that are required for patient/client management. Documentation should show that the physical therapist integrates the five elements of patient/client care--examination, evaluation, diagnosis, prognosis, and intervention--in a manner designed to maximize a patient's/client's outcome. Training therefore should provide a working knowledge of the following:

- APTA's Core Documents including: <u>Standards of Practice for Physical Therapy</u> and the Criteria, <u>Guidelines: Physical Therapy Documentation of Patient/Client Management</u>, <u>Code of Ethics</u>, <u>Guide for Professional Conduct</u>, <u>Standards of Ethical Conduct for the Physical Therapist Assistant</u>, <u>Guide for Conduct of the Physical Therapist Assistant</u>, and <u>Professionalism in Physical Therapy: Core Values.</u>
- *Guide to Physical Therapist Practice*.
- Chapter guidelines, when applicable.
- Functional assessment tools and various types of outcomes and their relationship (or lack of relationship) to functioning.
- Literature-based (including evidence-based) practice and functional outcomes, including APTA's Hooked on Evidence database and preferred practice patterns in the *Guide to Physical Therapist Practice*.

C. Billing and Coding

A physical therapist performing peer review must have an understanding of billing, coding and confidentiality, including but not limited to diagnostic classification systems, current or applicable Current Procedural Terminology (CPT) and Relative Value Resource Based System (RVRBS) guidelines, current Medicare and Medicaid regulatory guidelines, The Health Insurance Portability and Accountability Act (HIPAA) or other accepted codes or guidelines used for billing.

Training should be based on the following principles:

- Documentation must substantiate the number and description of CPT or other accepted codes used for billing.
- Contracts may include specific exclusions or limitation of the services to be provided. Application and interpretation of contracts is the responsibility of the payer. Physical therapist

peer review addresses medical necessity and appropriateness of care, not contractual agreements.

- The party requesting peer review may ask the reviewer to comment on the fees associated with the services or codes billed. The peer reviewer may choose to make recommendations concerning appropriate payment based on his or her knowledge of (a) the value of the services and (b) standardized and accepted payment methodologies (e.g., RVRBS). It is not the peer reviewer's role, however, to determine actual payment for services.

D. Record Review

A physical therapist performing peer review must have a working knowledge of record review. Training should address each step of record review. These steps include:

1. Organize and record the documents that are provided.
2. Determine whether the documents are adequate for the purpose of peer review, and request additional information when necessary.
3. Review the claims made.
4. Match the record to the billings.
5. Review the medical record and assess it relative to identified standards, guidelines, state laws, and regulations, including Standards of Practice for Physical Therapy and the Criteria, and the *Guide to Physical Therapist Practice*. (A checklist may be useful in organizing the review process.)
6. Evaluate findings, answering such key questions as:
   a) Were services provided by appropriate personnel?
   b) Is there evidence of coordination and communication with other health care professionals as appropriate?
   c) Does the record reflect timely patient/client-related instruction, including a home program and education of patient/client, family, significant other, and caregiver?
   d) Is there measurable, sustainable, and functional progress toward defined goals and outcomes, with reference to ongoing discharge planning?
   e) Does the record reflect appropriate changes in patient/client management strategy? Is there evidence of critical thinking, professional judgment, and skilled interventions?
   f) Does the documentation link impairment, activity limitation, and participation restriction to predicted functional outcomes and the physical therapy plan of care?
   g) Is the billing supported by the documentation?
7. Develop conclusions and recommendations based on evaluation of the record using the established standards, guidelines, state laws, and regulations.
8. Answer any specific or additional questions that have been posed by the party requesting the review.

E. Report Writing

A physical therapist performing peer review must have a working knowledge of report writing. Training should address each item of a peer review report, including, but not limited to:
- Basic identification information for each file (e.g., patient/client ID #, claim #).
- The list of records and claims received by the peer reviewer.
- Documents on which the review is based (e.g., Standards of Practice for Physical Therapy and the Criteria, Guidelines: Physical Therapy Documentation of Patient/Client Management, the *Guide to Physical Therapist Practice*, and state practice act).
- The results of the claims review and the medical review.
- Conclusions.
- Recommendations.
- Answers to specific questions and concerns.

- A disclaimer indicating that the payer is ultimately responsible for the payment or the denial of the claim.
- Invoice, if appropriate.

Training also should encourage the physical therapist reviewer to:
- Substantiate the findings of peer review by quoting from the preamble of APTA's <u>Standards of Practice for Physical Therapy</u> and the Criteria: "These Standards are the profession's statement of conditions and performance that are essential for provision of high-quality physical therapy. The <u>Standards</u> provide a foundation for assessment of physical therapy practice."
- Be as specific as possible, quoting the medical record, APTA's <u>Standards of Practice for Physical Therapy</u> and the Criteria, the *Guide to Physical Therapist Practice*, and state statutes to support conclusions.
- Assess overall quality of the physical therapy provided, but be very specific in the report itself regarding whether the physical therapy provided meets APTA's <u>Standards of Practice for Physical Therapy</u> and the Criteria and therefore, criteria for medical necessity and appropriateness of care.
- Use language that reflects that recommendations are based only on medical necessity and appropriateness of care. (Recommendations should <u>not</u> indicate whether a claim should be paid.)

F. Claims Appeals

A physical therapist performing peer review must have a working knowledge of the claims appeals process of each payer and should encourage payers to develop an appeals process if one does not exist. Training should emphasize the following:
- When an appeals process is initiated, the peer reviewer may review additional information and write an addendum to the original report.
- The appeals process should include the option for the provider to receive a review by another peer reviewer if the provider and the original reviewer are unable to reach agreement.

G. Communication With Payers

Physical therapists performing peer review should use communication with payers as an opportunity to educate them about the appropriate utilization of physical therapy. Training should emphasize that, at a minimum, communication must convey the following principles:
- Professional guidelines and standards used in peer review can be appropriately applied only by a physical therapist.
- It is critical for the payer requesting the review to supply the entire record, including referral, when applicable; initial examination and evaluation; daily notes; progress reports; billings; and background information from other providers.
- The terms physical therapy and physiotherapy should be used only in reference to services that are provided by or under the direction and supervision of a licensed physical therapist/physiotherapist and, when so used, these terms are synonymous.

Training should also instruct physical therapists in how to do the following as part of the peer review process:
- In all communications regarding the role of the physical therapist and the scope of physical therapist practice, emphasize that physical therapy can be provided or directed only by physical therapists.
- Provide pertinent documents to educate payers about the scope of physical therapist practice and about appropriate utilization of physical therapy (e.g., APTA's *Guide to Physical Therapist Practice*, and APTA's <u>Guidelines: Physical Therapy Claims Review)</u>.
- Encourage or support an appropriate appeals process.
- Promote positive communication among payers, reviewers, and providers.

- Encourage payers to inform physical therapy providers of the peer review process.

H. Communication with Providers

Communication with providers should have an educational focus. Training should address the following:
- Different types of review (retrospective, concurrent, prospective) require different means of communication.
- Communication should be based on established guidelines and should direct providers to pertinent resources.
- All conclusions and recommendations should be based on available physical therapy documentation and established standards, guidelines, state laws, and regulations.

I. Marketing the Value of Peer Review

A physical therapist performing peer review must have a working knowledge of how to market the value of peer review to payers and providers. Training should instruct the physical therapist to base marketing efforts on the following:
- The value of peer review, including the value of established guidelines and nationally accepted professional standards as applied by a trained peer reviewer.
- The value of peer review in (a) ensuring adherence to professional standards, (b) promoting appropriate utilization outcomes through the education of physical therapists, and (c) ensuring accountability to the community for the quality of physical therapy provided.

Training also should emphasize:
- The importance of networking to develop relationships, using various marketing vehicles (e.g., telephone, visits, letters, brochures).
- The legal ramifications involved in marketing peer review services.

J. Ethical and Legal Issues

A physical therapist performing peer review must have a working knowledge of ethical and legal issues, including:
- State practice acts both for physical therapists and for non-physical therapists.
- Other state, jurisdiction, and federal rules, regulations, and statutes regarding (a) data privacy, (b) patient/client bill of rights, and (c) confidentiality.
- Facility policies and procedures regarding release of information.
- Reviewer's responsibility for obtaining liability protection coverage for performance of external reviews.
- Confidentiality in all matters related to the review process, with the understanding that the physical therapist reviewer should access information only when there is a need to know. Adherence to The Health Insurance Portability and Accountability Act (HIPAA).
- Potential conflicts of interest, which might skew the reviewer's judgment.
- APTA's Code of Ethics, Guide for Professional Conduct, Standards of Ethical Conduct for the Physical Therapist Assistant, and Guide for Conduct of the Physical Therapist Assistant.
- Antitrust laws.
- Peer review contract negotiation with insurers, including clarification of (a) whether the reviewer is masked to the provider, (b) insurer expectations, and, (c) reviewer payment guidelines (i.e., paid per review or per hour).

Additional considerations:
- The reviewer should request that the review be referred to another reviewer when that review is beyond his or her own clinical expertise and body of knowledge.
- The reviewer should understand the ethical and legal dimensions of the claims appeals process.

IV. Training Methods

Suggested methods of peer review training (which does not have to be limited to a workshop) may include any of the following:
- Lecture and audiovisual presentations.
- Use of a training manual.
- Presentation of case studies during instruction or as part of post-course assessment.
- Use of self-assessment tools.
- Assignment of pre-program readings.
- Testing on course content.
- Small group discussions.
- "Test" reviews conducted with mentors and as a member of a review team.
- Use of interreviewer reliability determination as part of ongoing training.

When instructors are utilized, the following is suggested:
- The instructor, or at least one instructor of a training team, should be an experienced physical therapist peer reviewer.
- Instructors must ensure confidentiality throughout all sensitive material, regardless of whether that material is presented verbally or in writing.

The effectiveness of training efforts can be assessed through determination of interreviewer reliability.

V. Recommended Resources

Training should incorporate resources that include, but are not limited to:
- APTA's Guide to Physical Therapist Practice.
- APTA's Hooked on Evidence database
- APTA's Core Documents:
  - Code of Ethics and Guide for Professional Conduct.
  - Standards of Ethical Conduct for the Physical Therapist Assistant and Guide for Conduct of the Physical Therapist Assistant.
  - Standards of Practice for Physical Therapy and the Criteria.
  - Guidelines: Physical Therapy Documentation of Patient/Client Management.
- APTA's Resource Guide: Peer Review/Utilization Review (includes core documents).
- APTA's Guidelines: Physical Therapy Claims Review.
- Pertinent state practice acts.
- Pertinent state laws and regulations.
- Other related state and federal statutes (e.g., data privacy; liability protection, if available; patient bill of rights).
- Examples of release forms used and signed by patients/clients.
- Standards of utilization review accrediting bodies (e.g., American Accreditation HealthCare Commission/URAC).
- Confidentiality statements signed by reviewers.
- Bibliography of related topics in *Physical Therapy, PT--Magazine of Physical Therapy*, and other professional publications.
- Common Procedural Terminology (CPT Codes) (year specific) and CPT definitions.
- Diagnostic classifications systems (e.g., International Classification of Disease-9, Clinical Modification [ICD-9-CM]), [ICD-10-CM].
- Health Care Financing Administration Common Procedure Coding System (HCPCS).
- Various claim form samples.

Relationship to Vision 2020: Evidence Based Practice
(Practice Department, ext 3176)

[Document updated: 12/14/2009]

Explanation of Reference Numbers:
BOD P00-00-00-00 stands for Board of Directors/month/year/page/vote in the Board of Directors Minutes; the "P" indicates that it is a position (see below). For example, BOD P11-97-06-18 means that this position can be found in the November 1997 Board of Directors minutes on Page 6 and that it was Vote 18.
P: Position | S: Standard | G: Guideline | Y: Policy | R: Procedure

Utilizing the International Classification of Functioning, Disability, and Health (ICF) Model in Physical Therapy Documentation

CHAPTER OBJECTIVES

1. Compare and contrast the Nagi Model and the ICF Model.
2. Identify the utility of the ICF Model in clinical decision making in patient or client management.
3. Recognize the utility of the ICF Model in documentation.
4. Apply the use of the ICF Model in documentation of various clinical scenarios.

KEY TERMS

Activity limitations
Body functions and structures
Contextual factors

Disability
Functioning
Participation restrictions

Introduction

The primary focus of this chapter is to compare and contrast the Nagi Model and the ICF Model and to present clinical application of each to delineate how the ICF Model provides a framework for successful clinical documentation.

History of the ICF Model and the Nagi Model

The *International Classification of Functioning, Disability, and Health* (ICF), a conceptual framework intended to describe one's functioning in life, was created by the World Health Organization in 2001 from a revision of the *International Classification of Impairments, Disabilities,* *and Handicaps* (ICIDH) developed in 1980.[1] The ICF model represents a philosophical shift in the way in which a disease process and how it affects an individual are described. Most physical therapists and physical therapist assistants are familiar with the Nagi Disablement Model on which early versions of the American Physical Therapy Association's (APTA) *Guide to Physical Therapist Practice* was based.[2] The APTA officially endorsed the ICF Model, which defines one of the major constructs of the most recent version of the *Guide*, in 2008 when the APTA's House of Delegates voted unanimously during their annual meeting to acknowledge a model that "allows physical therapists and other health care providers to more accurately record and consider the many factors that contribute to a patient's treatment and recovery."[3] Both the Nagi model and the ICF model are rooted in biopsychosocial concepts indicating that one's level of disability is an accumulation of the characteristics of a pathologic process or medical condition, of personal qualities inherent to an individual, and of the social and physical aspects of one's environment.[4] The Nagi model is described as a "disablement" model indicating that there is an "impact of chronic and acute conditions on the functioning of specific body systems and on people's abilities to act in necessary, usual, expected and personally desired ways in their society."[5] The ICF model reorganizes the disablement framework into what can be termed an "enablement" model,[6] a term originally conceived in a report by the Institute of Medicine in 1997, to portray that disability is not the fundamental consequence of impairments and functional limitations. Rather disability exists on a continuum, the severity of which is determined by the individual and in many instances can be reversed with intervention.[7]

The Nagi Model Defined

The Nagi model (FIGURE 2-1) emphasizes the disability and limitations that remain in an individual when the pre-pathologic state cannot be achieved. The Nagi model is linear indicating that each component is separate and distinct. A unidirectional arrow links each component indicating an inherent sequence. In other words, the active pathology, or interruption of normal physiologic processes, determines impairments, or abnormalities, at the body systems level. These abnormalities define functional limitations at the level of the whole person, which in turn has an effect on one's level of disability, or performance in

the environment. Thus, in the Nagi model, one's level of disability is influenced by one's ability to achieve an expected status in society. Consider the following scenario.

Mr. A is an 86-year-old male who was admitted to an inpatient rehabilitation facility after experiencing a left middle cerebral artery cerebrovascular accident (CVA) 5 days ago. He has right-sided hemiparesis and global aphasia. He requires moderate assistance of one person as well as a standard walker to perform a stand-pivot transfer. He ambulates approximately 15 feet with a wide-base quad cane and maximum assistance of two people to advance the right lower extremity and to facilitate weight shifting at the pelvis. He is the primary caregiver to his wife who has Alzheimer's disease. He has an adult son however who lives in the area and has agreed to step in as the caregiver for his mother until Mr. A's recovery can be determined.

FIGURE 2-2 classifies Mr. A's current health status according to the Nagi model. This model allows for impairments and functional limitations that have occurred as a consequence of the active pathology. In addition, this model reveals that Mr. A has acquired a disability because of his current inability to assume the role as the primary caregiver to his wife who has Alzheimer's disease. The Nagi model assumes Mr. A will have some level of disability as a result of his active pathology, impairments, and functional limitations. Consider another scenario.

Ms. B is a 31-year-old working mother of two young children, ages 3 and 1, who has gradually experienced an increase in right shoulder pain over the last 2 weeks since rearranging furniture in her 3-year-old's room

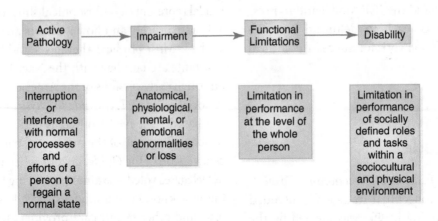

FIGURE 2-1 The Nagi Disablement Model.
Adapted from Snyder AR, Parsons JT, Valovich McLeod TC, Bay RC, Michener LA, Sauers EL. Using Disablement Models and Clinical Outcomes Assessment to Enable Evidence-Based Athletic Training Practice, Part I: Disablement Models. Journal of Athletic Training. 2008;43(4)428-436.

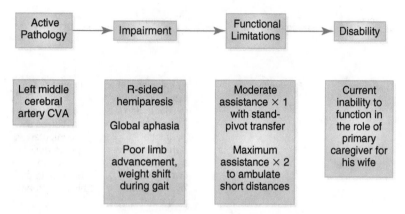

FIGURE 2-2 The Nagi Disablement Model Application – Mr. A.
Adapted from Snyder AR, Parsons JT, Valovich McLeod TC, Bay RC, Michener LA, Sauers EL. Using Disablement Models and Clinical Outcomes Assessment to Enable Evidence-Based Athletic Training Practice, Part I: Disablement Models. Journal of Athletic Training. 2008;43(4)428–436.

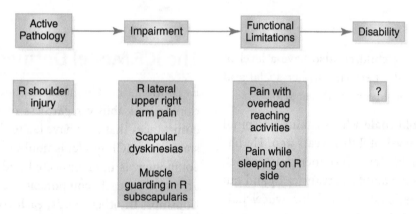

FIGURE 2-3 The Nagi Disablement Model Application – Ms. B.
Adapted from Snyder AR, Parsons JT, Valovich McLeod TC, Bay RC, Michener LA, Sauers EL. Using Disablement Models and Clinical Outcomes Assessment to Enable Evidence-Based Athletic Training Practice, Part I: Disablement Models. Journal of Athletic Training. 2008;43(4)428–436.

to accommodate a twin-size bed. She complains of pain with overhead reaching activities and notes pain into her lateral upper right arm. She notes that she has pain attempting to sleep on that side as well. She demonstrates scapular dyskinesias with overhead movements. Passive movement testing reveals muscle guarding in the right subscapularis and posterior glenohumeral joint hypomobility.

FIGURE 2-3 classifies Ms. B's current health status according to the Nagi model. Ms. B's active pathology, impairments, and functional limitations are clearly organized by this model. However, Ms. B's disability level based on the given information is difficult to comprehend. Several assumptions would have to be made regarding Ms. B's ability to carry out her responsibilities as a mother of two young children in order to make a clinical judgment regarding her level of disability. It is possible

that Ms. B would be limited in such a capacity that she would no longer be able to care for her children's everyday needs, perform her work duties, or care for herself. However, it is equally possible that Ms. B would have the capacity to carry out all of the activities required of her without any alteration in her social context despite her impairments and functional limitations.

In actuality, the disability level of each of the patients or clients in the above scenarios is difficult to determine because the details that would influence your clinical judgments about each individual's ability to perform in the environments described are lacking in the Nagi model. For example, consider Mr. A again. Details such as Mr. A's age, length of time between experiencing the cerebrovascular event and hospital admission, and the willingness of his adult son to step in as a caregiver for his wife will ultimately affect Mr. A's ability to perform in his environment. Likewise, Ms. B's age and the age and

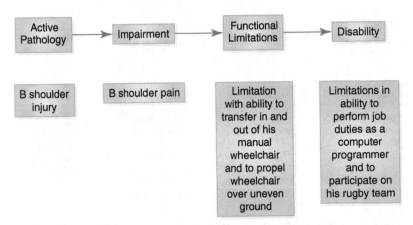

FIGURE 2-4 The Nagi Disablement Model Application – John.
Adapted from Snyder AR, Parsons JT, Valovich McLeod TC, Bay RC, Michener LA, Sauers EL. Using Disablement Models and Clinical Outcomes Assessment to Enable Evidence-Based Athletic Training Practice, Part I: Disablement Models. Journal of Athletic Training. 2008;43(4)428–436.

development of her young children also have a level of influence over the tasks she performs in her social and physical environment. Consider a third scenario.

John is a 42-year-old male who sustained a spinal cord injury at the level of T10 7 years ago. He has recently developed bilateral shoulder pain, which has interfered with his ability to transfer in and out of his manual wheelchair, propel his wheelchair over uneven ground, his job duties as a computer programmer, and his recreational activities on his rugby team.

FIGURE 2-4 classifies John's current health status based on the Nagi model. What becomes apparent in this scenario is the challenge of how to categorize John's spinal cord injury. The presence of this injury certainly has an influence on the development of John's shoulder pain, but is not the active pathology itself. It is more difficult to rationalize that John's active pathology, a bilateral shoulder injury, directly results in his impairments, functional limitations, and disability as the Nagi model suggests. The presence of John's spinal cord injury naturally influences the development of the physical therapy plan of care and is undoubtedly considered as a factor in John's recovery; however a mechanism to organize this information within the Nagi model does not exist. Furthermore, other factors such as John's age, the time frame since his spinal cord injury, the anatomic and neurologic level of the injury, and the type of assistive equipment he uses also influence his plan of care, but are not considered in the Nagi model framework.

The ICF Model Defined

By contrast, the ICF model **(FIGURE 2-5)** emphasizes functioning and ability regardless of the health-related circumstances that may have led to the individual's current status. The ICF model is nonlinear, indicating that each component is interconnected and unified. Bidirectional arrows link each component indicating dynamic relationships. In other words, each component is integrated such that each has an effect or impact on the other components. The specific **body functions and structures** implicated depend on the characteristics of the health condition. Similarly, the characteristics of the health condition impact which body functions and structures are affected. Likewise, an individual's execution of activities or participation in life events depend on the health condition, the body functions and structures involved, and the presence of environmental and personal factors, collectively termed **contextual factors**. Each of these terms is defined in **TABLE 2-1**.

There are two broad terms whose definitions can be implied by components of the ICF model: *functioning* and *disability*. The term **functioning** reflects the body functions and structures that permit an individual to experience activities and participate in life situations.[1] The term **disability** reflects the boundaries of functioning and describes decrements in impairments in body functions and structures, limitations in activities, and restrictions in participation of life events.[7] Therefore, an individual's characteristics, termed "categories of functioning,"[4] included in each of these three components represents the individual's

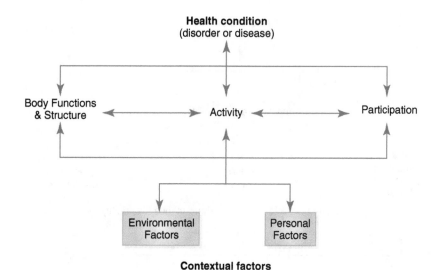

FIGURE 2-5 The International Classification of Function, Disability, and Health (ICF).
Reproduced from "Towards a Common Language for Functioning, Disability and Health ICF," World Health Organization, 2002. http://www.who.int/classifications/icf/training/icfbeginners guide.pdf

TABLE 2-1 Definitions of ICF Components

Component	Definition
Health Condition	Disease, disorder, or injury analogous to the medical diagnosis
Body Functions	Physiological functions of body systems (including psychological functions)
Body Structures	Anatomical parts of the body such as organs, limbs, and their components
Impairments	Problems in body functions or structures such as a significant deviation or loss
Activity	Execution of a task or action by an individual
Participation	Involvement in a life situation
Activity Limitations	Difficulties an individual may have in executing activities
Participation Restrictions	Problems an individual may experience in involvement in life situations
Contextual Factors - Environmental factors - Personal factors	The physical, social and attitudinal environment in which people live and conduct their lives

Reproduced from World Health Organization. International Classification of Functioning Disability and Health: ICF. Geneva, Switzerland: World Health Organization; 2001.

level of functioning on a continuum. For example, decreased muscle power is an impairment in body function and structure that could lead to a decreased ability to lift and carry a 20-pound load and restrict an individual from participating in necessary job-related tasks.[8] Thus, in the ICF model, one's level of disability is influenced by the ability to function and is described as **activity limitations** and **participation restrictions** (FIGURE 2-6).

ICF QUALIFIERS AND CORE SETS

In this text, the terms *functioning* and *disability* are added to the original graphical representation of the ICF model (Figure 2-6) to indicate that a person's level

of functioning and disability is influenced by associations and relationships among the main components of the ICF model. Thus, the ICF model is not based on the health condition despite its representation at the top of the original version of the ICF graphic. Rather, the model considers the severity of the identified impairments, an individual's ability to perform a task in a given environment with a given set of impairments, and an individual's capacity to execute a task at any time regardless of the current environment.[1] Severity, performance, and capacity are determined via qualifiers (Figure 2-6) that aim to convert the ICF framework into a classification system. Within the ICF model, a qualifier is applied to each impairment in body function and structure, activity

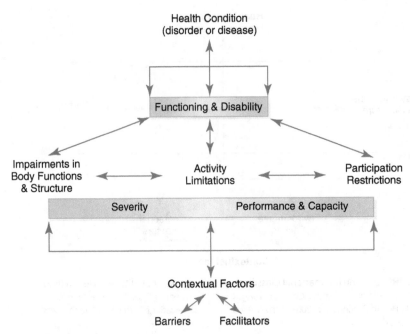

FIGURE 2-6 Adapted ICF Model.

Modified from "Towards a Common Language for Functioning, Disability and Health ICF," World Health Organization, 2002. http://www.who.int/classifications/icf/training/icfbeginnersguide.pdf

limitation, participation restriction, and as well as to contextual factors to further define severity, capacity, performance, and whether or not an individual's environment serves to facilitate or hinder the level of function and disability.[7] These qualifiers are numeric codes that specify the extent or magnitude of functioning or disability in a specific category.[9]

In addition to qualifiers, lists of categories called core sets are intended to serve as standardized directories for multidisciplinary description and assessment[10] of functioning and disability and to assist clinicians in describing all of the possible aspects of functioning and disability that can result from a certain health condition. For example, a comprehensive condition-specific core set for multiple sclerosis, consisting of 138 categories, was developed to represent the areas of functioning and health of people with multiple sclerosis that physical therapists believe should be assessed.[11] A core set consisting of 30 categories was developed for the physical health and engagement of older adults that are deemed relevant when examining this population and during re-examination to monitor changes.[12] A generic core set (TABLE 2-2), consisting of 28 categories, was found to provide a comprehensive description of functioning and was developed for use with patients or clients with multiple conditions and with those for whom a core set has not been developed.[4]

Applying the ICF Model to Patient or Client Management

Some authors have proposed using ICF qualifiers and core sets as templates for standardized and efficient documentation during an encounter with a patient or client.[4,8,13–15] Others have investigated how well ICF components are represented in existing outcome measures such as the Late-Life Function and Disability Instrument[16,17] and the Patient-Specific Functional Scale.[18] The actual utility and application of ICF qualifiers and core sets in clinical practice continue to be investigated for reliability and validity.[9,13,19,20] It is not the intention of this text to propose how to use the hierarchical coding structure, qualifiers, and core sets of the ICF model. Rather the aim is to facilitate proficiency applying ICF terminology to describing a patient or client whether that description is in the form of verbal communication as with colleagues and caregivers or if that communication is written as in documentation in a patient or client's health record. Clinicians must become more familiar with components of the ICF model and classifying impairments, actions, and experiences prior to implementing other details of the ICF model. By becoming proficient at identifying the characteristics of your patient or client for appropriate categorization within each of the ICF components, you can identify relationships that exist among impairments in body

TABLE 2-2 ICF Generic Core Set

Body Functions (b)	Activities and Participation (d)	Environmental Factors (e)
b130 Energy and drive functions	d1 Learning and applying knowledge	e450 Individual attitudes of health professionals
b134 Sleep functions	d230 Carrying out daily routine	
b140 Attention functions	d3 Communication	
b144 Memory functions	d410 Changing basic body position	
b152 Emotional functions	d415 Maintaining basic body position	
b210 Seeing	d430 Lifting and carrying objects	
b230 Hearing	d450 Walking	
b280 Pain	d455 Moving around	
b710 Mobility of joint functions	d510 Washing oneself	
b730 Muscle power functions	d530 Toileting	
	d540 Dressing	
	d640 Doing housework	
	d750 Informal social relationships	
	d760 Family relationships	
	d770 Intimate relationships	
	d850 Remunerative employment	
	d920 Recreation and leisure	
Any other body functions that the clinician may want to document outside of the generic Core Set (e.g., blood pressure, respiratory rate, skin integrity)	Any other activities and participation that the clinician may want to document outside of the generic Core Set (e.g., school)	Any other environmental factors that the clinician may want to document outside of the generic Core Set (e.g., assistive devices, home setting, work environment, health services)

Reprinted from Creating an Interface Between the International Classification of Functioning, Disability and Health and Physical Therapist Practice by Reuben Escorpizo, PHYS THER. 2010; 90:1053-1063, with the permission of the American Physical Therapy Association. © 2010 American Physical Therapy Association.

functions and structures, activity limitations, participation restrictions, and contextual factors. Furthermore, the patient or client's and caregiver's perceptions of his or her level of functioning and disability can be included as contextual factors since these items encompass the physical, social, and attitudinal environment in which people live and conduct their lives (Table 2-1).

To become more familiar with ICF terminology and using it to describe your patient or client, consider creating a graphical representation of the ICF model such as those depicted in Figure 2-6 and FIGURE 2-7 to help identify the relationships that exist among these components to guide your clinical decision making and to clarify your documentation.[8,14,15,21] Using a flow chart or conceptual map can help to portray seemingly arbitrary bits of information in an organized and structured fashion[22] so that additional information can materialize. This list could be generated concurrently or immediately after an initial or follow-up encounter with a patient or client based on a chart review, history, systems review, and collection of tests and measures. Subsequently, you can challenge yourself to move away

from creating a concurrent list or graphic and incorporate this language directly into your documentation.

Revisit Mr. A from the scenario above. Figure 2-7 classifies Mr. A's health status based on the ICF model. The additional details included in the ICF framework and not accounted for in the Nagi model that influence the overall plan of care include the contextual factors and potential relationships that exist among each of the components of the ICF model. The impairments in body functions and structures are detailed alongside each activity limitation and participation restriction. The ability to create links between why Mr. A requires assistance to transfer and ambulate and his ability to walk in his home or care for his wife is readily facilitated. Similarly, factors that may serve as barriers and facilitators during Mr. A's rehabilitation also become apparent. Why these items are listed as barriers and facilitators can also be explored. The identification of these relationships ultimately serves to facilitate thought processes and communications on behalf of your patient or client. For example, the environmental and personal factors listed here can shape the course of

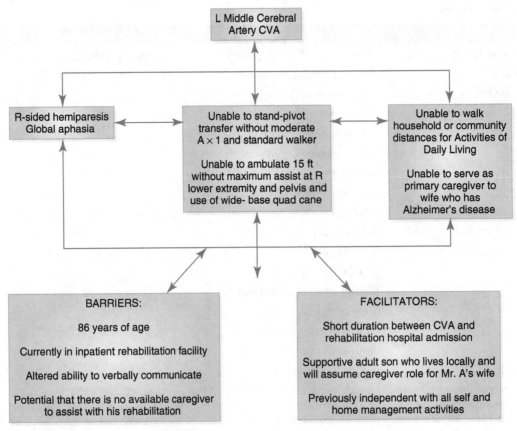

FIGURE 2-7 The ICF Model Application – Mr. A.
Data from Towards a Common Language for Functioning, Disability and Health (ICF). World Health Organization, 2002.

Mr. A's prognosis potentially influencing the mode, intensity, duration, frequency, and location of the care Mr. A receives. The short duration between the CVA and the rehabilitation hospital admission improves Mr. A's overall prognosis indicating that he may have a shorter inpatient rehabilitation hospital stay and quicker access to more intense outpatient rehabilitation services. Further, the presence of Mr. A's son may give Mr. A reassurance that his wife's needs will be met while he continues his recovery. This peace of mind may further accelerate Mr. A's recovery and subsequent return to his previous level of functioning. Similarly, Mr. A's age may indicate that he has certain age-related changes or comorbid conditions that delay his recovery process. The altered ability for Mr. A to communicate may indicate the need for additional outpatient services. Further, a new communication strategy that he can use with his wife may have to be developed in order to fulfill his prior role as her caregiver regardless of his physical recovery. Considering these contextual factors enables a healthcare team coordinating Mr. A's care to continuously assess the dynamic relationships that exist between the status of Mr. A's body functions and structures, activities, participation, and contextual factors that affect his recovery. Ultimately communication can be initiated with Mr. A and his son that reveals his own perceptions and helps to prioritize each of these factors. For example, Mr. A may have had a nonverbal communication strategy already in place with his wife indicating that his global aphasia is not a barrier to resuming his role as primary caregiver for his wife. Perhaps the presence of global aphasia becomes more of a barrier in communicating with his son or for executing other daily activities such as coordinating his wife's healthcare needs. Alternatively, identifying these relationships may reveal that Mr. A's physical recovery is not his primary concern because it gives him a respite from caring for his wife. This realization may come with some level of guilt for Mr. A, which potentially identifies a need for additional services for Mr. A and his family such as counseling. The interpretation provided here is simply one interpretation of any combination of the factors outlined in Figure 2-7. However, it is likely that Mr. A's perceptions of his health status would never be utilized to lead to prioritizing his plan of care and identifying members of the team to best

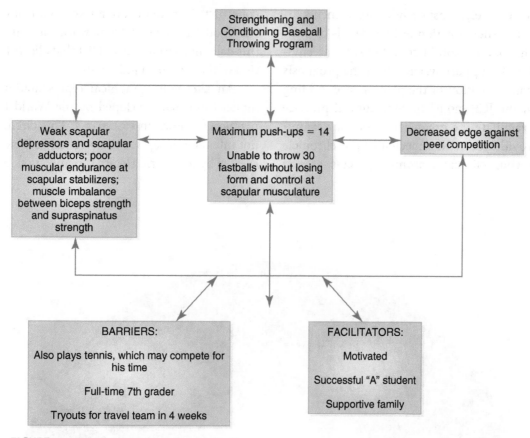

FIGURE 2-8 The ICF Model Prevention Application.
Data from Towards a Common Language for Functioning, Disability and Health (ICF). World Health Organization, 2002.

aid in Mr. A's recovery if the components of the ICF model are not explicitly considered.

UTILIZING THE ICF MODEL IN WELLNESS AND PREVENTION

It is important to note that an individual need not have a health condition to be classified according to the ICF model. Important relationships between the status of an individual's body functions and structures, abilities with activities and participation, and contextual factors can still be identified for an individual who is seeking health condition prevention or a wellness program. Perhaps in place of the term "health condition" it would be valuable to integrate the remaining components of the ICF model with an individual's "health goal" in mind instead. Consider the following scenario.

You receive an inquiry from an individual indicating that her son's baseball coach would like a baseball throwing conditioning and strengthening program to be developed by a physical therapist. You decide to use the ICF model to classify the findings from the initial examination with the client. The details of your classification are shown in **FIGURE 2-8**. This classification can help you identify not only the content of the throwing program but also how it might be integrated into his schedule so that he is successful.

Utilizing the ICF Model for Clinical Reasoning

Overall, it is the capacity of the ICF model to consider an individual's level of *functioning* and *disability* though elucidating relationships among each component of the ICF model that earns the descriptor of an "enablement" model and distinguishes it from traditional disablement models such as the Nagi model. A graphical illustration of the ICF model is meant to reinforce that many factors shape your interaction with your patient or client and is designed to help you organize and synthesize the data that you collect during encounters with your patient or client. Even if you have not yet had the opportunity to utilize the ICF model in your clinical practice, it is very likely that you routinely consider how impairments affect a patient or client's function or how details of one's past medical history, comorbid conditions, home environment, or family support system affect the prognosis and the ultimate execution of the plan of care. Adding concepts from the ICF model to your clinical practice however, will facilitate the organization of your examination and provide you with a mechanism to chronicle or document your clinical reasoning process as you construct the plan of care for your patient or client. The ICF model provides a framework for you to categorize this data into a well-ordered list that allows for prioritization of these clinical judgments.

An alternative graphical representation of the ICF model from that developed by the World Health Organization is shown in **FIGURE 2-9**. This circular graphic is not intended to replace the original graphic (Figure 2-5) created by the World Health Organization, but rather has

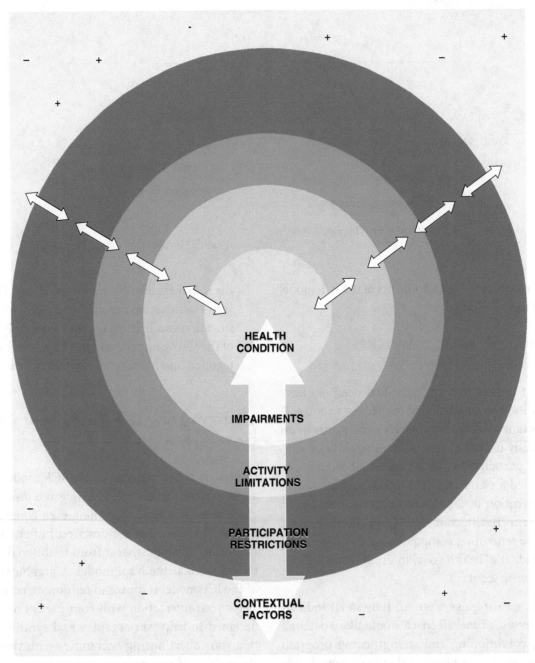

FIGURE 2-9 Circular Representation of the ICF Model.
Data from Towards a Common Language for Functioning, Disability and Health (ICF). World Health Organization, 2002.

been developed for use as an adjunctive tool in a clinical setting to help integrate ICF terminology into conceptualizing the unique characteristics of a patient or client whether for verbal discussion or written documentation. The circular depiction of each component of the ICF model is intended to portray that each component is continuous with no beginning or end. No significance is given to the acuity, chronicity, or hierarchy of any of the components. However, the magnitude of the contribution of each component to the overall model is implied by the size of each concentric circle. The health condition is represented in the center by the smallest circle followed by impairments. The health condition is the initial stimulus for becoming aware of impairments in body functions and structures, but one need not have a diagnosed health condition to benefit from the services you provide as a physical therapist or a physical therapist assistant. Activity limitations precede participation restrictions and contextual factors, respectively, and are represented as progressively larger circles to depict that the context of a person and his or her life situation has exponential influence on each of the other components. The plus and minus symbols that occupy the space designated for contextual factors represent the designation of each environmental and personal factor as either a barrier or a facilitator to one's level of functioning and disability. Each circle ultimately adds layers of detail to exemplify an individual's health-related status. The large bidirectional arrow reinforces the notion that each component impacts the other components of the model. The smaller bidirectional arrows that span each circle represent the idea that one's level of functioning and disability is determined by the relationships and associations created by the presence of the details in each component. FIGURE 2-10 classifies Mr. A's health status using this circular graphical representation of the ICF model. This graphical representation may allow the relationships that exist between each component of the ICF model to be more readily perceived as you improve your ability to incorporate ICF terminology into your clinical decision-making and documentation.

Utilizing the ICF Model for Documentation

Once you have completed classifying the results of the encounter with your patient or client into an ICF framework,

you can then begin to identify relationships among the components of the ICF by asking yourself the following questions:

1. What are the patient or client's activity limitations and participation restrictions and how should these be prioritized?
2. How do these activity limitations and participation restrictions relate to the impairments identified during the examination?
3. How does each contextual factor relate to the identified activity limitations and participation restrictions, the impairments in body functions and structures, and other contextual factors?
4. Why are certain contextual factors listed as facilitators or barriers?
5. What relationships can you generate to use in the development of your:
   a. Choice of tests and measures and outcome measures during the examination?
   b. Diagnosis and clinical impression?
   c. Prognosis?
   d. Anticipated goals and expected outcomes?
   e. Frequency and duration of the episode of care?
   f. Intervention plan?

Consider the following scenario to elaborate more on each of these questions.

Your patient or client is a 15-year-old boy who had an open reduction internal fixation of his tibia and fibula after experiencing a fracture when snow skiing with his family. A well-respected, world-renowned surgeon operated on your patient or client's leg and gave him a specific rehabilitation protocol that he presented to you at his initial examination in outpatient physical therapy 4 weeks after surgery. Your patient or client indicates that he is worried because not only does his leg still hurt where he believes the fracture occurred, but he is also experiencing pain at his knee and ankle where the surgeon inserted a rod into his bone. He notes that he thinks that the surgeon may have "messed up" his patella because it seems more elevated than his other knee and it hurts to bend the knee. He mentions to you that he is eager to walk without his crutches and that he started walking around his house using one crutch. He notes that his surgeon asked that he wait until he started physical therapy before putting weight through his

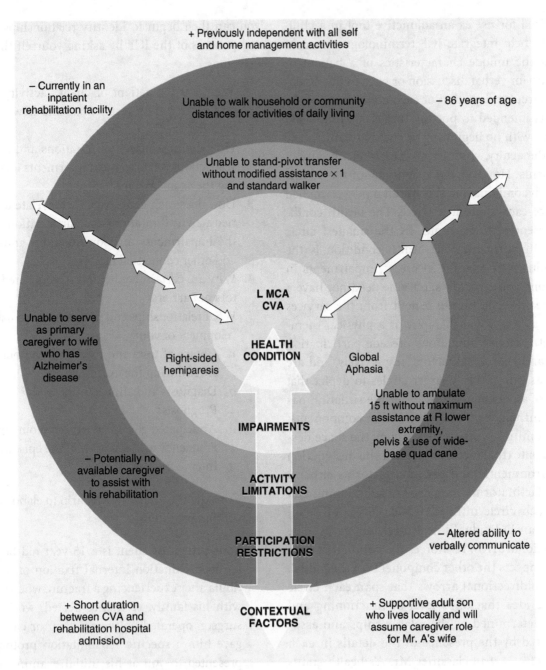

FIGURE 2-10 Circular Representation of the ICF Model–Mr. A.
Data from Towards a Common Language for Functioning, Disability and Health (ICF). World Health Organization, 2002.

leg, but he figured it was okay because it did not hurt to walk in this manner. He states that he doesn't hang out or sleep in his room because it is upstairs, and that he doesn't attend a full day of school because his leg aches too much if he can't lie down and prop it up. He states that he is frustrated and that he just wants to be ready for football practices, which start in 3 months. Your initial examination reveals two approximated and well-healed ½-inch incisions at the distal insertion of the vastus lateralis and the distal lateral lower leg anterior to the lateral malleolus. You note mild circumferential edema at the right knee, decreased patellar mobility, decreased active and passive range of motion at the tibiofemoral joint, decreased muscle activation at the vastus medialis oblique, and decreased muscle strength of the gluteus medius, hamstrings, gluteus maxiumus, anterior tibialis and fibularis muscles.

IDENTIFYING RELATIONSHIPS AMONG THE COMPONENTS OF THE ICF MODEL

Using the questions above as a guide to determining the details of the ICF graphic, first identify your patient or client's primary activity limitations and participation restrictions. To objectify your patient or client's perceptions of these components, apply the Patient-Specific Functional Scale (PSFS) (FIGURE 2-11). The PSFS is a self-report outcome measure that has been found to represent the activity component of the ICF model[18] and can be used to gather this information directly during the history,

helping you to immediately identify your patient or client's perception of his functioning and disability for consideration in the overall plan of care.

FIGURE 2-12 and FIGURE 2-13 illustrate how each detail from the scenario above is captured within the ICF framework using the original graphical representation created by the WHO and the circular graphical representation, respectively. These types of illustrations can be used to identify how each activity limitation and participation restriction relates to impairments identified during the examination. For example, decreased ambulation speed may be present due to pain, decreased knee range of motion,

---

Initial Assessment:

I am going to ask you to identify up to three important activities that you are unable to do or are having difficulty with as a result of your _____ lower leg _____ problem. Today, are there any activities that you are unable to do or having difficulty with because of your _____ lower leg _____ problem? (Clinician: Show scale to patient and have the patient rate each activity.)

Follow-Up Assessments:

When I assessed you on (state previous assessment date), you told me that you had difficulty with (read all activities from list at a time). Today, do you still have difficulty with: (read and have patient score each item in the list)?

Patient-Specific Activity Scoring Scheme (point to one number):

| 0 | 1 | 2 | 3 | 4 | 5 | 6 | 7 | 8 | 9 | 10 |

| Unable to perform activity | | | | | | | | | | Able to perform activity at the same level as before injury or problem |

ACTIVITY	Initial Score/Date	Reassessment Score/Date	Discharge Score/Date
1. Unable to sit for a full day in school.	4		
2. Unable to walk without crutches.	0		
3. Unable to get to his room (climb stairs).	0		
4. Unable to run.	0		
5. Unable to play football.	0		
Additional			
Additional			
Total Score	0.8		

Total score = sum of the activity scores/number of activities

Minimum detectable change (90%CI) for average score = 2 points

Minimum detectable change (90%CI) for single activity score = 3 points

PSFS developed by Stratford P, Gill C. Westaway M, Binkley J. Assessing disability and change on individual patients: a report of a patient specific measure. *Physiotherapy Canada*. 1995;47:258–263.

FIGURE 2-11 The Patient-Specific Functional Scale to Objectify a Patient/Client's Perceptions of Activity Limitations and Participation Restrictions.
© 1995, P. Stratford, reprinted with permission.

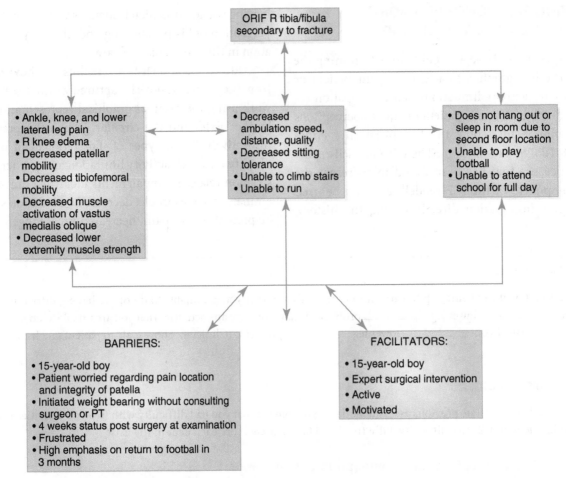

FIGURE 2-12 The ICF Model Application – Patient with ORIF R LE.
Data from Towards a Common Language for Functioning, Disability and Health (ICF). World Health Organization, 2002.

decreased muscle performance, or some combination of these impairments in body functions and structures. Decreased sitting tolerance in school may be due to edema at the knee or to the sitting position required such as a desk with a left-sided opening and right-sided closure limiting the ability to adjust the position of the right leg. The inability to climb stairs or run is likely related to decreased lower extremity muscle performance. The inability to access his bedroom on the second floor, play football, and attend a full day at school are important participation restrictions to consider when investigating the magnitude of each impairment identified. For example, the amount of active knee range of motion required to achieve a three-point stance as a defensive lineman is greater than that needed to sit in desk at school. In other words, different demands will be placed on the knee depending on if your patient or client is to return to his role as a student or if he is to return to his role on his football team. Further investigation into the etiology of each impairment can

also occur. For example, knee pain may be present due to decreased mobility of the surgical incisions, decreased patellar mobility, decreased tibiofemoral mobility, decreased support from the quadriceps, or the patient or client's fear that his surgeon compromised his patella.

Identifying how each contextual factor relates to each other and to other components of the ICF model may help you clarify findings from your examination or why certain activity limitations and participation restrictions exist. For example, the fact that your patient or client decided to initiate weight bearing may contribute to the level of pain that he is experiencing at his knee and ankle or the level of edema present at the knee. Similarly, the fact that your patient or client is only 4 weeks from the date of his surgery gives you insight as to the level of tissue healing that has occurred and why he is unable to efficiently ambulate or climb stairs.

Next, identifying how each contextual factor relates to the other components of the ICF model will help to

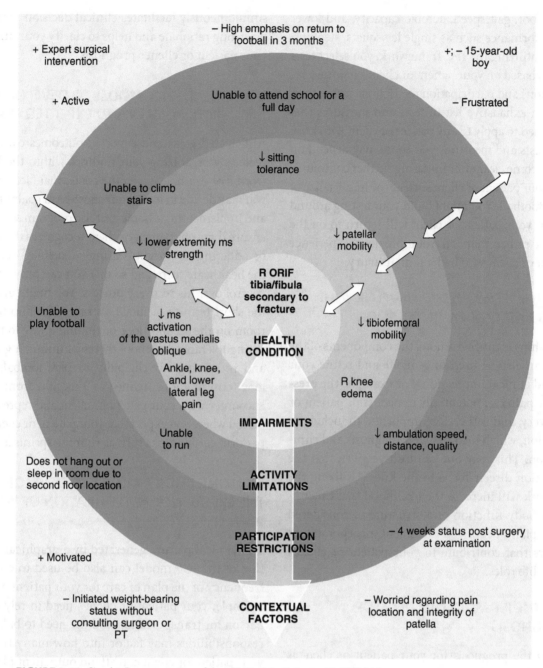

FIGURE 2-13 Circular Representation of the ICF Model – Patient with ORIF R LE.

clarify why you chose to list certain factors as barriers or facilitators. For example, listing your patient or client's age as both a barrier and a facilitator could prompt you to gather more information about his attitude, expectations, and contribution to his rehabilitation. In addition, identification of the etiology of your patient or client's fear may stimulate education that his right patella appears altered due to quadriceps muscle atrophy rather than a mistake on the part of his surgeon.

UTILIZING THE ICF MODEL TO DEVELOP TESTS AND MEASURES AND OUTCOME MEASURES

Once you have identified relationships among each component of the ICF model, identify tests and measures or outcome measures you may have omitted from your examination. For example, as your patient or client achieves full weight-bearing status, it would be relevant to assess lower extremity proprioception and kinesthesia, mobility at the joints of the foot, gait speed, aerobic capacity, and lower extremity performance such as single leg squats, step ups, or lunges. By utilizing the IFC framework, you select tests and measures based on your patient or client's reported activity limitations and participation restrictions rather than performing an exhaustive list of tests and measures that you have learned to apply to any patient or client with knee pain. Other tests and measures you chose may depend on details that become clear after initiating further communication with your patient or client such as the importance of returning to football. You might build your testing around what position your patient or client will return to on the football team rather than on your previous experience with a patient or client who had a similar injury.

UTILIZING THE ICF MODEL TO DEVELOP YOUR DIAGNOSIS AND CLINICAL IMPRESSION

The relationships identified among the components of the ICF model can also be used to generate and refine your diagnosis and clinical impression. For example, the presence of ankle pain can potentially impact your patient or client's recovery, and is therefore important to include in your evaluation, which includes your diagnosis and clinical impression. This may not be intuitive given that the health condition directs focus to the knee. Utilizing the ICF framework will increase the likelihood that this impairment in body function and structure is considered and that the plan of care you document incorporates all of the factors that contribute to your patient or client's return to his life roles.

UTILIZING THE ICF MODEL TO DEVELOP YOUR PROGNOSIS

Determining the prognosis for your patient or client is also facilitated by outlining the data you collect during interactions. For example, you might determine that it will take longer than 3 months to build muscle strength and power based on your findings that your patient or client has deficits activating the vastus lateralis oblique as well as additional strength deficits in his affected lower extremity. Simultaneously, you may decide your patient or client's motivation to return to football as well as his active lifestyle help to accelerate his recovery time. Alternatively, this motivation could potentially interfere with your patient or client's recovery if tissue healing is delayed because of early weight bearing. Considering these factors

simultaneously facilitates clinical decision making based on strong rationale and helps to clarify your impression of your patient or client's prognosis.

UTILIZING THE ICF MODEL TO DEVELOP YOUR ANTICIPATED GOALS AND EXPECTED OUTCOMES

Anticipated goals and expected outcomes can also be directed by organizing your findings within the ICF framework. For example, given the contextual factors identified, you may decide to focus your short-term goals on education and implementing a home exercise program so that you can ensure that your patient or client recognizes the importance of adhering to weight-bearing guidelines established by the healthcare team and so that you can provide him some control over his recovery process. You might also decide in the short term to facilitate a strategy for him to get to his room on the second floor or finding a way to improve his sitting tolerance in school thereby minimizing his absence and preserving his eligibility to play football. Similarly, long term might be defined as 3 months from your initial encounter with your patient or client and represents a time period where you expect that your patient or client be able to perform certain tasks such as running sprints and jumping.

UTILIZING THE ICF MODEL TO DEVELOP THE FREQUENCY AND DURATION OF YOUR PLAN OF CARE

The clinical picture generated by a graphical representation of the ICF model can also be used to construct the frequency of the plan of care for your patient or client. For example, your patient or client's need to rely on another person for transportation and the need to balance school responsibilities may factor into how many times a week your patient or client can attend outpatient physical therapy. Similarly, your patient or client's goal of returning to football may facilitate a conversation with his coach to implement a program that can be incorporated with his team once or twice a week in place of coming to the physical therapy clinic.

UTILIZING THE ICF MODEL TO DEVELOP YOUR INTERVENTION PLAN

Intervention plan development is also facilitated by delineating relationships among the components of the ICF model. The concept that a physical therapist or physical therapist assistant treats a patient or client with a certain diagnosis, disease, or health-related problem solely based on an intervention protocol or past experience with individuals with a similar diagnosis, disease, or health-related problem is eliminated by the ICF model. Rather, the ICF model facilitates the notion that each individual is affected uniquely by a particular health condition thereby forcing a physical therapist to construct a plan of care exclusively for that individual. Therefore, revealing the relationship between your patient or client's inability to tolerate sitting in school and knee pain may stimulate conversation about the possibility of temporarily changing where or how your patient or client sits in the classroom to facilitate a more tolerable position. In addition, the initial home exercise program may focus on interventions that directly address your patient or client's pain and patellar mobility because of the knowledge that he is worried about how these impairments might affect his recovery.

The list of questions used above to facilitate your identification of relationships among the components of the ICF can be modified to apply to situations where you are working towards prevention and wellness rather than mitigating the effects of a health condition. These questions are:

1. How does the health goal relate to the patient or client's current activities and participation in life events?
2. How do the impairments identified at the initial examination affect the health goal and any identified activity limitations and participation restrictions?
3. Were there any impairments identified that indicate that the patient or client's health goal is not feasible at this time and that the individual is more appropriate for increased frequency and duration of physical therapy care?
4. How does each contextual factor relate to the identified activity limitations and participation restrictions, the impairments in body functions and structures, and other contextual factors?
5. Why are certain contextual factors listed as facilitators or barriers?
6. What relationships can you generate to use in the development of your:
   a. Choice of tests and measures during the examination?
   b. Clinical impression of how long it may take to achieve the health goal?
   c. Anticipated goals and expected outcomes?
   d. Frequency and duration of the episode of care?
   e. Interventions?

The identified relationships can ultimately assist you to identify if a preventative or wellness program is feasible or if more detailed and frequent physical therapy intervention is warranted. The details derived above could serve to assist you with communication to your patient or client and his family, and with documentation to your patient or client's healthcare providers, your employer, a third-party payer, or the legal system to help show why physical therapy services are medically necessary and justified.

Summary

Many expert clinicians demonstrate superior clinical skills that generate positive clinical outcomes and satisfied patients or clients. But not every clinician is able to translate his or her expertise into his or her documentation. It is the ability to capture your clinical reasoning in writing that produces successful documentation. Escorpizo and colleagues point out that the ICF model represents the framework for "what" information to gather during an encounter with a patient or client.[4] Using the ICF framework to practice extracting the "what" from your interactions with your patients or clients will assist you in making your thoughts and reasons behind your clinical decisions tangible. Research continues on how to best integrate the content revealed by the ICF model into documentation for physical therapists and physical therapist assistants. The efficacy of classifying a physical therapy encounter with a patient or client using the ICF framework and terminology is unknown. Similarly, it is not known if the clinical utility of core sets and qualifiers to determine outcomes is superior or adjunctive to other tools used to ascertain outcomes. As we move towards mandatory electronic health records, a working knowledge of ICF model terminology and conceptual framework will be paramount for facilitating your ability to collaborate with colleagues to create user-friendly ICF-based electronic documentation materials and templates that interface with current systems. How the details of the ICF model are displayed will ultimately depend on the details of the electronic documentation system itself. Nevertheless, those details will be determined by clinicians with a strong understanding of the operational definitions of the ICF components and the working knowledge of how to apply this information when conducting a history and systems review, prioritizing the contents of an initial examination, formulating a diagnosis and clinical impression, developing a prognosis, setting goals, and designing interventions. What is clear is that the ICF model has infiltrated the physical therapy profession as a superior framework to the Nagi model as the instrument for facilitating the reintegration of a patient or client into his or her life roles regardless of any perceived level of functioning or disability. Remember, that successful documentation is defined as that which delineates such a clear clinical representation of your plan of care with your patient or client that little to no clarification about what you have documented is necessary. By utilizing ICF model terminology in your documentation, you can provide patients or clients and families, physical therapist colleagues, patient or client's healthcare providers, third-party payers, and policy makers with a mechanism to communicate health information across the health continuum to advance health care.

Discussion Questions

1. Discuss how you would or do use the ICF model in clinical practice.
2. Compare and contrast the characteristics of a "disablement" model and an "enablement" model of an individual's health status.
3. What is meant by the term *disability* according to the Nagi model? The ICF model?
4. In each of the following scenarios complete the following:
   a. Classify the details of the scenario into each component of the Nagi model.
   b. Classify the details of the scenario into each component of the ICF model using the WHO version of the ICF model and the circular ICF model presented in this chapter.
   c. In each scenario, what relationships were you able to define among the components of the Nagi model? The ICF model? Did you identify different relationships depending on which graphical representation of the ICF model you used?
   d. Utilize the Patient-Specific Functional Scale in each scenario to identify activity limitations and participation restrictions.

   Scenario A: Frank is an 82-year-old male who suffered a middle cerebral artery CVA 1 week ago. He was found by his adult son on the floor in the bathroom after he heard him fall. He was admitted to the hospital immediately and had a 3-day length of stay before transferring to the inpatient rehabilitation hospital where you work. During your initial examination you learn that he is the primary caregiver to his wife who suffers from severe osteoporosis and chronic obstructive pulmonary disorder (COPD). He states that his son was only visiting for the weekend but has been able to stay with his wife until further plans can be arranged. Your patient appears worried and has many questions about what he can do to regain the use of his right arm and leg.

   Scenario B: Jerry is a 32-year-old male who was throwing around the football in his backyard with his sons when he stepped awkwardly in a hole. He heard a horrible cracking sound and fell to the ground when he felt a sharp searing pain in his calf and foot. He was unable to put weight through his foot to walk so he decided that he should go to the emergency room right away. After an evaluation and imaging at the emergency room he was diagnosed with an Achilles tendon tear, was immobilized in a boot, and given a pair of axillary crutches.

   Scenario C: Ann is a 73-year-old female who is receiving home health physical therapy after having a 5-day stay at an acute care hospital. She was admitted with a urinary tract infection but subsequently developed a blood infection, which left her very weak and not able to move very well. She has a 7-year history of Parkinson's disease with related postural imbalance and a history of falls for which she was receiving outpatient physical therapy services prior to her hospitalization.

5. Explain how using a graphical representation of the ICF model to organize information you gather from an encounter with your patient or client might assist you with your clinical reasoning as you develop a plan of care for your patient or client.
6. You receive an inquiry from a 40-year-old male who would like to start on a comprehensive conditioning program to improve his overall health. You gather from your conversation with him that he has an older brother who died in his mid-50s from cardiac issues. He states that he has two school-aged children and is a full-time bank executive. He notes that he has never exercised before beyond being active with his

kids on the weekends. He appears to be moderately overweight.

   a. How would you proceed with developing an exercise program for this individual?

   b. How can you use the ICF model to help plan the components of the exercise program? Consider using a graphical representation of the ICF model to fill in the details you have from your brief conversation with the man.

7. Choose a patient or client with whom you have recently worked in the clinic. Classify the details you can recall about this individual into the components of the ICF model without looking at the health record. Once you have completed this, go to the health record and compare your classification of the patient or client using the ICF model to the data that was actually collected and documented in the health record.

   a. Is the clinical representation of the patient similar? Different? How?

   b. Is there any information that you identified as being important about the patient or client that you did not initially document in the health record? What do you think are the reasons that you did not include these details in the documentation of your original encounter with the patient or client?

Case Study Questions

1. Sue is a 64-year-old female who is receiving home health physical therapy services after having a right total knee arthroplasty. You see her for the initial examination 4 days status-post surgery. At her initial home health visit you learn that she is very active in her church and is looking forward to getting back to her job there as the Coordinator of Volunteer Services. She notes that she will probably still have to use a cane since her left knee is also painful. She notes that after her rehabilitation for her current surgery, her surgeon advised her to have a knee replacement on the left knee as well. Her current medications include Percocet (oxycodone/acetaminophen), Lasix (furosemide), and Prinivil (lisinopril). Sue lives in a two-story home with three steps with a handrail to enter. Her active knee range of motion is 10 to 85 degrees. She has a poor ability to recruit her right vastus medialis oblique via your observation. Manual muscle testing reveals a 3/5 strength in the right gluteus medius and a 4/5 in the left gluteus medius muscle.

   You find the following details during your systems review and collection of tests and measures and outcome measures:

   ○ Aerobic Capacity and Endurance: 6-Minute Walk Test = 403 feet

   ○ Anthropometric Characteristics: BP rest = 161/91 mmHg; HR rest = 62 bpm; RR rest = 15 breaths/minute

   ○ Assistive Devices: standard walker, single point cane, shower chair in walk in shower, raised toilet seat

   ○ Peripheral Nerve Integrity and Sensory Integrity: Decreased light touch at skin 1 inch (2.54 cm) to the right and left of surgical incision at right knee, intact to light touch superior and inferior to incision; sharp/dull discrimination intact at right lower extremity; decreased kinesthesia at right knee and ankle; intact kinesthesia at bilateral hips, left knee and left ankle

   ○ Gait, Locomotion, and Balance: Timed Up and Go with walker = 24 sec; Timed Up and Go without walker = 31 sec; One-Leg Stand Test on Right = 3 sec; One-Leg Stand Test on left = 5 sec; Functional Gait Assessment = 14/30

   ○ Integumentary Integrity: Healing incision; 12 staples in place held with Steri-Strips; nonpitting edema noted 3 cm above the superior border of patella at right knee

   ○ Muscle Performance: poor ability to recruit vastus medialis oblique—palpable trace contraction; Five Times Sit to Stand Test = 34 seconds with use of upper extremity for last three repetitions; 19-inch (48.3 cm) height kitchen chair

   ○ Pain: at rest with pain medication = 2/10; at worst with pain medication = 6/10 (transition from sit to stand and when walking)

   ○ Posture: sits with right leg kicked out in front or elevated on foot rest of recliner; currently sleeps in recliner

   ○ Other: Western Ontario and McMaster Universities (WOMAC) = 69%

   a. Classify the details of the scenario above into the components of the ICF model.

   b. What are Sue's activity limitations and participation restrictions and how should these be prioritized?

   c. How do these activity limitations and participation restrictions relate to the impairments identified during the examination?

   d. How does each contextual factor relate to the identified activity limitations and participation restrictions, the impairments in body functions and structures, and other contextual factors?

   e. Why are certain contextual factors listed as facilitators or barriers?

   f. What relationships can you generate to use in the development of your:

     i. Choice of tests and measures during the examination?

     ii. Diagnosis and clinical impression?

     iii. Prognosis?

     iv. Anticipated goals and expected outcomes?

     v. Frequency and duration of the episode of care?

     vi. Intervention plan?

2. Martin is a 41-year-old male who comes to your outpatient physical therapy practice with complaints of right leg pain. He states that his pain started while hiking on vacation in the Smoky Mountains with his wife 2 weeks ago. He notes that he and his wife hiked a total of 30 miles over 2 days. By the end of the second day, he was feeling sore and asked his wife to stretch his leg. He describes that a passive stretch was applied to his quadriceps while he was in prone. He states that the stretching may have been too aggressive since he felt pain during the stretching that has been present ever since. He reports a 3/10 pain and tenderness at the right lateral thigh at rest that increases to a 7/10 pain at the right knee during ambulation of any distance. He states that ibuprofen decreases his pain to allow him to get some sleep but does not eliminate it. He notes that he is anxious to return to his job duties as biologist stating that he took an extra week off to rest his knee before returning to his field work. Your examination reveals the following:

    ○ Tenderness to palpation at the lateral right knee joint line, and at the insertion and distal one-third of the right iliotibial band

    ○ Decreased knee joint passive range of motion 0 degrees to 95 degrees

    ○ Positive Ober's Test, negative McMurray's Test, negative Anterior Drawer Test, negative Ely's Test

    ○ Decreased stance time on the right lower extremity during gait with decreased knee extension range of motion at heel contact

    ○ Decreased patellar mobility

     a. Classify the details of the scenario above into the components of the ICF model.

     b. What are Martin's activity limitations and participation restrictions and how should these be prioritized?

     c. How do these activity limitations and participation restrictions relate to the impairments identified during the examination?

     d. How does each contextual factor relate to the identified activity limitations and participation restrictions, the impairments in body functions and structures, and other contextual factors?

     e. Why are certain contextual factors listed as facilitators or barriers?

     f. What relationships can you generate to use in the development of your:

       i. Choice of tests and measures during the examination?

       ii. Diagnosis and clinical impression?

       iii. Prognosis?

       iv. Anticipated goals and expected outcomes?

       v. Frequency and duration of the episode of care?

       vi. Intervention plan?

References

1. World Health Organization. *Towards a Common Language for Functioning, Disability, and Health: The International Classification of Functioning, Disability and Health*. Geneva: World Health Organization; 2002.

2. American Physical Therapy Association (APTA). *Guide to Physical Therapist Practice*, 2nd ed. Alexandria, VA: American Physical Therapy Association; 2001:27/S19-29/S21.

3. APTA. HQ Press Release. Alexandria, VA: American Physical Therapy Association; July 8, 2008. Available at: www.apta.org/Media/Releases/APTA/2008/7/8/. Accessed on September 5, 2012.

4. Escorpizo R, Stucki G, Cieza A, et al. Creating an interface between the *International Classification of Functioning, Disability, and Health* and physical therapist practice. *Phys Ther.* 2010;90:1053–1063.

5. Verbrugge LM, Jette AM. The disablement process. *Soc Sci Med.* 1994;38:1–14.

6. Brandt EN Jr., Pope AM. *Enabling America: Assessing the Role of Rehabilitation Science and Engineering*. Washington, DC: National Academy Press; 1997:62-80.

7. Jette AM. Towards a common language for function, disability, and health. *Phys Ther.* 2006;86:726–734.

8. Rundell SD, Davenport TE, Wagner T. Physical therapist management of acute and chronic low back pain using the World Health Organization's *International Classification of Functioning, Disability, and Health. Phys Ther.* 2009;89:82–90.

9. Jette AM. Invited commentary. *Phys Ther.* 2010;90: 1064–1065.

10. Cieza A, Ewert T, Üstün B, et al. Development of ICF Core Sets for patients with chronic conditions. *J Rehabil Med.* 2004;(44 suppl):9–11.

11. Conrad A, Coenen M, Schmalz H, et al. Comprehensive ICF Core Sets for multiple sclerosis from the perspective of physical therapists. *Phys Ther.* 2012;92:799–820.

12. Ruaro JA, Ruaro MB, Guerra RO. International Classification of Functioning, Disability and Health Core Sets for physical health of older adults. *J Geriatr Phys Ther.* 2014;37:147–153.

13. Rausch A, Escorpizo R, Riddle DL, et al. Using a case report of a patient with spinal cord injury to illustrate the application of the *International Classification of Functioning, Disability, and Health* during multidisciplinary patient management. *Phys Ther.* 2010;90:1039–1052.

14. Helgeson K, Smith RA. Process for applying the *International Classification of Functioning, Disability and Health* model to a patient with patellar dislocation. *Phys Ther.* 2008;88:956–964.

15. Steiner WA, Ryser L, Huber, E et al. Use of the ICF model as a clinical problem solving tool in physical therapy and rehabilitation medicine. *Phys Ther.* 2002;82:1098–1107.

16. Jette AM, Haley SM, Coster WJ, et al. Late-Life Function and Disability Instrument, I: development and evaluation of the disability component. *J Gerontol A Biol Sci Med Sci.* 2002;57:M209–M216.

17. Haley SM, Jette AM, Coster WJ, et al. Later-Life Function and Disability Instrument, II: development and evaluation of the function component. *J Gerontol A Biol Sci Med Sci.* 2002;57:M217–M222.

18. Fairbairn K, May K, Yang Y, et al. Mapping Patient-Specific Functional Scale items to the *International Classification of Functioning, Disability, and Health (ICFDH). Phys Ther.* 2012;92:310–317.

19. Starrost K, Geyh S, Trautwein A, et al. Interrater reliability of the extended ICF Core Set for stroke applied by physical therapists. *Phys Ther.* 2008;88:841–851.

20. Grill E, Mansmann U, Cieza A, Stucki G. Assessing observer agreement when describing and classifying functioning with the *International Classification of Functioning, Disability, and Health. J Rehabil Med.* 2007;39:71–76.

21. Wahlgren A, Palombaro K. Evidence-based physical therapy for BPPV using the *International Classification of Functioning, Disability, and Health* model: a case report. *J Geri Phys Ther.* 2012;35:1–6.

22. Shepard KF, Jensen GM. Strategies for teaching in academic settings. In: Shepard KF, Jensen GM, eds. *Handbook of Teaching for Physical Therapists.* Boston: Butterworth-Heinemann; 1997:73–118.

Physical Therapy Documentation Content

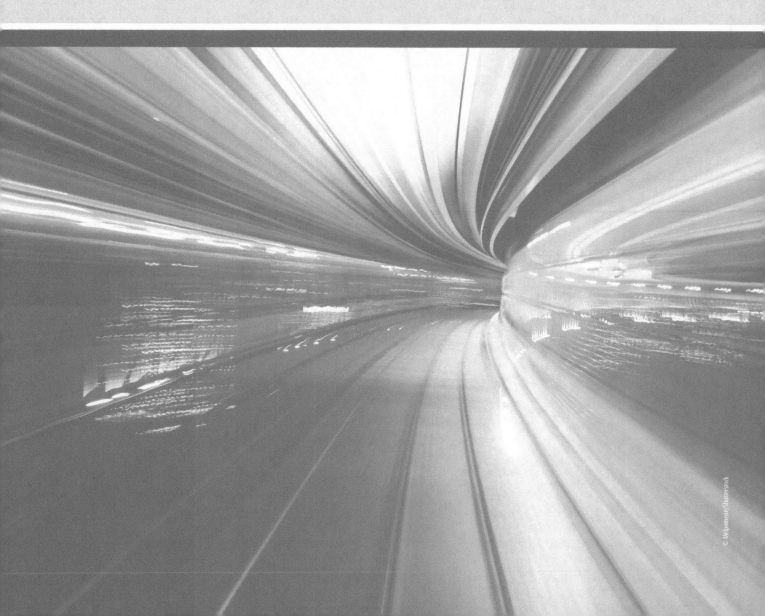

CHAPTER 3

Documenting the Initial Examination

CHAPTER OBJECTIVES

1. Recognize the components of the initial examination.
2. Determine the documentation content of each component of the initial examination
   a. History
   b. Systems review
   c. Tests and measures/outcome measures
   d. Evaluation
      i. Diagnosis
      ii. Clinical impression
   e. Prognosis
   f. Anticipated goals and expected outcomes
   g. Frequency and duration of the episode of care
   h. Intervention plan
3. Identify the differences between the terms *initial examination* and *evaluation*.
4. Identify the differences between the terms *clinical impression* and *diagnosis*.
5. Recognize the clinical reasoning framework behind creating the content of the initial examination note.

KEY TERMS

Clinical impression
Diagnosis
Evaluation

Initial examination
Outcome measures

Introduction

Since the quality of the initial examination helps to determine the quality of the rest of the documentation that follows, the primary focus of this chapter is to divide the initial examination into its component parts and to provide clinical examples of how the content of each component is represented in physical therapy documentation.

The **initial examination** is the cornerstone of your physical therapy documentation. In other words, the quality of its contents directly affects the way in which the initial examination is interpreted and subsequently used either by you and your physical therapy colleagues or other consumers of the health record such as members of your patient or client's healthcare team, your client and their family members or caregivers, your organization's audit team, external auditors, third-party payers,

or the legal system. It would be futile to attempt to alter the contents of your initial examination documentation based upon who you think might use the note to make decisions. Rather you should assume that all of the parties mentioned above will at some point utilize your documentation. Therefore, you should determine a framework for creating the contents of a well-written initial examination that would simultaneously satisfy the needs of any user of your documentation. For example, the Centers for Medicare & Medicaid Services have rules and regulations that define what detail supports that the services rendered were reasonable and medically necessary depending on the setting in which the documentation is created. However, if your documentation follows a sound clinical reasoning framework then all of the components

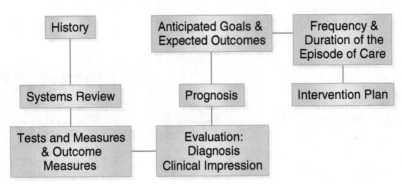

FIGURE 3-1 Components of the Physical Therapy Initial Examination.

that deem a piece of documentation as acceptable according to a third-party payer will be present. Remember, that a third-party payer is a funding source, not a standard of practice. Therefore, the framework for creating your documentation need not be an outline of the rules and regulations mandated by a third-party payer, but rather should follow a framework that has sound clinical reasoning at its core.

The details of your initial examination (**FIGURE 3-1**) should be collected in a way that leads you through a process of synthesizing, analyzing, and interpreting data with your patient or client. For example, it would be challenging to write objective, measurable, and functional goals for your patient or client without first determining his or her prognosis. Similarly, it would be a challenge to develop your intervention plan without first developing an understanding of your patient or client's impairments in body structures and functions, activity limitations, participation restrictions, and contextual factors. Consider that you work in an inpatient rehabilitation facility and you are conducting an initial examination of a 56-year-old male who is recovering from a total knee arthroplasty 3 days ago. Would you attempt to create this patient or client's intervention plan based on this information alone because you have experience working with this population in this setting? Would you create your goals and determine your prognosis based on what you perceive to be the interventions you should do with similar patients or clients? Or, would you collect more detail regarding this unique patient or client's impairments in body structures and functions, activity limitations, and participation restrictions so that you could not only determine your intervention plan, but also create a unified prognosis, anticipated goals and

expected outcomes, and frequency and duration of the episode of care?

The components of the initial examination can be collected in the order presented in Figure 3-1 to utilize as a framework around which to structure your initial examination documentation. The history is an information gathering process where you determine not only if your patient or client is appropriate to receive physical therapy services, but also where you determine the information you would like to collect as a screen in your systems review or in your more detailed tests and measures. In your **evaluation**, you would formulate your **diagnosis** and relay your **clinical impression** of your patient or client regarding the impairments in body functions and structures, activity limitations, participation restrictions, and contextual factors assembled from the information you have gathered from your history, systems review, and tests and measures. The diagnosis and clinical impression that you have determined in your evaluation is synthesized with further clinical judgment to determine a prognosis for your patient or client. Creating your anticipated goals and expected outcomes after determining your prognosis should assist you with formulating a clinical picture in your mind of how you expect your patient or client to recover by the conclusion of the episode of care. This understanding should lead you to define the frequency and duration of the episode of care and the subsequent creation of your intervention plan.

History

The content of the history section of your examination documentation is the foundation of the rest of your initial examination note. Because of the vast amount of

TABLE 3-1 History Content of the Initial Examination

Current status, condition, concern, complaint
Patient or client's perception of health, abilities
Patient or client's and/or family members' goals
Demographic information such as age, gender, race
Past medical history
Past surgical history
Past physical therapy, other medical or pharmacologic interventions
Lab results or imaging study results
Prior level of function
Current and past exercise history
Current level of function including use of equipment or devices
Comorbid conditions or syndromes such as falls or incontinence history
Current medications
Pain or other symptom description
Social history such as cultural or religious beliefs, limitations, or participation restrictions with certain social activities
Family history including relevant medical history, support, caregiver
Living environment
Work status
Hobbies and recreational activities
Communication style, learning style, mental status
Precautions or contraindications to movement or activity

information that could comprise a history (**TABLE 3-1**) it is important that you develop a strategy for organizing these details within this section. The American Physical Therapy Association (APTA) *Guide to Physical Therapist Practice* offers a comprehensive list of the types of information that may be generated from a patient or client history.[1] As indicated above, the quality of the information you collect in this section can help you build a well-structured and completely documented initial examination encounter. The details included in the history are also where you can start to formulate your patient or client's activity limitations, participation restrictions, and contextual factors so that relationships can be discerned with the information you gather regarding impairments in body functions and structures during your systems review and when collecting tests and measures and outcomes measures. It is important to keep track of these details for eventual inclusion in your evaluation and your goals. It is the relationships between these components of the World Health

Organization's (WHO) *International Classification of Functioning, Disability, and Health* (ICF) model that can help you to relay to the note's user the need for your medically necessary physical therapy intervention to optimize your patient or client's level of functioning and health.

The content of the history can be gathered from multiple sources depending on the setting in which you practice. The details of your history may not only come from a direct interview with your patient or client and the patient or client's caregivers, but also from any additional health records provided by the patient or client, intake or admission paperwork, documentation from other members of your patient or client's healthcare team, or information available from the previous level of care the patient or client received. Access to your patient or client's health history can help you to streamline and systematically direct your interview process during your initial examination.

One approach to documenting a history could be to create a free-text narrative based on the direction the interaction with your patient or client leads you. Consider the following narrative history from a patient or client in an outpatient setting.

> Mr. A is a 56-year-old male who experienced a R total knee arthroplasty 16 days ago. He reports a 7/10 pain currently and has been using a four-wheeled rolling walker. His goals include wanting to drive, getting back to work as a middle school teacher, and attending his son's baseball games. See history and intake form for further details.

Is there enough detail in this history to build the rest of your initial examination? Do you know if Mr. A has ever experienced a surgery before and how he responded to it? Do you know the details of Mr. A's hospital stay and if it was uneventful or if there were complications? Do you know when he was discharged from the hospital and if he has had home health physical therapy services? Do you know how he has been functioning at home over the last 16 days? Do you know if or how he is managing his pain? Do you know if Mr. A uses his walker in his home and what type of physical environment he has at home? Do you know if Mr. A was able to drive prior to his surgery? Do you understand the logistics involved in Mr. A attending his son's baseball games? What details of the history and intake paperwork are of interest? Are there any details reported in the paperwork that warrant further investigation? Are you aware of where to access this information in Mr. A's health record?

You may be aware of these details because of the interaction you actually had with Mr. A. However, if your documentation does not reflect the actual content of your interaction than it will be assumed that you are not aware of these important details. Furthermore, any other user of your note will not be able to gather relevant information from your history to make decisions. In other words, the lack of detail provided in the above history facilitates the use of assumptions regarding your patient or client's actual level of functioning and ability as well as his actual need for your physical therapy services. As you know, the use of assumptions to guide clinical decision making is not an evidence-based approach to the comprehensive care of your patient or client.

Now consider this history for the Mr. A.

> Mr. A is a 56-year-old male who is accompanied today by his wife to this physical therapy examination. He ambulated into the clinic with a four-wheeled rolling walker using a step-to and antalgic gait pattern. He appeared out of breath when ambulating 50 feet from the waiting room to the initial examination room. He states that he had a right total knee arthroplasty 16 days ago and that he feels that this is way too early to start physical therapy after such a surgery. He states that he has never had physical therapy before and is concerned because despite taking his pain medication he is experiencing a lot of pain. Mr. A reports a 9/10 pain in the right knee while sitting and a 5/10 pain when walking. He states that he is annoyed because he can't drive currently and this is significantly affecting his independence. Mr. A states that he has not had physical therapy before but that he received corticosteroid injections approximately three times per year over the last 2 years. He states that he had a previous bicycle accident where he twisted his right knee although he did not have any surgery or physical therapy after the accident, which was 10 years ago. He notes that over time his knee had become more and more painful and had started to interfere with his job as a middle school teacher. Mr. A notes that in addition to not being able to drive he is on leave from his job until he recovers. He states that he is unsure of when that will be or how long his recovery will take. He notes that he is unable to sleep in his bed due to experiencing pain in his knee when he attempts to roll or move his right leg. Therefore, he sleeps in the recliner in his living room, which seems to be irritating his back. Mr. A notes that he has episodic low back pain, which he has been able to control in the past with Advil (ibuprofen) and stretching. He states that he takes medication for hypertension but otherwise has no other medications or medical history except osteoarthritis. He states that he has had to alter everything that he does in his daily routine. He states that he sits to get dressed because his leg is painful to stand on. He states that he is not able to wear socks and that he must wear slip-on shoes, which he feels may not be safe for him in his home. He also states that he has difficulty getting off a low seat such as his couch or commode. Mr. A lives in a single story home with his wife and two teenage sons. He notes that he would like to get back to walking without pain as soon as possible so that he can attend his son's baseball games. He states that he is returning

to see his surgeon at the end of this week (in 4 days) for his second follow-up visit.

While this history for Mr. A seems comprehensive, it is actually unorganized. It contains valuable information but it is not presented in a format that would facilitate the ability to easily find specific information. It is difficult to identify quickly what relevant information might be missing and it does not give a clear sense of what information you might proceed with in your systems review or when collecting your tests and measures and outcome measures. Therefore, an alternative approach to creating a free-text narrative entry for documenting the history includes following a framework or an outline that enables you to direct your interview with your patient or client.

Consider the framework in TABLE 3-2 based on the scenario above.

Table 3-2 outlines the content of the history with suggested headings so that information is easily organized in a consistent location within the initial examination note. This organization can serve to improve your efficiency as you progress through your history with your patient or client as well as provide a framework so that any other user of your documentation can easily locate information. The "history of current status" section details information regarding your patient or client's complaint(s) and reason(s) for seeking physical therapy services. This is also where you can report your patient or client's subjective perception of his or her health and current status. Discerning current status early in your encounter with

TABLE 3-2   Framework for Creating the History Section of the Initial Examination Documentation

History of Current Status: Mr. A is a 56-year-old male who experienced a R total knee arthroplasty 16 days ago. He states that he is experiencing a lot of pain and is concerned about the length and speed of his recovery. He notes that he is significantly limited at this time since he is not able to drive and has had to alter how he performs his ADLs. Following up with surgeon at end of week on 6/7/2013.

Patient or Client Goals: return to driving, decrease pain, walk without a walker and without pain, improve ability to get up off low seat like commode, perform dressing and hygiene tasks, sleep in own bed without waking due to pain, attend two teenage sons' baseball games, return to work as a middle school teacher.

Past Medical History and Past Surgical History: R total knee arthroplasty on 5/20/2013; bicycle accident 10 years ago in which Mr. A "twisted" his R knee. Mr A. reports full recovery from this accident. Skin cancer (melanoma) removed from R ear and R shoulder on 1/14/2013. Did not receive radiation or chemotherapy. Also see medical history and intake form; additional details of social history and exercise habits included here.

Concurrent Conditions: low back pain (episodic) – reports currently aggravated due to sleeping in a recliner due to R knee pain.

Precautions or Contraindications to Movement or Activity: none.

Past Interventions: no prior physical therapy for knee or low back pain; corticosteroid injections at R knee three times per year over the last year.

Lab Results or Imaging Study Results: none since 2-day hospital stay.

Prior Level of Function: active and independent with all ADLs.

Current Level of Function: using four-wheeled rolling walker in home for all transfer and ambulation tasks; using four-wheeled rolling walker for ambulation in community to attend medical appointments; modified I for dressing, grooming, and showering tasks due to increased length of time to complete tasks, pain, poor control and balance; unable to sleep in bed.

Current Medications: Lortab (hydrocodone/acetaminophen), Mobic (meloxicam), Robaxin (methocarbamol), ibuprofen discontinued at this time; patient/client reports that he is taking medications as prescribed but he is having breakthrough pain.

Pain or Other Symptom Description: anterior R knee pain from distal 1/3rd of upper leg to tibial tubercle; R posterior and medial knee pain; tight and aching; feels better when standing and walking than when sitting or trying to sleep; low back feels tight like it needs to stretch after sitting >20 minutes; denies lower leg cramping or foot/ankle pain.
Worst pain = 9/10 in knee after sitting >20 minutes
Best pain = 2/10 after taking pain meds
Average pain = 5/10
Current pain = 9/10 in knee after sitting >20 minutes; 5/10 in knee when walking

Family History: attended session with wife; supportive family; lives with wife and two teenage sons; hypertension; osteoarthritis, lung cancer, Parkinson's disease.

Living Environment: one-story home with two steps to enter in front; no railing; one step into home from garage; pool with handrails.

Work Status: on medical leave until 7/1/2013.

Hobbies and Recreational Activities: going to sons' baseball games.

Communication Style, Learning Style, Mental Status: prefers visual representation of HEP; cognitively intact.

your patient or client can help you determine if your patient or client is in fact appropriate for physical therapy services either in the setting in which you are conducting your history, in an alternative setting, or if your patient or client requires a referral to an entirely different service altogether before physical therapy services can commence. Consider the following scenario.

You are working in an inpatient rehabilitation setting and you are attempting to conduct an initial examination on an 18-year-old male who sustained a closed head injury in a motor vehicle accident 3 weeks ago. According to the patient or client's hospital admission paperwork, you expect to encounter a patient or client who is medically stable with a Glasgow Coma Scale rating of 12 (moderate head injury with spontaneous eye opening response, confused conversation but able to answer questions, withdraws in response to pain). However, as you proceed with your examination you find that after 10 minutes your patient or client has difficulty staying awake and only intermittently responds to your inquiries with appropriate words. Furthermore, there are several points during your history with the patient or client that you have to redirect his attention to you or provide tactile stimulation to hold his attention and keep him awake. After 30 minutes of attempting to progress your initial examination, you decide to meet with your team to discuss your concerns that this patient or client may not be appropriate for physical therapy intervention at this time.

Your history documentation of this encounter may appear in the health record as follows.

Attempted physical therapy initial examination at 10:00 am. The patient had extreme difficulty staying awake and required constant tactile cuing to arouse. The patient was intermittently able to respond to verbal questions with appropriate responses. The patient required the total assistance of one person to transfer to a wheelchair and required the wheelchair to be reclined at least 45 degrees to stay positioned in the chair. Will attempt further examination this afternoon after discussion with healthcare team.

The "patient or client goals" section is an area of your history that can assist you to identify your patient or client's activity limitations and participation restrictions.

You can objectify this section by applying the Patient-Specific Functional Scale (PSFS) for example. Your documentation of this section for Mr. A might appear as follows.

Patient or Client Goals per Patient-Specific Functional Scale

ACTIVITY	Initial Score/Date	Reassessment Score/Date	Discharge Score/Date
1. Unable to drive	0		
2. Unable to walk without device	0		
3. Difficulty getting dressed especially lower body (socks and shoes)	5		
4. Unable to sleep in bed due to pain	3		
5. Unable to attend son's baseball games	0		
6. Unable to return to work as a middle school teacher	0		
Additional			

© 1995, P. Stratford, reprinted with permission.

Later in the initial examination note, you can incorporate the score of the PSFS as well as the specific items in the scale into your anticipated goals and expected outcomes.

The "past medical history and surgical history" section is an opportunity for you to refer to data that may have already been collected via intake paperwork prior to your face-to-face encounter with your patient or client. It is your responsibility however to ensure that you review this information and clarify any of its contents with the patient or client. It is equally important to reiterate content from this paperwork in this section that will impact your patient or client's plan of care. In the case of Mr. A, it is relevant to report in your history the presence of skin cancer given the potential for metastatic disease to indicate that you are aware and have considered the potential impact of this condition on the plan of care. On the other hand, it is not necessary to report other details regarding Mr. A's medical or surgical history such as a left ankle sprain 20 years ago or laser eye surgery 5 years ago since these conditions do not impact the plan of care.

The "concurrent conditions" section is intended to list the patient or client's current conditions that have a direct impact on the plan of care such as hypertension, osteoporosis, fall history, or deconditioning due to a lengthy and complicated hospital stay. This detail will lead you to explicitly list any precautions or contraindications that should be elucidated. The "past interventions" section should not only include past medical, pharmacological, or physical therapy interventions, but should also include details such as the benefit of these interventions to the patient or client and if any other future interventions are planned. The "lab and imaging study results" is a section in which you can refer to any reports that your patient or client shares with you. Like the intake paperwork, it is your responsibility to review the provided results and carry forward into the history any relevant details that could potentially impact your plan of care. The "prior" and "current level of function" sections allow for a direct comparison of your patient or client's status at two points in time and can stimulate your insight to the development of your prognosis. This section will also help you to generate the need for medically necessary care since you will include the specific limitations your patient or client currently has with his functioning and abilities.

The "current medications" section can give you insight to any conditions for which the patient or client is receiving pharmacologic intervention as well as potential side effects of these medications that might impact the patient or client's current status and ultimately the plan of care. Furthermore, you can detail if the patient or client is taking these medications as prescribed and if they are effective. In Mr. A's case, this information can help you determine the need to communicate with the surgeon on Mr. A's behalf or help you to communicate to Mr. A the details that he should talk with the surgeon about at the next follow-up appointment. The "pain and symptom description" section is the area where you can capture more details other than pain ratings regarding your patient or client's pain such as the location and description of pain, activities that improve or worsen pain, the frequency and duration of pain, as well as other symptoms such as paresthesias or dizziness that the patient or client could be experiencing that may impact the plan of care.

The "family history" section is the area where you would indicate your patient or client's living arrangements to discern the level of support available during the plan of care. Additionally, you could determine if your patient or client has responsibilities to other family members such as caring for an aging parent or a child. Furthermore, you can indicate any family medical history to heighten your awareness of the potential impact on your patient or client's plan of care such as undiagnosed hypertension. The "living environment" section allows for the inclusion of details regarding your patient or client's home environment so that you can consider these details in your plan of care. The "work status" section can help you to track details such as your patient or client's expected return to work as well as any alterations or restrictions on work load from your patient or client's employer that you might need to consider in creating your plan of care. The "hobbies and recreational activities" is an additional opportunity to identify other activities that interest your patient or client so that you can use this information to connect with your patient or client and incorporate it into your plan of care.

The "communication/learning style/mental status" section serves to record your thoughts on your patient or client's capacity to be an active participant in his or her own care, how your patient or client might learn or be able to incorporate a home exercise program, and if you will need to conduct further testing regarding cognitive status. You may alternatively decide to include this section in your systems review. It is presented in the history section in this framework, however, to facilitate an understanding of your patient or client's ability to communicate and make decisions prior to collecting too much information that may not be accurate or useful. Thus, the headings provided to create Mr. A's history in Table 3-2 are intended as a suggested list to create a framework for organizing the information you gather from your history. For example, a history taken in an inpatient or skilled nursing setting might include headings such as "admission date" or "community services" being received. Ultimately, the intention of utilizing headings or an outline format to organize your history is so that a solid foundational framework is in place for the construction of the next components of your initial examination documentation, the systems review and collection of tests and measures and outcome measures.

Systems Review

The systems review is a short examination process that has a dual purpose. First, the systems review helps you to rule out conditions that may be beyond the scope of your practice as a physical therapist. Second, the systems review serves to help you identify those signs and symptoms as well as other contextual factors that will potentially affect the plan of care you develop for your patient or client. The systems review is not intended to be an optional part of the examination. Rather it is intended to be a component of the examination process that further helps you to consider your patient or client holistically. It also serves as a mechanism to help you convey the tests and measures and outcome measures you will proceed with in the next section of your initial examination. The *Guide to Physical Therapist Practice* suggests that the systems review be organized according to four biological systems in the human body and encompass information regarding a patient or client's communication and language abilities, cognitive and mental status, and learning style (**TABLE 3-3**).[1]

A review of the cardiovascular and pulmonary systems includes a vital sign assessment and assessing the extremities for edema. Because you will be engaging your patients or clients in some form of movement, activity, or exercise as a physical therapist or physical therapist

assistant, it is your obligation to be aware of your patient or client's cardiovascular and pulmonary status both at baseline and in response to activity regardless of the setting in which you practice. In the example above, it would

TABLE 3-3   Systems Review Components and Content

Cardiovascular and Pulmonary Systems
○ Vital signs
○ Edema
Integumentary System
○ Skin integrity
○ Scars and incisions
○ Wounds
Musculoskeletal System
○ Gross postural assessment
○ Gross range of motion
○ Gross strength
Neuromuscular System
○ Gross coordination
○ Movement quality
○ Motor control
○ Motor learning
Communication, language, cognition, learning style
○ consciousness
○ orientation
○ emotional and behavioral responses
○ learning preferences

Data from The American Physical Therapy Association's Interactive Guide the Physical Therapist Practice 3.0, 2014.

be valuable to know prior to initiating any movement or exercise program with Mr. A, his cardiovascular response to movement especially because of his family history of hypertension and the fact that he reports a high level of pain. Thus, it would be more appropriate for you to rule out undiagnosed hypertension with your assessment than it would be to assume that Mr. A does not have hypertension based on the fact that he does not report it and does not report taking anti-hypertensive medications. Remember, if you assess it but neglect to record it, the assumption by the user of your note is that the assessment was not completed. The systems review documentation

for Mr. A in **TABLE 3-4** verifies that Mr. A is safe to proceed with exercise based on his baseline vital signs. It will be important at some point in your interaction with Mr. A however to verify and document his response to exercise.

A review of the integumentary system includes any skin abnormalities, including hair and nails, you observe on your patient or client regarding skin integrity, color, scar formation, or wounds. The documentation of the quick assessment of Mr. A's integumentary system indicates that you discussed a potential problem area on Mr. A's right shoulder and verified that he is aware of it (Table 3-4). This is important given his prior history of melanoma on

TABLE 3-4 Framework for Creating the Systems Review Content of the Initial Examination Documentation

Cardiovascular and Pulmonary Systems
- Vital signs:
  - BP rest = 131/76 mmHg
  - HR rest = 72 bpm bounding, regular pulse (radial)
  - RR rest = 15 breaths per minute
- Edema:
  - R knee = peripatellar; appears consistent with surgical intervention.
  - None observed distal to knees or at feet and ankles bilaterally.

Integumentary System
- Skin integrity – appears to have a small irregularly shaped mole on posterior right shoulder lateral to scar where prior melanoma was removed. Mr. A reports that he is aware of this growth and relays that he has an appointment with his dermatologist next week. No other disruptions noted. No skin discolorations noted except for bruising at posterior medial R knee that appears to be healing and consistent with total knee arthroplasy due to yellowish-green skin hue.
- Scars – none observed other than dime-shaped scar on posterior medial R shoulder due to melanoma removal.
- Wounds – healing surgical incision anterior R knee (see tests and measures); no other wounds observed; Mr. A denies history of wounds.

Musculoskeletal System
- Height = 71 inches; Weight = 192 pounds
- Gross postural assessment
  - Pes planus observed at L foot; Mr. A notes that he wears a custom orthotic in his L shoe; this has not been reassessed for approximately 2 years.
- Gross range of motion
  - Bilateral upper extremities – no gross limitations
  - Spine – no gross limitations
- Gross strength
  - Grip – R = 109#; L = 101# (R hand dominant)

Neuromuscular System
- Gross coordination – intact and equal bilaterally via lower extremity heel-to-shin test and repeated alternating toe taps.
- Movement quality – slow cautious movement of the R knee due to pain.
- Motor function
  - Deep tendon reflexes = intact and equal bilaterally
  - Clonus = negative bilaterally
  - Babinski = negative bilaterally
  - Light touch and pinprick sensation intact bilaterally

Communication, Language, Cognition, Learning Style
- Able to follow multi-step commands.
- Intact cognition based on interaction and awareness of person, place, time, and event.
- Prefers visual demonstration and visual representation of exercises.

Data from The American Physical Therapy Association's Interactive Guide the Physical Therapist Practice, 2003.

the right shoulder and because of the potential impact to your plan of care should Mr. A's visit with his dermatologist lead to more significant future findings such as metastatic disease. Also acknowledged here is that the surgical incision at the right knee is healing and that further examination of the incision is documented elsewhere in the note. Consider that the content of the integumentary component of Mr. A's systems review note was left blank. In this case, it would be important to ensure that you fully document data regarding Mr. A's skin in your tests and measures section of your examination documentation. Even if Mr. A's surgical incision is healing perfectly, it is important that you document this ideal baseline status. In the event that a compromise to the surgical site manifests, your thorough documentation will enable you to precisely indicate when this problem occurred, which may lead to determining further intervention and prevention.

A review of the musculoskeletal system includes your patient or client's height and weight as well as gross observations of axial and extremity postures, range of motion, and strength that might potentially impact the plan of care. The systems review of this section for Mr. A indicates the presence of pes planus at the left foot, which may have the potential to impact Mr. A's low back pain or ambulation status and is therefore relevant to document in this section (Table 3-4).

A review of the neuromuscular system includes a quick assessment of your patient or client's movement quality as well as varied components of a neurologic screen. Based on the history you have gathered to this point, you may decide to defer documenting further coordination, movement quality, and motor function details until the tests and measures section of the note. In Mr. A's case, it is pertinent to ensure that he lacks neurologic involvement to rule out these signs and symptoms as potential complications of his surgery as well as to verify that a concurrent neurologic issue is not occurring.

The communication, language, cognition, and learning style section of the systems review is an opportunity in the initial examination documentation for you to record the ability of your patient or client to interact and participate in the plan of care you create on his or her behalf.

It is just as important in the systems review section of your initial examination documentation as it is in the history section to be organized and systematic regarding the information you collect and subsequently document. It is the content in this section that will enable you to

> ### BOX 3-2 The Electronic Health Record: Systems Review
>
> The systems review section in an electronic health record may be a straightforward list of body systems with relevant headings to represent the content. Alternatively, the systems review section could be a free-text box in which you create a narrative of the information you want to include in this section. Therefore, it is important for you to have an understanding of the purpose of the systems review so that the appropriate detail can be included based on the particular features of your electronic health record documentation.

investigate further any preliminary findings with more detailed and comprehensive tests and measures and outcome measures, or to facilitate communication on behalf of your patient or client regarding unexpected findings that may be unrelated to the reason your patient or client sought physical therapy services. By documenting this information you are upholding your responsibility to "provide high-quality professional service to society"[2] as well as relaying your ability to function effectively as a point of entry for your patient or client into the healthcare system.

Tests and Measures and Outcome Measures

By the end of the history and systems review process you should have gathered enough information to generate an initial clinical impression regarding your preliminary hypotheses for the etiology of your patient or client's current status. It is this impression that you use to develop the rest of your examination. The data generated from the selected tests and measures and outcome measures can then be used to refine your clinical impression for inclusion in the evaluation portion of your initial examination documentation. There are many tests and measures and outcome measures available to you as a physical therapist or physical therapist assistant as indicated by the *Guide to Physical Therapist Practice*.[1] A test and measure is a mechanism used to gather data regarding some characteristic of your patient or client. Collating the results that you gathered on your patient or client via tests and measures leads to the clinical determination of the expected outcomes you have for your patient or client. This is not to be confused with an **outcome measure**, which is a tool that has established validity and can be used to determine the efficacy of an intervention by measuring change over time.[3] Therefore, not all tests and measures are outcome measures. In other words, tests and measures inform the outcome measures you might employ with your patient or client to measure change over time. For example, testing the quadriceps muscle via manual muscle testing is a test and measure. The Five Times Sit to Stand Test is an outcome measure of functional lower extremity strength because a minimum amount of change that occurs over time in the Five Times Sit to Stand Test, or responsiveness, has been established.[4,5]

The way in which you choose to organize the tests and measures and outcome measures you select in your initial examination documentation should follow a structured sequence so that the data you collect is easy to subsequently locate for clinical decision making. For example, you may decide to categorize the tests and measures you select for your examination as screening-, diagnostic-,

or impairment-based tests and measures. The Neer Test can be used to screen for the presence of shoulder pathology. Similarly, the Wells criteria can be applied to screen for the presence of deep vein thrombosis. Diagnostic or health condition-related tests and measures are those that may help you to rule in or out a certain diagnosis or health condition such as a Lachman Test for an anterior cruciate ligament rupture or an upper limb tension test for cervical radiculopathy. Impairment-based tests and measures are those used to collect data related to impairments in body functions and structures such as range of motion, visual observation of postural alignment, light touch sensation, or deep tendon reflexes.

Like the documentation strategy you implement for recording tests and measures, it can be valuable to organize your documentation of the outcomes measures you choose to help inform further detail regarding your evaluation, prognosis, goals, frequency and duration of the episode of care, and intervention plan. There are two primary categories of outcome measures: self-report and performance based (**FIGURE 3-2**). In other words, if you are not asking

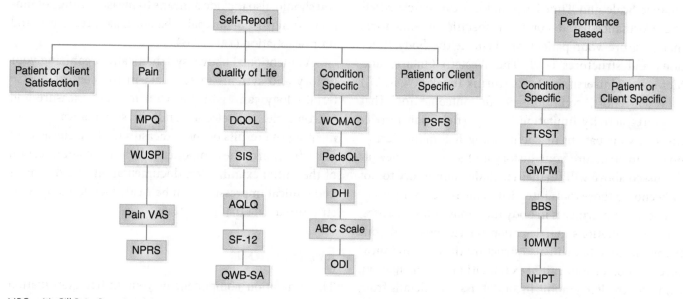

MPQ = McGill Pain Questionnaire
WUSPI = Wheelchair Users Shoulder Pain Index
Pain VAS = Pain Visual Analog Scales
NPRS = Numeric Pain Rating Scale
DQOL = Diabetes Quality of Life Measure
SIS = Stroke Impact Scale
AQLQ = Asthma Quality of Life Questionnaire
SF-12 = 12 Item Short Form Health Survey
QWB-SA = Quality of Well Being – Self Administered
WOMAC = Western Ontario and McMaster Universities Index

PedsQL = Pediatric Quality of Life Inventory
DHI = Dizziness Handicap Inventory
ABC Scale = Activities-Specific Balance Confidence Scale
ODI = Oswestry Disability Index
PSFS = Patient-Specific Functional Scale
FTSST = Five Times Sit to Stand Test
GMFM = Gross Motor Function Measure
BBS = Berg Balance Scale
10MWT = 10-Meter Walk Test
NHPT = Nine-Hole Peg test

FIGURE 3-2 Outcome Measures Framework.

your patient or client or your patient or client's caregiver to report certain information, such as pain or perception of the ability to complete certain tasks, then you are observing performance. Self-report measures can be further classified to include patient or client satisfaction, pain, quality of life, and condition-specific and patient- or client-specific measures. For an outcome measure to be patient- or client-specific, the patient or client should self-identify the factors being measured. For example, activities included in the Patient-Specific Functional Scale are offered by the patient or client. Performance-based measures can also be further classified as condition- or patient- or client-specific. Theoretically, performance-based, patient- or client-specific outcome measures may be valuable in the examination of your patient or client; however, there exists a gap in the evidence regarding this category of outcome measures. More abundant evidence exists for self-report measures and performance-based, condition-specific outcome measures.

Rather than select tests and measures and outcome measures from a long alphabetical list, it may be helpful to employ ICF model terminology once again to provide an organized framework. For example, the Berg Balance Scale and Timed Up and Go can be classified as performance-based, condition-specific outcome tools that measure your patient or client at the body functions and structures level. The Western Ontario and McMaster Universities Osteoarthritis Index (WOMAC) is a self-report, condition-specific outcome tool that measures activity limitations and participation restrictions in your patient or client. Using ICF model terminology to structure your history and systems review as discussed above will further facilitate your ability to not only choose those tools intended to measure your patient or client's impairments in body functions and structures, activity limitations, participation restrictions, and contextual factors, but will also structure the tests and measures section of your initial examination documentation. Consider the ICF graphic in **FIGURE 3-3**. The details from Mr. A's history and systems review were referenced to populate the health condition, activity limitations, participation restrictions, and contextual factors sections of the ICF graphic. This information can be subsequently used to support your clinical judgment and reasoning to populate the impairments in the body functions and structures section of the ICF graphic. In this way, the ICF graphic ultimately lends support to how you proceed with your initial examination and how you document the tests

and measures and outcome measures you select. In other words, each entry into the graphic should be represented by a means to measure and track it. For example, Mr. A's activity limitations include his inability to drive or sleep in his own bed, his need for assistance with dressing, hygiene, and showering tasks, as well as for getting off the commode, and his need for an assistive device for household and community ambulation. Since these items represent activities and participation in life events that Mr. A would like to change, you will likely decide to direct your interventions to improve these activity limitations and participation restrictions. However, it would not be appropriate to implement interventions with your patient or client if you have not measured them. At this point in your initial examination process with Mr. A you have only collected this data. You have not yet determined how you will measure change in this data. Therefore, a mechanism to measure change in these domains must be employed. For example, the WOMAC is an appropriate outcome tool to issue to Mr. A during his initial examination to measure change in his activity limitations. Similarly, the data entered into the ICF graphic indicates that you should also include a means to measure range of motion, strength, edema, pain, balance, gait, transfers, and stair negotiation (**TABLE 3-5**).

As mentioned above, systematically organizing your history and systems review data in the context of ICF terminology can assist you with test and measure and outcome measure selection and with systematically documenting the results of these measures. Thus, subsequent identification of the components of the evaluation section of the initial examination documentation, the diagnosis and clinical impression, can be easily facilitated by well-structured data that precedes it.

Evaluation

The evaluation component of your initial examination documentation can be thought of as a synopsis of the data collected on the patient or client's behalf including the response to tests and measures and outcome measures. This information is then integrated with data collected during the history and systems review to develop your diagnosis and clinical impression. This is the area of your initial examination documentation that a user of your note would go to first to find out why your patient or client is receiving physical therapy services. The components of

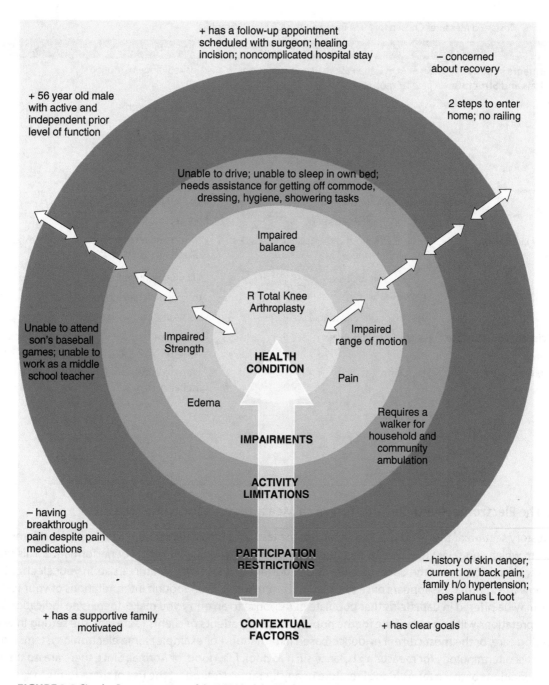

FIGURE 3-3 Circular Representation of the ICF Model – Mr. A.

Data from Towards a Common Language for Functioning, Disability and Health (ICF). World Health Organization, 2002.

the evaluation section of your initial examination documentation include the diagnosis or diagnoses and your clinical impression. It is important to note that the APTA *Guide to Physical Therapist Practice* further defines the evaluation as the process by which physical therapists determine the prognosis and develop the remaining components of the plan of care.[1] While developing the remaining components of the plan of care requires knowledge of data previously collected, the actual content of the

prognosis, the anticipated goals and expected outcomes, the frequency and duration of the episode of care, and intervention planning are presented separately to facilitate the psychomotor skills of actually creating the content of these components. Ultimately, it is the content of the diagnosis and clinical impression that must permeate the core of your evaluation for the remaining components of the plan of care to cohesively represent why your patient or client is seeking physical therapy services.

TABLE 3-5   Tests and Measures Chosen for Mr. A Based on the ICF Model Graphic

ICF Category	Test and Measure or Outcome Measure	Entry into ICF Graphic for Mr. A
Impairments in Body Functions and Structure	Knee Active and Passive Range of Motion, patellar mobility testing	Impaired range of motion
	Quadriceps, hamstring, gluteus medius manual muscle testing	Impaired strength
	Heel Rise Test	Impaired strength
	Circumferential Measurement at the Knee	Edema
	Numeric Pain Rating Scale	Pain
	Single Limb Stance	Impaired balance
	Functional Gait Assessment	Impaired balance
Activity Limitations	Western Ontario and McMaster Universities Osteoarthritis Index	Pain, getting off commode, dressing tasks, walking, lying in bed
	Five Times Sit to Stand	Difficulty getting off the commode
	10-Meter Walk Test	Ambulation limitations
	Patient-Specific Functional Scale	Unable to drive, unable to sleep in bed
Participation Restrictions	Patient-Specific Functional Scale	Unable to attend sons' baseball games, unable to return to work as a middle school teacher
Contextual Factors	Stair Climb Test	2 steps to enter home; desire to attend sons' baseball games

---

BOX 3-3 The Electronic Health Record: Tests and Measures and Outcome Measures

Like the history section of the electronic health record, the tests and measures section may simply be a comprehensive list from which you select to input the results of your patient or client's self-report or performance. This section may also list interpretations of the data you enter. It is important to know if this feature exists in your electronic system and how the information appears once this section is completed. Even though interpretations of your tests and measures may be offered in data fields that populate in response to an entry you make, there is no indication that these interpretations will be appropriate for the population your patients or clients represent, the setting in which you are delivering care, or the most current evidence-based information. For example, some electronic systems use non-evidence-based terminology for measuring balance such as poor, fair, good, or normal. Since there are no universally accepted definitions of these terms in the literature or any literature to support the use of these terms to quantify a balance impairment, then it becomes difficult to interpret how these findings actually translate to the true level of functioning and ability of your patient or client. Therefore, it is important for you to have an understanding of what tests and measures you want to collect for your patient or client as well how to interpret each so that you can relate your findings back to your unique patient or client. Furthermore, if a test and measure or outcome tool that you want to use is not listed in your documentation system, it is important to resist the urge to select one that only closely represents what you wish to measure. It would be more appropriate to utilize a free-text or "Other" category to input the exact test and measure or outcome tool you desire. Lastly, the drop-down menus provided in this section should not be "browsed" to determine the content of your tests and measures section of the initial examination. Rather, you should have already developed a preliminary clinical impression of your patient or client based on the data you collected from the history and systems review and have a well-developed understanding of the tests and measures you will use to initiate this portion of your initial examination.

Consider that as a physical therapist or physical therapist assistant, you provide interventions to improve or rectify your patient or client's impairments in body functions and structures, activity limitations, and participation restrictions rather than to change a medical diagnosis or diagnostic label.[6] Therefore, it is appropriate to describe your patient or client's diagnosis or diagnoses in these terms (TABLE 3-6). In Mr. A's case, it may be tempting to define the diagnosis as a right total knee arthroplasty. However, if your goal in providing physical therapy services is to remediate deficits and recover functioning and ability for your patient or client then this categorization is inappropriate. Mr. A's right total knee arthroplasty will never be eliminated or lessened, but the deficits associated with it will. It is appropriate however to indicate the health condition, in this case osteoarthritis, that led to the need for the total knee arthroplasty.

The clinical impression component of your initial examination documentation represents the synthesis of all of the data you have collected thus far into a narrative that answers one important question: Why does your patient or client need your skilled services? Simply reporting that your patient or client has experienced a "decline in function" does not include enough detail to support the need for your skilled services. The detail of your answer should instead include specific details from your history and systems review when you organized these findings using ICF terminology. Relaying the answer to this question in a narrative format will underscore the medical necessity of your services in one specific location in the initial examination documentation. Consider the evaluation for Mr. A's initial examination below.

Mr. A experienced a right total knee arthroplasty on 05/20/2013 due to longstanding knee osteoarthritis. His impairments in body functions and structures include pain, edema, impaired range of motion and patellar mobility, impaired lower extremity muscle strength, poor lower extremity muscle performance, and impaired dynamic standing balance. His activity limitations include the inability to drive or to sleep in his own bed, his need for assistance to get off the commode and for dressing, hygiene, and showering tasks, as well as the need for assistance with a walker for community and household ambulation. Mr. A's participation restrictions include the inability to attend his son's baseball games and his inability to work as a middle school teacher. The contextual factors that affect Mr. A's recovery include the fact that he has clear goals, a supportive family, and an active lifestyle. Mr. A has a history of melanoma on the right shoulder. An area on the right shoulder was identified during this examination that Mr. A notes he is having evaluated by his dermatologist next week. In addition, he reports that he is experiencing breakthrough pain at the right knee despite taking his medications as prescribed. Mr. A was educated to report this information to his surgeon at his follow-up visit in 4 days or to call his surgeon's office to report his concerns if the breakthrough pain continues to worsen prior

TABLE 3-6 Content of the Diagnosis and Clinical Impression Components of the Initial Examination Documentation

Diagnosis	Clinical Impression
What is your patient or client's health condition and reason for seeking physical therapy services?	Why would your patient or client benefit from skilled physical therapy care? ○ What are the patient or client's impairments in body functions and structures that indicate the need for physical therapy intervention? ○ What are the patient or client's activity limitations and participation restrictions that indicate the need for physical therapy intervention? ○ What are the contextual factors that may impact your patient or client's recovery?
	Are there any details that exist that indicate that physical therapy services are not warranted at this time?
	Are there any details that exist that indicate the need for a referral to an alternative service?

to his appointment. In addition, I will place a call on Mr. A's behalf to his surgeon's office to relay this concern by the end of business today.

It is also relevant in this section to include any details that you would want to highlight to your patient or client's referral source or to anyone who may be using the note to make decisions. For example, if you were concerned after performing your initial examination that Mr. A might have an infection at his incision site, not only would you have documented your findings in the appropriate previous sections of your systems review and tests and measures and outcome measures sections of the initial examination, but you would also indicate in your clinical impression your concerns about Mr. A's incision, your recommendations, and the actions you took to address the problem. The evaluation of this situation might appear as follows.

> Mr. A experienced a right total knee arthroplasty on 05/20/2013 due to longstanding knee osteoarthritis. His impairments in body functions and structures include pain, edema, warmth, significant inflammation and redness around the surgical incision at the right knee, impaired range of motion and patellar mobility, impaired lower extremity muscle strength, poor lower extremity muscle performance, and impaired dynamic standing balance. His activity limitations include the inability to drive or to sleep in his own bed, his need for assistance to get off the commode and for dressing, hygiene, and showering tasks, as well as the need for assistance with a walker for community and household ambulation. Mr. A's participation restrictions include the inability to attend his son's baseball games and his inability to work as a middle school teacher. The contextual factors that affect Mr. A's recovery include the fact that he has clear goals, a supportive family, and an active lifestyle. Based on the findings from the initial examination above Mr. A may have delayed healing secondary to a possible infection at his surgical incision site at the right knee. A call was placed to Mr. A's surgeon's office during this physical therapy examination and arrangements were made for Mr. A to go to see his surgeon this afternoon.

It is important to recognize that your clinical impression of your patient or client can change based on new information that you learn or based on the changes that your patient or client makes over time as long as your documentation reflects these changes. It is appropriate to keep track of your patient or client's progress throughout the documentation of your plan of care such as in daily notes, progress notes, and re-examination notes. However, an addendum would be appropriate if you became aware of new information prior to reassessing your patient or client that affects the plan of care. Consider that a week goes by before Mr. A's first follow-up visit since the initial examination. Upon his return he shares with you that he followed up with his surgeon at the end of last week who was pleased with his progress. However, over the weekend Mr. A sprained his right ankle when he stepped awkwardly down the step into his garage. He states that he went to urgent care and x-rays taken were negative for any fracture at the right ankle. He states that the right ankle pain is better today, but it is fairly swollen and interferes with his mobility. It would be appropriate in this situation to create in entry in the intervention section of the daily note for that visit that refers to an addendum to your initial examination documentation that would then be used to communicate to Mr. A's surgeon. This addendum might appear as follows.

> Mr. A returns to physical therapy today for his first follow-up visit since the initial examination on 06/03/2013. He reports that he has visited with his surgeon on 06/07/2013 who is happy with his progress. However, on 06/08/2013 Mr. A stepped awkwardly down the step into his garage and sprained his right ankle. He states that he was walking with his cane at the time and did not fall. However he notes that his ankle is very swollen and interferes with his mobility. Mr. A reports that x-rays taken of the ankle and foot at an urgent care center are negative for a fracture.
>
> Additional and re-measured tests and measures:
> ○ Pitting edema: 2+ at right sinus tarsus and dorsal lateral aspect of right foot;
> ○ AROM Right: Dorsiflexion = 4 degrees (pain), Plantarflexion = 23 degrees (tight), Inversion = 15 degrees (pain), Eversion = 25 degrees (pain)
>
> Additional and re-measured outcome measures:
> ○ Single Leg Stance on Right = 4 seconds (pain)
> ○ Functional Gait Assessment = 14/30
> ○ Five Times Sit to Stand = not able

○ Heel Rise Test = not able

○ Stair Climb Test = not able

Adjusted evaluation: Mr. A's additional impairments in body function and structures based on the new findings from his ankle sprain include ankle and foot edema, decreased ankle and foot active range or motion, impaired dynamic standing balance, impaired muscle control and performance at the right ankle due to pain, which further impairs Mr. A's ability to stand from a low seat, negotiate steps, and walk over even and uneven surface with and without an assistive device.

In addition, this addendum will also include an adjusted prognosis, additional goals and expected outcomes, and adjusted frequency and duration of the episode of care and an additional intervention plan. Ultimately, details of the ICF graphic created in Figure 3-3 and the questions presented in Table 3-6 were used to construct the details of the evaluation documentation above and can be used as templates in creating the content of the evaluation for any patient or client in any setting with any situation. See **APPENDIX 3-A** for additional information that would be included in the initial examination for a workers' compensation patient or client. This organized structure of the diagnosis and clinical impression then leads directly into the next component of your initial examination documentation: the prognosis.

BOX 3-4 The Electronic Health Record: Evaluation

The evaluation section in an electronic health record may simply be a free-text data field in which you input relevant information. Alternatively, this section could be a comprehensive list of many possible impairments in body functions and structures, activity limitations, participation restrictions, and contextual factors from which you select. It is important to ensure that the information you select actually represents the information you collected in the rest of your initial examination documentation so that an accurate reflection of your patient or client's need for reasonable and medically necessary physical therapy care is depicted.

Prognosis

The prognosis component of your initial examination documentation includes your interpretation of the level of improvement or outcome your patient or client will achieve.[6] In the evaluation component of your initial examination documentation, you described your patient or client in terms of functioning and ability using ICF terminology. Similarly, you can use your patient or client's current level of functioning and ability to make a professional judgment regarding his or her ability to improve this level. It is important to make an explicit statement regarding your patient or client's capacity to improve and what details you are using to make this judgment. In this way, you will be supporting the need for physical therapy services for your patient or client. Consider the following prognosis added to a version of Mr. A's evaluation that eliminates the presence of breakthrough pain.

> Mr. A's prognosis is excellent based on his ability to progress through the initial examination, his response to interventions provided during the initial examination (see attached home exercise program), as well as his high level of motivation and previous active lifestyle.

Consider the following prognosis statement for the evaluation that relays Mr. A's breakthrough pain.

> Assuming that Mr. A's breakthrough pain is addressed, his prognosis for improving the impairments, activity limitations, and participation restrictions indicated above is good. Currently Mr. A's level of irritability is high given the pain he is experiencing and his inability to sleep comfortably in his bed. This pain will potentially slow his ability to meet his goals indicated below.

In addition to providing your interpretation of the level of improvement or outcome your patient or client will achieve, it is also important to indicate your judgment of the time frame your patient or client will take to achieve it. You may decide to include the time it takes to improve your patient or client's level of functioning and ability in the prognosis section of your initial examination documentation, or you might decide to include it in the frequency and duration of the episode of care section of your note after you establish your anticipated goals and expected outcomes. It is important to realize that the content of the prognosis component of your initial examination can change as your patient or client changes, as long as you update your documentation to reflect this change. Assume that on the first follow-up visit after the initial examination Mr. A reports that he has an infection at his surgical incision site. He states that he has been given antibiotics and has been advised to continue physical therapy; however he is concerned regarding the pain he experiences with movement. It would be appropriate at this time to create an addendum to the prognosis component of your initial examination documentation to reflect this new information, which might appear in the health record as below.

> Addendum to prognosis: Mr. A reports at his first follow-up visit since his initial examination 2 days ago that he has an infection at his incision site that is now being treated with antibiotics. He reports that he has been advised by his surgeon to continue with physical therapy but he is concerned regarding the level of pain he feels at his right knee with any movement. Mr. A's impairments in body functions and structures, activity limitations, and participation restrictions are further affected by the presence of this infection. Therefore, the prognosis for Mr. A is good assuming that the antibiotics eliminate the infection and Mr. A can proceed with the plan of care as indicated. The presence of the infection may potentially delay Mr. A's progress with the goals as established in this plan of care. If no positive change occurs in the level of Mr. A's pain or in his level of functioning and ability in 1 week, his surgeon will be contacted to relay his delayed progress.

BOX 3-5 The Electronic Health Record: Prognosis

This section of the EHR may be represented by a drop-down menu that simply indicates "excellent," "good," "fair," or "poor." If there is not an additional location in the EHR where you can substantiate your selection, you must identify an alternative location in the initial examination documentation to support your claim. It is also important to consider that if you chose to indicate that your patient or client has a "poor" or "fair" prognosis that these choices could be interpreted as the patient or client not being appropriate to receive physical therapy services.

Anticipated Goals and Expected Outcomes

Measuring goals and outcomes for any program is the basis for determining that program's value. It should be clear to you, your colleagues, your patient or client, your patient or client's caregivers, and any other user of your documentation what you are striving for within the plan of care that you have created for your patient or client. The quality of the goals you create within your plan of care will help determine the efficacy of your interventions and facilitate the management of your patient or client's progression through the plan of care. Consider the following goals.

1. Improve active shoulder flexion range of motion by 20 degrees.
2. Report decreased low back pain when sitting to drive.
3. Demonstrate improved dynamic balance when walking using the least restrictive device.
4. Improve strength of right gluteus medius from 3/5 to 4/5.

Do you consider these goals to be useful, or do they simply represent a to-do list? For a goal to be useful for guiding your interventions and for demonstrating the medical necessity of your physical therapy services, it must be patient- or client-centered, objective, measurable, functional, and include a time element for meeting the goal (TABLE 3-7). Now consider the rewritten goals below.

1. In 2 weeks, improve active shoulder flexion range of motion by 20 degrees to allow patient or client to reach overhead shelf in bathroom.
2. In 4 weeks, report at least a 2-point improvement in Numeric Pain Rating Scale during 30-minute drive to work.
3. In 8 weeks, achieve at least a 22/30 on the Functional Gait Assessment to indicate a decreased fall risk when turning during household ambulation.
4. In 8 weeks, demonstrate the ability to perform a One-Legged Stance on the right leg for at least 5 seconds to facilitate increased stance time on the right when stepping over obstacles during gait.

These patient- or client-centered, objective, measurable, functional, and time-dependent goals can be used to determine progress and allow for subsequent adjustment of your clinical impression, prognosis, duration

TABLE 3-7   Criteria for Creating Useful and Effective Goals

Criteria	Definition
Patient or client-centered	Tailored or customized to the unique needs of an individual
Objective	Unbiased and based in fact
Measurable	Quantifiable
Functional	Relating to a particular use or purpose
Time-dependent	Held accountable to a determined interval

and frequency of the episode of care, conclusion of care plan, and intervention plan. The tests and measures and outcome measures that you collect during your initial examination are the blueprint for the content of your goals. Therefore, there should never be new information regarding your patient or client revealed in your goals. In other words, each goal should depict a characteristic you already measured. Consider the ICF graphic created for Mr. A in Figure 3-3. Modeling your goals after your patient or client's impairments in body functions and structures, activity limitations, participation restrictions, and contextual factors, and considering the subsequent tests and measures and outcome tools you selected for your patient or client will assist you in meeting the criteria for writing useful and effective goals (Table 3-7). Consider the following goals created for Mr. A based on the details of his above examination.

1. In 2 weeks, achieve at least 0–110 degrees of active knee flexion range of motion to facilitate ability to get in and out of the passenger side of the car.
2. In 2 weeks, decrease edema at peripatellar region of the right knee to be within 1 cm of the left knee's circumferential measurement to allow for improved motor control and comfort during position changes such as rolling in bed.
3. In 2 weeks, demonstrate the ability to ambulate household distances (at least 100 feet) with equal step length without an assistive device with safety and independence.
4. In 4 weeks, demonstrate an increase in gait speed of at least 0.05 m/s without an assistive device to indicate improved mobility.
5. In 4 weeks, improve Five Times Sit to Stand time by at least 2.5 seconds to indicate a significant improvement in lower extremity functional strength for standing from low surface.

6. In 4 weeks, improve Functional Gait Assessment score by at least 8 points to indicate a significant improvement in dynamic balance when turning during gait.
7. In 4 weeks, improve WOMAC score by at least 21% to indicate a significant improvement in ability to perform dressing tasks, to walk on even surfaces, and to lie in bed.
8. In 6 weeks, improve average score on Patient-Specific Functional Scale by at least 2 points to indicate a significant improvement in ability to drive and attend son's baseball games.
9. In 6 weeks, achieve at least 0–135 degrees of active knee flexion range of motion to facilitate ability to get in and out of the driver's side of patient or client's sports car.

Each goal is tailored to Mr. A's unique needs and is therefore considered patient or client-centered because each is based on his level of functioning and ability according to the ICF terminology applied when gathering data during his initial examination. Each goal is unbiased, and therefore objective, because each was created using tangible facts collected during the examination process. Each goal is quantifiable because each can be measured to determine progress. Each goal relates to a particular use or purpose and is therefore considered functional. Lastly, the achievement of each goal depends an anticipated timeframe. It is important to consider the descriptors that you use when developing your goals for your patient or client. For example, rather than suggesting a range for improvement on a measure or an assistance level with a functional task, use your clinical judgment to formulate clearly measurable goals. For example, goals written such as those below should be avoided.

1. In 8 weeks, demonstrate the ability to reach overhead to retrieve between 10 and 20 pounds from an overhead shelf.

> ## BOX 3-6 The Electronic Health Record: Anticipated Goals and Expected Outcomes
>
> Because the anticipated goals and expected outcomes are the basis of the efficacy of the interventions you implement with your patient or client, it is important that you do not yield to the drop-down menus and prefabricated sentence structure of an electronic health record when writing goals. Unfortunately, these features of an EHR do not always allow for the complete creation of patient- or client-centered, objective, measurable, functional, and time-dependent goals. Therefore, it is imperative that you add additional information to any prefabricated goals to ensure that each is complete and well written. Some electronic systems may have an "other" data field that allows you to skip any prefabricated, generic goals and create in a free-text style your anticipated goals and expected outcomes.

2. In 6 sessions, perform stand-pivot transfers to and from the wheelchair and commode with minimum to moderate assistance.
3. Between initial examination and discharge, improve gluteus medius strength such that patient or client can maintain a single-limb stance position on right or left leg for at least 10 seconds without a pelvic drop.

It is equally relevant to note here that while Mr. A's goals are patient- or client-centered, time-dependent, and were created to objectively measure improved functional outcomes, not all of the goals were written using outcome measures. For example, goals 1–3 and 9 utilize tests and measures to meet a certain anticipated outcome, while goals 4–8 utilize outcome measures with known responsiveness and their associated change scores: minimal detectable change or minimal clinically important difference.

Frequency and Duration of the Episode of Care

An important part of your initial examination documentation is ensuring that you indicate the frequency and duration of the episode of care. The frequency is how often you will provide physical therapy services to your patient or client: 2 × per day, three times per week, daily. The duration refers to the amount of time the episode of care will cover: 4 weeks, 8 weeks, 6 months. It may also be valuable to relay the actual duration of time within each session that physical therapy services will be delivered: 30-minute, 45-minute, 1-hour sessions. The frequency and duration of the episode of care may be estimated based on many different factors including the setting in which you practice, the capacity of your patient or client to participate in the plan of care, the patient or client's transportation and caregiver needs, and limitations mandated by third-party payers. Regardless of these limitations it is important to include your patient or client and their families in this decision to ensure a patient- or client-centered approach to the delivery of your physical therapy services. The frequency and duration of the episode of care may appear in your initial examination documentation as an entry after the prognosis or after the anticipated goals and expected outcomes components of your initial examination documentation such as 3 × week for 4 weeks. This information could also appear as a statement such as the following.

1. Physical therapy interventions will be delivered for two 45-minute sessions daily for 3 weeks.
2. Begin plan of care 3 × week for 2 weeks; then decrease to 2 × week for an additional 8 weeks after pain is controlled.
3. Initiate physical therapy intervention 1 × per week for 2 weeks; then increase to 3 × week for 8 weeks after weight-bearing restrictions are lifted.

Just as when creating your goals, it is important to use your clinical judgment along with evidence and your unique patient or client to commit to a specific frequency and duration of the episode of care, rather than reporting a range.

An additional detail in this section includes content regarding your preliminary impressions of the conclusion of the episode of care plan for your patient or client. For example, it will be important to consider this plan when coordinating with the rest of your patient or client's care team for the inclusion of additional services for your patient or client or for recommending a transition to an alternative setting such as a different school or an assisted living facility. Therefore, an explicit statement in your initial examination documentation

(FIGURE 3-4)

BOX 3-7 The Electronic Health Record: Frequency and Duration of the Episode of Care

Like the prognosis section, this component of the initial examination documentation in an electronic health record may simply be drop-down menus of frequencies and duration from which you select. Some systems will not allow for a written statement that is explicitly labeled, "Frequency and duration of the episode of care." Therefore, it would be necessary for you to ensure that this information is added in some location of the note that has a free-text option such as the evaluation component. In addition, any detail regarding information about the conclusion of the episode of care plan would also have to be added into a free-text area such as the evaluation component of the note.

is warranted to show that this planning has been anticipated from the very beginning of the episode of care. Such a statement may appear in your documentation as follows.

1. Begin plan of care 3 × week for 2 weeks then decrease to 2 × week for an additional 8 weeks after removal of surgical sutures with plan to return to work in 6 weeks.
2. Physical therapy interventions will be delivered for two 45-minute sessions daily for 3 weeks with plans to return to own home to live with husband. Patient or client's husband will need to attend caregiver training for wheelchair to bed, commode, and car transfers. Patient or client will likely require home health physical therapy services and subsequent outpatient physical therapy services.

Intervention Plan

Documenting the intervention plan in the initial examination can be thought of as the conclusion or summary statement for the narrative that is your plan of care. This is the area of your note where you would indicate the broad areas of intervention that are medically necessary for your patient or client. The intervention plan for Mr. A

might appear in the initial examination documentation as follows:

> Mr. A would benefit from skilled physical therapy interventions to address the impairments in body functions and structures, activity limitations, and participation restrictions identified in this initial examination. Recommended interventions include transfer training, gait training, therapeutic exercises, balance training, and modalities as indicated.

More specific details of your intervention plan might appear in a flow sheet (FIGURE 3-4) that is linked in some way to the rest of the initial examination documentation. It would be valuable to create this flow sheet when creating the rest of the documentation rather than wait until your patient or client's first follow-up visit so that your clinical rationale is still fresh in your mind. Furthermore, any interventions that you delivered at the initial examination can be recorded here as well as interventions that you plan on completing in the future. These entries in the flow sheet can then be adjusted, added, or omitted as your patient or client progresses with the intervention plan. Remember, if you did not measure a particular characteristic in your patient or client, then you cannot

BOX 3-8 The Electronic Health Record: Intervention Plan

Relaying the intervention plan component of the initial examination documentation in an electronic health record is similar to other components of the note that are more clearly delivered using a free-text space such as the evaluation, prognosis, anticipated goals and expected outcomes, and frequency and duration of the episode of care. It is important to include this section as a narrative component of the documentation rather than to refer the user of the note to the flow sheet to ensure that the intervention plan delineated is medically necessary for your patient or client. The APTA *Guidelines: Physical Therapy Documentation of Patient/Client Management* indicate that "flow sheets or charts are considered a component of the documented health record but do not meet the requirements of documentation in and of themselves."[7]

Primary Health Condition	Osteoarthritis resulting in R total knee arthroplasty
Comorbid Conditions	Episodic low back pain; skin cancer—questionable location on posterior R shoulder
Precautions/Contraindications	None
Visit Count	1 of *insert visit number here*
Next Progress/Status Note Due	*insert date here*
Outcome Measures to Track	Five Times Sit to Stand; Functional Gait Assessment, 10-Meter Walk Test, One-Legged Stand Test
Patient/Caregiver Education	
Home Exercise Program (HEP)	Provided per attached

MANUAL THERAPY
  Soft Tissue Techniques
    Deep tissue mobilization
  Joint Oscillations
  Joint Mobilizations
  Neurodynamics	

THERAPEUTIC EXERCISE/NEUROMUSCULAR RE-EDUCATION
  Mobility/Symptom Relief/Tissue Health
    Ice
    Quad Sets (supine, small pillow under knee)
    Active Heel Slides (supine)
    Recumbent Bike
  Motor Control/Coordination
    Straight Leg Raise
  Endurance
    Standing Mini-Squats
  Strengthening
    Leg Press
    Side-lying Hip Abduction
  Power
	
	Educated patient or client re: use at home (See HEP)
	3 × 50 reps (also for HEP)
	3 × 25 reps 5 sec hold (also for HEP)
	1/2 turns; seat #6

THERAPEUTIC ACTIVITIES
  Functional Performance Training
    Sit to Stand from bed height (25 inches)
    Sit to Stand from commode height (18.5 inches)
  Balance Activities
    Static
      One-Legged Stance – EO
    Dynamic
      Backwards walking
      Side stepping
    Center of Mass Perturbations
    Base of Support Perturbations
    Vestibular Training	

GAIT TRAINING Overground with quad cane	

FIGURE 3-4 Clinical Reasoning Flow Sheet – Mr. A.

track its improvement and therefore should not include an intervention related to it in your intervention plan.

Additional content in this section includes communication regarding how the intervention plan is to be delivered: by a physical therapist/physical therapist assistant team, by a team that will include an aide or a student, or by a physical therapist who is different from the therapist who conducted and documented the initial examination. In this case, information identifying the physical therapist of record is warranted.

Summary

The components of the initial examination can be organized in a structured sequence that imparts a consistent framework to creating successful initial examination documentation. The data collected from the history and systems review can be used together to formulate the initial clinical impression of your patient or client and subsequently inform the selection of your tests and measures and outcome measures. The evaluation, which includes your diagnosis and clinical impression, can be constructed by levying an interpretation of all of the data collected regarding the need for physical therapy services using your clinical judgment, evidence from the literature, and your unique patient or client. The evaluation can be expanded to include your prognosis, which further helps to guide the timing of the outcomes you expect for your patient or client. Collecting high-quality information from your tests and measures and outcome measures can facilitate you in creating well-structured and effective goals as well as accurately determining the frequency and duration of the episode of care. Furthermore, the time that you think it will take to meet these goals helps to relay information regarding the plans for the conclusion of the episode of care for your patient or client. Finally, the intervention plan relies on the quality of the information that precedes it to convey that the delivery of physical therapy services was medically necessary for your patient or client. See **Appendix 3-B** for a complete compilation of Mr. A's initial examination documentation. The commonality that unites each of the components of the initial examination into a cohesive document in the patient or client's health record is the use of ICF terminology to convey the unifying message that the skilled care recommended is medically necessary.

Discussion Questions

1. What is the difference between the terms:
   a. *Initial examination* and *evaluation*?
   b. *Clinical impression* and *diagnosis*?
2. Create a framework for documenting a history that would facilitate further creation of the initial examination documentation note in the following settings:
   a. Outpatient
   b. Inpatient
   c. Home health
   d. Skilled nursing
   e. School
3. Exchange the history section of your initial examination documentation with your colleague. Are you able to discern details regarding the patient or client's activity limitations, participation restrictions, and contextual factors? Why or why not?
4. Exchange the history section of your initial examination documentation with your colleague. Are the details present enough to help you formulate what you would include in the systems review or tests and measures? What are these details? What information is missing that you would include to make subsequent decisions?
5. Exchange the systems review and tests and measures sections of the same initial examination documentation as your above history with your colleague. Did there seem to be a clinical rationale based on the history behind the data collected in the systems review and the tests and measures section of the note? What are the details that led you to the clinical rationale? What information is missing from the systems review and tests and measures that you would have included based on the prior history?
6. Refer to your initial examination documentation for one of your patients or clients.
   a. What tests and measures did you collect as part of this examination?
   b. Are you able to identify details in the history and systems review documentation that support why each test and measure was collected? If so, delineate the details of why each was collected in the examination. If not, what details are missing?
7. Exchange the same documentation from the previous question with your colleague.
   a. What tests and measures were collected as part of this examination?
   b. Are you able to identify details in the history and systems review documentation that support why each test and measure was collected? If so, delineate the details of why each was collected in the examination. If not, what details are missing?
   c. Compare your results with your colleague.
8. Exchange initial examination documentation with your colleague. Identify the tests and measures collected and what category of the ICF model each one represents.
9. Refer to your initial examination documentation. Use the information from your history and systems review to populate an ICF graphic.

a. Have you documented enough detail to complete this task?

b. If not, what information is missing?

c. What tests and measures would you collect based on the details entered into the ICF graphic?

d. Compare the list you generated from the ICF graphic to the actual tests and measures you collected in your initial examination documentation.

e. Are there any differences between the two lists of tests and measures?

10. Refer to the evaluation section of your initial examination documentation for one of your patients or clients.

a. What information did you use to create this section?

b. Did you relay your patient or client's health condition and the reason for seeking physical therapy services?

c. Did you use ICF terminology to relay why your patient or client would benefit from skilled physical therapy care?

d. Is there any information missing? If so, rewrite the evaluation to reflect the appropriate information.

11. Exchange the evaluation section of your initial examination documentation with one of your colleagues. Critique the evaluation based on the information provided in TABLE 3-6.

12. Exchange initial examination documentation with one of your colleagues. Identify the prognosis. Where was it located in the note? Can you determine the clinical rationale for the indicated prognosis?

13. Exchange initial examination documentation with one of your colleagues.

a. Deconstruct the goals and determine if each meets the criteria for a useful and effective goal as outlined in TABLE 3-7.

b. Rewrite each goal if necessary to reflect this criteria.

14. Exchange initial examination documentation with your colleague. Identify the frequency and duration of the episode of care plan in the note. How is it written? Is there evidence in the documentation that the conclusion of the episode of care planning occurred during the initial examination?

Case Study Questions

1. Consider the following history in an outpatient setting.

    Mrs. B is a 45-year-old female who slipped off the edge of her rolling office chair at home and landed on her buttocks on a tile floor 2 weeks ago. Since that time she has had pain in her low back radiating into her right buttock and posterior thigh. She self-treated with Advil and hot packs, but after a week with no relief, she saw her primary care physician. Radiographic imaging of the pelvis and lumbar spine were negative. The physician prescribed a muscle relaxant and pain medication and referred her to physical therapy.

    a. What history content is missing?

    b. Create headings for the content that is missing.

2. Consider the following history in a skilled nursing setting.

    Mr. G is a 72-year-old male admitted to _____ Nursing Facility yesterday after a 2-week hospital stay at _____ Rehabilitation Hospital. He was admitted to inpatient rehabilitation with worsening CHF and was found to have a new diagnosis of Parkinson's disease. He was treated at that time with IV diuretics and started on a regimen of anti-Parkinson's medications. He states that he is still in the trial period of determining if the medications are beneficial for him. He states that his tremor that was in the left hand seems to be less and that he is less stiff than he was last week although he feels that the improvement in these symptoms is minimal at this point. He has a history of atrial fibrillation and COPD. Mr. G lives in a two-story home with his wife and has three steps to enter without a handrail. He states that he made good progress in inpatient rehabilitation, but feels that he still needs help with walking and getting into and out of a low chair. He states that he becomes very short of breath and finds that walking is much more challenging now than it was before he was admitted to the hospital. He states that he used to be able to walk into and out of his house with his cane and now he has a hard time using his cane and his walker.

    a. What history content is missing?

    b. Create headings for the content that is missing.

3. Consider the following history in an inpatient rehabilitation setting.

    Mrs. H is a 55-year-old female status post right basal ganglia intracranial hemorrhage 3 weeks ago on 6/17/2013. Her past medical history is significant for respiratory failure, hypertension, Type II diabetes mellitus, obesity, hypoxia, pneumonia, and breast cancer. She has a tracheostomy with supplemental oxygen and complains of double vision, left-sided weakness that includes her face and right foot drop from diabetic neuropathy. She tests positive for a MRSA infection. She reports constant and burning pain in her right ankle and foot. She reports right hip and low back pain that is dull, aching, and constant that is worse when she tries to roll over in her bed. Her medications include Vancocin (vancomycin), Zyvox (linezolid), Lopressor (metoprolol), Cozaar (losartan), Lipitor (atorvastatin), Desyrel (trazodone), Depakote (divalproex sodium), Glucophage (metformin), and calcium with Vitamin D. Her primary goal is to return home to live with her two sisters. Her home is a one-story wheelchair-accessible home with a ramp to enter. She has a tub bench, a 3-in-1 commode chair, a sliding board for transfers, a power scooter, a rollator with a seat, and a right ankle foot orthosis with bilateral metal uprights. She has a history of falls prior to this hospital admission and her primary means of mobility in her home was her scooter. She enjoys reading and being with her sisters.

a. Organize the details of this history using a framework with headings.

b. Is there any history information missing? If so what is it?

c. What details will you collect in your systems review?

d. What tests and measures and outcome measures will you collect and why?

4. Consider the following history in an outpatient setting.

Ms. Z is an 18-year-old female with cerebral palsy. She states that she had Botox injections in her left hamstrings about 2 weeks ago and has since experienced deterioration in her ability to walk. She states that she used to be able to walk with bilateral Lofstrand crutches but is now able to only walk with her posterior walker. She states that she is planning to enroll in classes next month so that she can get her high school diploma. She states that her goal is to be able to walk with her Lofstrand crutches in her graduation ceremony, which is 8 months from now. She also notes that she was able to sit on the edge of her bed to dress herself and now she finds that she has much more difficulty with this task. She reports that she has to lie on her back to dress her lower body unless she has someone next to her to help support her in a sitting position. She also states that she used to be able to climb into her bed or around on the floor on her hands, which was helpful if she had to fix her covers on her bed or if she had to pick something off the floor. However, since she received the Botox injections she is not able to complete these tasks independently.

Use the Patient-Specific Functional Scale to list the patient/client's personal goals, activity limitations, and participation restrictions.

5. Consider the following history and systems review in an outpatient setting.

HISTORY

Mrs. R is a 74-year-old female who presents to your outpatient clinic approximately 1 month after experiencing a left ischemic stroke. She did not receive inpatient rehabilitation following her CVA but did have home health physical therapy for 4 weeks. She arrived being pushed in a manual wheelchair and is accompanied by her daughter.

Past medical history: hypertension, hypercholesterolemia, NIDDM (non-insulin dependent diabetes mellitus), osteoarthritis, depression

Past surgical history: cholecystectomy 2004

Medications: Coumadin (warfarin), Elavil (amitriptyline), Tenormin (atenolol), Glucophage (metformin), Aleve (naproxen)

Social history: Patient lives with her daughter and son-in-law and their three children in a single-story home with one step to enter. She was a housewife but her husband passed away 2 years ago. She does not smoke or drink alcohol. She does not drive. She attends church every Sunday and belongs to a ladies church group that makes rosaries but has not been able to participate in this activity since she experienced this stroke.

Prior level of function: Patient or client did not perform any exercise. She helped with light housework and did most of the cooking and laundry for the family. She was independent with all activities of daily living. She ambulated without an assistive device. Daughter states that Mrs. R currently gets around the house using the wheelchair and only walked with the supervision of the home physical therapist. Daughter states that Mrs. R's goal is to get back to walking within the home, cooking meals, and attending church services again.

SYSTEMS REVIEW

Cardiovascular/Pulmonary: In sitting: BP rest = 134/78 mmHg, HR rest = 84 bpm, RR rest = 18. No edema noted.

Integumentary: Not impaired.

Musculoskeletal: Gross passive range of motion in lower extremities bilaterally, left upper extremity: not impaired; right upper extremity: impaired; gross strength: impaired right upper extremity and right lower extremity. Posture: kyphotic thoracic spine, rounded shoulders and forward head. Height: 61 inches. Weight: 137 lbs.

Neuromuscular: Gross coordinated movements all impaired in right and left upper extremities and lower extremities; motor function impaired on right.

Communication: Patient or client is awake, alert, and oriented to person, time, place, and event. Spanish is primary language. Patient or client speaks some English and understands simple commands in English. Daughter can translate. Patient or client wears glasses and has a mild hearing deficit but does not use hearing aids. She is pleasant and cooperative but affect is flat. Patient or client and family will need education re: safety, home exercise program, and use of assistive devices. Family requests that all information regarding what patient or client should be doing at home be provided in both Spanish and English, with illustrations and large font.

a. Is there any information missing from the history or systems review sections above?

b. What information would you add?

c. Would you reorganize this information in any way? If so, how?

d. What tests and measures and outcome measures will you collect based on the information presented above?

6. Organize the data from the history and systems review section above into an ICF graphic.

a. Determine the tests and measures and outcome measures you would collect based on the ICF graphic.

b. Compare the list generated here with the list generated in the previous question.

c. Create an evaluation based on the examination provided above. What information did you use to create this content?

d. Create a prognosis statement based on the information above.

7. Assume that on the day of the initial examination for your patient or client, who was admitted to inpatient rehabilitation after a mitral valve replacement, there were circumstances beyond your control that interrupted your initial examination. In this case, your patient or client had to use the bathroom, which required you and the assistance of a nurse. As a result, you did not get to collect all of the data that you were intending to include such as ambulation, stair negotiation, or dynamic standing balance and are forced to continue the examination on a subsequent day.

a. Write the evaluation component of your initial examination to reflect this situation.

b. How would you document your prognosis for this patient or client?

c. Create your anticipated goals and expected outcomes to include in the initial examination.

d. Create the frequency and duration of the episode of care.

e. Determine your initial conclusion of the episode of care plan.

f. Now assume that the next day, you were able to complete your patient or client's initial examination and you want to incorporate the following findings into your initial examination: Timed Up and Go = 21 seconds; 6-Minute Walk Test = 390 feet with four-wheeled rolling walker (average RPE = 15; required six standing rest breaks); Stair Ascent Time = 23 seconds; eight steps step-over-step with bilateral hand rails and minimum assistance $\times$ 1; Berg Balance Test = 41/56. Create an addendum to your initial examination documentation to reflect this additional information. What information would you include in this addendum?

8. Consider the goals below and answer the following questions for each.

a. Do you think that this goal is a well-written goal? Why or why not?

b. Compare your analysis of each goal with a colleague. Did you agree on your analysis of each goal?

○ In the next five visits, report the ability to obtain an average of at least 8 hours of sleep per night without interruption due to low back pain.

○ In 2 weeks, demonstrate the ability to perform a stand-pivot transfer from the wheelchair to the commode with the least restrictive assistive device.

○ In 2 weeks, propel wheelchair on level surface with right upper extremity and right lower extremity for 50 feet.

○ In 6 weeks, improve standing balance to maximum attainable level.

○ Improve the Patient-Specific Functional Scale to 8/10 in order to demonstrate significant return to prior level of function.

○ In 1 week, ambulate 30 feet $\times$ 4 with stand by assistance using a large base quad cane.

○ In 6 weeks, patient or client will demonstrate the ability to lift 5 pounds, 10 times in order to place and retrieve dishes on overhead shelf.

○ Demonstrate the ability to walk between 250 and 500 feet with a straight cane to enable patient or client to safety walk to car in driveway.

○ In 1 week, patient will roll with maximum assistance.

○ In 3 weeks, demonstrate the ability to ambulate at least 50 feet with a four-wheeled rolling walker with supervision/independence.

References

1. American Physical Therapy Association (APTA). Principles of physical therapist patient and client management; Figure 2-4. *Guide to Physical Therapist Practice* 3.0. Alexandria, VA: American Physical Therapy Association; 2014. Available at: guidetoptpractice.apta.org/content/1/SEC2.body. Accessed on October 18, 2014.

2. APTA. *Standards of Practice for Physical Therapy.* Alexandria, VA: American Physical Therapy Association; last updated October 1, 2013. Available at: www.apta.org/uploadedFiles/APTAorg/About_Us/Policies/Practice/StandardsPractice.pdf. Accessed on October 18, 2014. [Standard]

3. Portney LG, Watkins MP. *Foundations of Clinical Research: Applications to Practice.* Upper Saddle River, NJ: Pearson Prentice Hall; 2009, 109-110.

4. Jones SE, Kon SS, Canavan J.L., et al. The five-repetition sit-to-stand test as a functional outcome measure in COPD. *Thorax.* 2013;68(11):1015–1020.

5. Meretta BM, Whitney, SL, Marchetti G.F., et al. The five times sit to stand test: responsiveness to change and concurrent validity in adults undergoing vestibular rehabilitation. *J Vestib Res.* 2006;16(4–5):233–243.

6. APTA. *Defensible Documentation: Components of Documentation within the Patient/Client Management Model.* Alexandria, VA: American Physical Therapy Association; last updated March 8, 2012. Available at: www.apta.org/Documentation/DefensibleDocumentation/. Accessed on October 18, 2014.

7. APTA. *Guidelines: Physical Therapy Documentation of Patient/Client Management.* Alexandria, VA: American Physical Therapy Association; last updated March, 2005. Available at: www.apta.org/uploadedFiles/APTAorg/About_Us/Policies/BOD/Practice/DocumentationPatientClientMgmt.pdf. Accessed on October 18, 2014.

Appendix 3-A Additional Initial Examination Documentation for Workers' Compensation Patients or Clients

History	○ Work history with current employer ○ Work history in job with similar requirements ○ Current work status ○ Current work load restrictions ○ Work goal: return to same position; alternative job? ○ Perception of current physical job demands ○ Mechanism of injury
Systems Review	--
Tests and Measures	○ Work disability self-report measures (Quick DASH) ○ Testing related to job demands
Evaluation	○ Consider barriers or facilitators to recovery. ○ Provide impression of correlation between mechanism of injury, work risk factors, and clinical findings. ○ Consider impairments in body functions and structures, activity limitations, and participation restrictions that limit performance of work duties and provide correlation between these factors and work-related limitations.
Prognosis	--
Anticipated Goals and Expected Outcomes	○ Must be clear regarding job/employer patient/client is returning to. ○ Must be related to physical requirements of the job.
Frequency and Duration of Episode of Care	--
Intervention Plan	○ Must include work-related tasks designed to facilitate safe return to work.

Data from the APTA's Defensible Documentation: Setting Specific Considerations in Documentation (2011).

Appendix 3-B Initial Examination Documentation for Mr. A

History

History of Current Status: Mr. A is a 56-year-old male who experienced a R total knee arthroplasty 16 days ago. He states that he is experiencing a lot of pain and is concerned about the length and speed of his recovery. He notes that he is significantly limited at this time since he is not able to drive and has had to alter how he performs his ADLs. Following up with surgeon at end of week on 6/7/2013.

Patient/Client Goals: Return to driving, decrease pain, walk without a walker and without pain, improve ability to get up off low seat like commode, and perform dressing and hygiene tasks, sleep in own bed without waking due to pain, attend two teenage sons' baseball games, return to work as a middle school teacher.

Past Medical History and Past Surgical History: R total knee arthroplasty on 5/20/2013; bicycle accident 10 years ago in which Mr. A "twisted" his R knee. Mr A. reports full recovery from this accident. Skin cancer (melanoma) removed from R ear and R shoulder on 1/14/2013. Did not receive radiation or chemotherapy. Also see medical history and intake form; additional details of social history and exercise habits included here.

Concurrent Conditions: Low back pain (episodic)—reports currently aggravated due to sleeping in a recliner due to R knee pain.

Precautions or Contraindications to Movement or Activity: none.

Past Interventions: No prior physical therapy for knee or low back pain; corticosteroid injections at R knee three times per year over the last year.

Lab Results or Imaging Study Results: None since 2-day hospital stay.

Prior Level of Function: Active and independent with all ADLs.

Current Level of Function: Using four-wheeled rolling walker in home for all transfer and ambulation tasks; using four-wheeled rolling walker for ambulation in community to attend medical appointments; modified I for dressing, grooming, and showering tasks due to increased length of time to complete tasks, pain, poor control and balance; unable to sleep in bed.

Current Medications: Lortab (hydrocodone/acetaminophen), Mobic (meloxicam), Robaxin (methocarbamol), ibuprofen discontinued at this time; patient/client reports that he is taking medications as prescribed but he is having breakthrough pain.

Pain or Other Symptom Description: Anterior R knee pain from distal 1/3rd of upper leg to tibial tubercle; R posterior and medial knee pain; tight and aching; feels better when standing and walking than when sitting or trying to sleep; low back feels tight like it needs to stretch after sitting > 20 minutes; denies lower leg cramping or foot/ankle pain.
Worst pain = 9/10 in knee after sitting > 20 minutes
Best pain = 2/10 after taking pain meds
Average pain = 5/10
Current pain = 9/10 in knee after sitting > 20 minutes; 5/10 in knee when walking

Family History: Attended session with wife; supportive family; lives with wife and two teenage sons; hypertension; osteoarthritis, lung cancer, Parkinson's disease.

Living Environment: One-story home with two steps to enter in front; no railing; one step into home from garage; pool with handrails.

Work Status: On medical leave until 7/1/2013.

Hobbies and Recreational Activities: Going to son's baseball games.

Communication Style, Learning Style, Mental Status: Prefers visual representation of HEP; cognitively intact.

Systems Review

Cardiovascular and Pulmonary Systems
- Vital signs:
  BP rest = 131/76 mmHg
  HR rest = 72 bpm bounding, regular pulse (radial)
  RR rest = 15 breaths per minute
- Edema:
  R knee = peripatellar; appears consistent with surgical intervention
  None observed distal to knees or at feet and ankles bilaterally

Integumentary System
- Skin integrity – appears to have a small irregularly shaped mole on posterior right shoulder lateral to scar where prior melanoma was removed. Mr. A reports that he is aware of this growth and relays that he has an appointment with his dermatologist next week. No other disruptions noted. No skin discolorations noted except for bruising at posterior medial R knee that appears to be healing and consistent with total knee arthroplasy due to yellowish-green skin hue.
- Scars – none observed other than dime-shaped scar on posterior medial R shoulder due to melanoma removal.
- Wounds – healing surgical incision anterior R knee (see tests and measures); no other wounds observed; Mr. A denies history of wounds.

Musculoskeletal System
- Height = 71 inches; Weight = 192 pounds
- Gross postural assessment
  Pes planus observed at L foot; Mr. A notes that he wears a custom orthotic
  in his L shoe; this has not been reassessed for approximately 2 years.
- Gross range of motion
  Bilateral upper extremities – no gross limitations
  Spine – no gross limitations
- Gross strength
  Grip – R = 109#; L = 101# (R hand dominant)

Neuromuscular System
- Gross coordination – intact and equal bilaterally via lower extremity heel-to-shin test and repeated alternating toe taps.
- Movement quality – slow cautious movement of the R knee due to pain.
- Motor function
  Deep tendon reflexes = intact and equal bilaterally
  Clonus = negative bilaterally
  Babinski = negative bilaterally
  Light touch and pinprick sensation intact bilaterally

Communication, Language, Cognition, Learning Style
- Able to follow multi-step commands.
- Intact cognition based on interaction and awareness of person, place, time, and event.
- Prefers visual demonstration and visual representation of exercises.

Tests and Measures and Outcome Measures

ICF Category	Test and Measure or Outcome Measure	Entry into ICF Graphic for Mr. A
Impairments in Body Functions and Structure	Knee active and passive range of motion, patellar mobility testing	Impaired range of motion
	Quadriceps, Hamstring, Gluteus Medius Manual Muscle Testing	Impaired strength
	Heel Rise Test	Impaired strength
	Circumferential Measurement at the Knee	Edema
	Numeric Pain Rating Scale	Pain
	Single Limb Stance	Impaired balance
	Functional Gait Assessment	Impaired balance
Activity Limitations	Western Ontario and McMaster Universities Osteoarthritis Index (WOMAC)	Pain, getting off commode, dressing tasks, walking, lying in bed
	Five Times Sit to Stand	Difficulty getting off the commode
	10-Meter Walk Test	Ambulation limitations
	Patient-Specific Functional Scale	Unable to drive, unable to sleep in bed
Participation Restrictions	Patient-Specific Functional Scale	Unable to attend son's baseball games, unable to return to work as a middle school teacher
Contextual Factors	Stair Climb Test	Two steps to enter home; desire to attend son's baseball games

Evaluation

Mr. A experienced a right total knee arthroplasty on 05/20/2013 due to longstanding knee osteoarthritis. His impairments in body functions and structures include pain, edema, impaired range of motion and patellar mobility, impaired lower extremity muscle strength, poor lower extremity muscle performance, and impaired dynamic standing balance. His activity limitations include the inability to drive or sleep in his own bed, his need for assistance to get off the commode and for dressing, hygiene, and showering tasks, as well as the need for assistance with a walker for community and household ambulation. Mr. A's participation restrictions include the inability to attend his son's baseball games and his inability to work as a middle school teacher. The contextual factors that affect Mr. A's recovery include the fact that he has clear goals, a supportive family, and an active lifestyle. Mr. A has a history of melanoma on the right shoulder. An area on the right shoulder was identified during this examination that Mr. A notes he is having evaluated by his dermatologist next week. In addition, he reports that he is experiencing breakthrough pain at the right knee despite taking his medications as prescribed. Mr. A was educated to report this information to his surgeon at his follow-up visit in 4 days or to call his surgeon's office to report his concerns if the breakthrough pain continues to worsen prior to his appointment. In addition, I will place a call on Mr. A's behalf to his surgeon's office to relay this concern by the end of business today.

Prognosis

Assuming that Mr. A's breakthrough pain is addressed, his prognosis for improving the impairments, activity limitations, and participation restrictions indicated above is good. Currently Mr. A's level of irritability is high given the pain he is experiencing and his inability to sleep comfortably in his bed. This pain will potentially slow his ability to meet his goals indicated below.

Anticipated Goals and Expected Outcomes

1. In 2 weeks, achieve at least 0 to 110 degrees of active knee flexion range of motion to facilitate ability to get in and out of the passenger side of the car.
2. In 2 weeks, decrease edema at peripatellar region of the R knee to be within 1 cm of the L knee's circumferential measurement to allow for improved motor control and comfort during position changes such as rolling in bed.
3. In 2 weeks, demonstrate the ability to ambulate household distances (at least 100 feet) with equal step length without an assistive device with safety and independence.
4. In 4 weeks, demonstrate an increase in gait speed of at least 0.05 m/s without an assistive device to indicate improved mobility.
5. In 4 weeks, improve Five Times Sit to Stand time by at least 2.5 seconds to indicate a significant improvement in lower extremity functional strength for standing from low surface.
6. In 4 weeks, improve Functional Gait Assessment score by at least eight points to indicate a significant improvement in dynamic balance when turning during gait.
7. In 4 weeks, improve WOMAC score by at least 21% to indicate a significant improvement in ability to perform dressing tasks, to walk on even surfaces, and to lie in bed.
8. In 6 weeks, improve average score on Patient-Specific Functional Scale by at least two points to indicate a significant improvement in ability to drive and attend son's baseball games.
9. In 6 weeks, achieve at least 0 to 135 degrees of active knee flexion range of motion to facilitate ability to get in and out of the driver's side of patient or client's sports car.

Frequency and Duration of Episode of Care

Begin plan of care three times per week for 2 weeks; then decrease to two times per week for an additional 8 weeks after pain is controlled.

Intervention Plan

Mr. A would benefit from skilled physical therapy interventions to address the impairments in body functions and structures, activity limitations, and participation restrictions identified in this initial examination. Recommended interventions include transfer training, gait training, therapeutic exercises, balance training, and modalities as indicated.

CHAPTER 4

Writing Daily Notes

CHAPTER OBJECTIVES

1. Recognize the need to provide a sound clinical rationale for each component of a daily note.
2. Recognize the architecture of a meaningful daily note.
3. Construct a daily note based on a clinical scenario.
4. Recognize how to utilize clinical rationale in creating an intervention flow sheet.
5. Recognize federal rules and regulations that reinforce the importance of utilizing clinical reasoning within the daily note.
6. Define special considerations to differing daily note types such as documenting group therapy, co-treatments, maintenance therapy, prevention and wellness, and worker's compensation daily notes.
7. Apply a guide to assist with self-examination of daily note writing skills.

KEY TERMS

Co-treatments
Group therapy
Maintenance therapy
Prevention and wellness

SIRP
SOAP
Workers' compensation

Introduction

Writing daily notes is an important component of physical therapist practice. This chapter begins by challenging you to consider how you use daily notes in your clinical practice. Next, the data-driven SOAP format, commonly used to generate the contents of a daily note, is introduced as well as SIRP, an alternative decision-driven format. Next, a clinical reasoning flow sheet is presented to further improve the ability to use the data generated from the daily encounter with a patient or client. Next, federal rules and regulations are presented to reinforce the notion that every daily note should include meaningful and decision-driven information regardless of the payer source. In addition, special circumstances such as documenting

group therapy, co-treatments, maintenance therapy, prevention and wellness, or workers' compensation in a daily note is introduced. Lastly, a guide to assist with self-examination of daily note writing skills is offered.

A daily note should be constructed such that it answers the following question: What is it about this patient or client's unique health condition that mandates that only a qualified physical therapist or physical therapist assistant could effectively deliver this plan of care? You should be able to answer this question during every clinical encounter with a patient or client. In other words, your daily note should reflect your professional judgment at every clinical session. Just as you should evaluate your clinical decision making during or after your interaction with your patient or client as a mechanism to further develop your skills as an expert clinician, you should also evaluate or reflect on the value of what you are including in your daily note. The American Physical Therapy Association (APTA) has adopted the position that documentation with focus primarily on clinical reasoning and decision making should occur in the provision of physical therapy services.[1] If you view a daily note as simply a necessary consequence of your interactions with your patient or client, then it will likely not be successfully written. In other words, you will likely not be able to use its contents as an adjunct to your clinical skills as a physical therapist or physical therapist assistant. On the other hand, if you view a daily note as the vehicle that guides your plan of care from session to session, then you will likely create a useful product in your daily note.

The daily note is an important component of the health record that is utilized by many more professionals than solely you as the note's author. The daily note serves to assist other healthcare providers involved in delivering the plan of care to your patient or client. It serves as an educational tool used by internal reviewers, external auditors, and third-party payers to identify intervention outcomes and patterns of clinical practice, and to make programmatic and reimbursement decisions. Third-party payers also review daily notes as well as progress notes to determine continued medical necessity, progress within the plan of care, and any remaining impairments, activity limitations, and participation restrictions that impact your patient or client's daily functioning. Furthermore, well-written daily notes serve to protect you as the provider as evidence that you met or exceeded the standard of care. Alternatively, a poorly written note can be called into question if legally reviewed to address the physical therapy care delivered.[2] As the creator of the note, reflect for a moment on its purpose. How do you use a daily note? Consider the following scenario.

You are working in a busy outpatient clinic. You are reviewing your caseload for the day and you see an individual on your schedule with whom you are not familiar. You determine that she is one of your colleague's patients or clients who is in the fifth week of her 8-week plan of care after a total knee arthroplasty. As you review the health record, you see the following daily note.

No new complaints to report.
See flow sheet.
Patient tolerated treatment well.
Continue POC.

Flow Sheet	Date:
Recumbent bike	10 min
Proprioceptive activities	10 min
Leg raises – 4 ways	Standing 4# cuffs 3 × 12
Mini squats	2 × 25
Seated leg press	3 × 10 75# L only
Dynamic balance activities	10 min
Ice as needed	10 min

Is there any information from this daily note you can use to supplement your clinical skills as a physical therapist or physical therapist assistant? Is there any information you can use to plan your interventions with your colleague's patient or client? You might decide to reproduce the activities indicated in the flow sheet. However, reflect for a moment about why you might to do this. Is it because you have reviewed additional content from this patient or client's health record such as prior daily notes, re-examinations, and the initial examination and deemed that the most recent flow sheet is appropriate to repeat? Or, is it because there is no other meaningful information in the current daily note from which to make any further judgments or decisions? Suppose that you intend on starting the patient or client on the recumbent bike, but when you greet her in the waiting room you see that she wears a solid ankle foot orthosis on one foot and ambulates with a quad cane. Furthermore, you learn that the patient or client perceived the recumbent bike to increase her low back pain so she has not used the recumbent bike for the last two visits. Is this the patient or client you expected? You may find yourself questioning if you reviewed the record of the correct patient or client. On the other hand, you may have been completely aware of the patient or client's history of stroke, the need for assistive devices, the concurrent low back pain, and the hold on the recumbent bike since a prior daily note reported this change. Justifiably, *one* daily note is only *one* piece of the health record. Similarly, the most recent daily note is not the document on which you should base *all* of your clinical decisions. However, the content of each daily note should relay information that complements the documentation that precedes it. Doing this will allow you to document the implementation of the entire plan of care as established by the physical therapist[3] from the initial examination to the final session. Consider an alternative daily note from the scenario above.

> Patient reports soreness at her left lower extremity after the addition of the leg press last session. Pt states that she was able to sleep without pain. Her complaint of low back pain has resolved since eliminating the recumbent bike last session.
>
> Implemented dynamic stretching in knee flexion via a mini squat (10 × 10 sec hold) to replace the recumbent bike and ensure continued increase in knee ROM.
>
> Patient required minimal verbal cues to avoid compensations (forward trunk flexion) during mini squats; required minimal assistance to avoid loss of balance during turning activities designed to simulate getting object out of refrigerator.
>
> Continue to focus on lower extremity functional strength (repeated sit to stands) and improving balance reactions. Add mini squat to HEP when patient can perform without compensations.

Is there any information from this daily note you can use to supplement your clinical skills as a physical therapist or physical therapist assistant? Is there any information you can use to plan your interventions with your colleague's patient or client? Is there detail in the note that helps you to formulate a clinical picture of this patient or client? Is there a difference from the mental image you may have attempted to form after reading the first note above? Consider that the daily note should contain enough information that you can begin to formulate a clinical representation of the patient or client before you meet and begin communicating with them. With the detail of this note, you as this patient or client's physical therapist or physical therapist assistant for the session have a great deal of information from which to generate judgments and clinical rationale as you start your interaction. Furthermore, the detail in this note warrants its use as an educational tool for other users of the note.

No universal standard or guideline exists that when utilized, consistently produces the meaningful content of a daily note regardless of the varied clinical situations of physical therapy practice. Universally, however, creating a successful daily note should be decision-driven rather than data-driven regardless of the practice setting or type of encounter: group therapy, maintenance therapy, or prevention and wellness. In other words, the content of the daily note should be derived from the synthesis of collected data with a critical analysis of each decision made while collecting and interpreting that data. Most commonly, in physical therapy documentation, the **SOAP** note format, a data-driven format, is used to populate the contents of a daily note. Clinical reasoning is largely absent because of an emphasis on the content that belongs in each section rather than an emphasis on understanding the relationships between each section.

The SOAP note format is part of a problem-oriented medical record (POMR) framework[4] used for creating a daily note (**TABLE 4-1**). "S" represents *subjective* information about the problem from the patient or client's or caregiver's perspective[5] such as reports of how the patient or client feels, a description of the patient or client's signs and symptoms, and the patient or client's perception of progress.[6] "O" represents *objective* information collected, measured, and recorded during the encounter with the patient or client and was originally intended to include a physician's physical and laboratory findings.[7] "A" represents judgments or analysis of identified problems based on the subjective and objective information gathered regarding the patient or client's response to the session. Finally, "P" represents the plan that will continue in the future and is based on the assessment. Revisit the previous note:

S: No new complaints to report.

O: See flow sheet.

A: Patient tolerated treatment well.

P: Continue plan of care.

TABLE 4-1   Definition of SOAP Note Components

S: Subjective	Patient or client's or caregiver's perception of the problem How the patient or client feels Self-reported signs and symptoms
O: Objective	Data measured and collected during the encounter ○ Results of physical assessments ○ Results of laboratory testing
A: Assessment	Analysis of problems identified based on the "S" and "O"
P: Plan	Future interventions planned based on the "A"

Do you think that this note meets the definitions of the SOAP terms detailed above? You might assume that "no new complaints" indicates that the patient or client's perception of his or her problem is improving and that he or she is progressing well. Making assumptions however is an inappropriate approach not only for conducting your clinical practice,[8] but also for creating the content of a daily note. For the objective portion of this note, you could argue that the flow sheet contains all of the information you collected or measured in the session. This is appropriate as long as the flow sheet shows progression over time and changes along with your patient or client's progress. Still, the flow sheet provided in this scenario does not relay complete information about the dosing of the interventions thus increasing the difficulty of implementing the intentions of the evaluating physical therapist or interpreting the services that were actually delivered. Reporting that your patient or client tolerated treatment well could be interpreted to mean that the patient or client is in a state where he or she no longer requires your skilled services. Lastly, indicating simply that the plan of care should be continued does relay the future plan for the patient or client; however, it is not clear if this means that the next session should be a repeat of the flow sheet or if there are other elements of the plan of care that should be continued. Furthermore, there is no indication of how the plan of care is progressing since its implementation. Overall, there is no evidence that a clinical reasoning or decision-making process underlies the content of this note. Now consider the revised SOAP note from above.

> Patient reports soreness at her left lower extremity after the addition of the leg press last session. She states that she was able to sleep without pain. Her complaint of low back pain has resolved since eliminating the recumbent bike last session.
>
> Implemented dynamic stretching in knee flexion via a mini squat (10 × 10 sec hold) to replace the recumbent bike and ensure continued increase in knee range of motion.
>
> Patient required minimal verbal cues to avoid compensations (forward trunk flexion) during mini squats; required minimal assistance to avoid loss of balance during turning activities designed to simulate getting object out of refrigerator.

Continue to focus on lower extremity functional strength (repeated sit to stands) and improving balance reactions. Add mini-squat to HEP when patient can perform without compensations.

Can you detect an underlying clinical reasoning process from the details provided in this note? What relationships can be established among the components of this note? TABLE 4-2 offers some potential associations that you as the intervening therapist or assistant might begin to develop that may influence your subsequent session with your colleague's patient or client. Not only do you gather meaningful information about this patient or client from the detail in this revised note, but you are able to access your colleague's clinical reasoning without ever having a verbal conversation with your colleague to "learn" about the patient or client prior to the session.

The SOAP note is only one of several parts of a POMR. Therefore, using it in isolation in physical therapy documentation is another fundamental limitation of the SOAP note format. The POMR, originally developed by a physician for physicians, is intended to start with what is termed "the database," followed by the problem list generation, treatment plan development, and utilization of the SOAP note format.[7] In the medical field, the database includes the patient or client's medical history, which is a narrative composed by the physician,[7] and physical and laboratory data.[9] From these data, the patient or client's problem list of health conditions is created.[10] A treatment plan is developed for every problem in the problem list and is created using the SOAP note format.[5,9] For example, a physician's note for a patient or client with a complaint of knee pain may look like the note presented in FIGURE 4-1. Furthermore, the SOAP note format was intended to be used as the format for a physician's initial encounter with a patient or client as well as to update progress notes. This is a very different model than those that exist within physical therapy practice where a patient or client encounter occurs on a daily or three times weekly basis at a minimum.

It can be helpful to conceptualize a daily note in sections as is suggested by the SOAP note format. However for this approach to be successfully used as a framework for creating a comprehensive daily note in physical therapy practice, each section should be considered within the context of a physical therapy session. The skill in creating

TABLE 4-2 Clinical Reasoning Underlying a Daily Note

Section of Note	Potential Issues to Consider After Reviewing the Note	Potential Relationships Among Sections of the Note
Patient or client reports soreness at her L lower extremity after the addition of the leg press last session. Patient or client states that she was able to sleep without pain. Her complaint of low back pain (LBP) has resolved since eliminating the recumbent bike last session.	○ Needs possible education on delayed onset muscle soreness (DOMS). ○ DOMS did not seem to interfere with function indicating that leg press intensity could be increased. ○ LBP does not seem to be interfering with function. ○ Recumbent bike was likely related to LBP.	○ Response to exercise on function (ability to sleep, ability to rise from chair) ○ DOMS and intensity of exercise dosing ○ Response to exercise and increasing intensity dose ○ Exercise dosing and balance abilities ○ Knee range of motion and ability with balance reactions ○ Knee range of motion and ability to perform sit to stands and dynamic balance activities ○ Triggers of future LBP episodes and continue progress in plan of care ○ Compensatory strategies during exercise and knee range of motion ○ Compensatory strategies during exercise and poor balance
Implemented dynamic stretching in knee flexion via a mini-squat (10 × 10 sec hold) to replace the recumbent bike and ensure continued increased in knee range of motion.	○ Inquire about how mini-squats affected LBP. ○ Is the stretching dose enough for the goal of continuing the gain already made in knee range of motion?	
Patient or client required minimal verbal cues to avoid compensations (forward trunk flexion) during mini-squats; required minimal assistance to avoid loss of balance during turning activities designed to simulate getting object out of refrigerator.	○ Are compensations still present during the mini-squats? ○ Is there any LBP during the mini-squat when performed with or without the compensations? ○ In which direction does LBP occur when turning? ○ Is patient or client able to perform similar turning activity without LBP now? ○ What other similar activities could be included?	
Continue to focus on lower extremity functional strength (repeated sit to stands) and improving balance reactions. Add mini-squat to home exercise program (HEP) when patient can perform without compensations.	○ Can sit to stands be attempted without upper extremity assistance. ○ Was a measure of functional lower extremity strength assessed initially? ○ May start with a Five Times Sit to Stand Test to reassess ability since initial examination. ○ Is adding the mini-squat to the home exercise program appropriate at this time?	

this meaningful content lies in the ability to convert the substance of the session into useful documentation and ultimately tie the note's data to more meaningful and usable information. The following perspective may help you organize the session's content so that you can use the note to complement your clinical reasoning skills.

1. What is the patient or client's current status?
    a. What gains did the patient or client make since the last session?
    b. Were there any negative consequences of the last session?

2. What did you do about it?
3. What was your interpretation of what happened during the session?
    a. How did the patient or client respond to your interventions?
    b. What are the patient or client's remaining deficits?
4. What are you going to do next time?

The fundamental purpose of a daily note for you as a clinician is to provide a record of your patient or client's current **status**, to describe the **interventions** completed during your interaction, to convey your patient or client's

Subjective (S)

Patient presents with complaint of R knee pain after stepping on uneven terrain and twisting her knee when walking her dog 6 days ago.

Objective (O)

Palpable pain present and muscle guarding present at anterior and medial R knee and at medial joint line; peripatellar edema noted; decreased active knee range of motion; instability noted with physical exam; AP and lateral x-ray series obtained.

Assessment (A)

X-ray series negative for internal derangement or fracture of R knee; rule out meniscus tear.

Plan (P)

Start on 500 mg naproxen 2 x daily for pain and inflammation; educate on use of rest, ice, elevation, and compression; MRI of R knee; refer to physical therapy.

FIGURE 4-1 Example of Physician's SOAP Note.

response to the interaction, and to communicate the **plan** for the subsequent session, or **SIRP** (TABLE 4-3). The SIRP acronym is intended to re-conceptualize the daily note as different from that of the SOAP acronym as a documentation format to help you apply the context of a clinical encounter into a daily note using a clinical reasoning

TABLE 4-3   Alternative Daily Note Acronym

Conventional SOAP Note Terminology	Alternative Language
S: Subjective	S: Status
O: Objective	I: Intervention
A: Assessment	R: Response
P: Plan	P: Plan

process. In doing so, the content of the daily note reflects a decision-driven process versus a data-driven process. There are similarities between the SIRP note terminology and the traditional SOAP note terminology. The terminology used in the SIRP note is consistent with terminology endorsed by the APTA for completing documentation of a physical therapy encounter.[11] The interpretation for what each component of the SIRP note represents however warrants further discussion (FIGURE 4-2).

Status

The "status" section of the daily note details information regarding how your patient or client has been managing since the last session. This may include an update regarding a recent physician's office visit, information about how

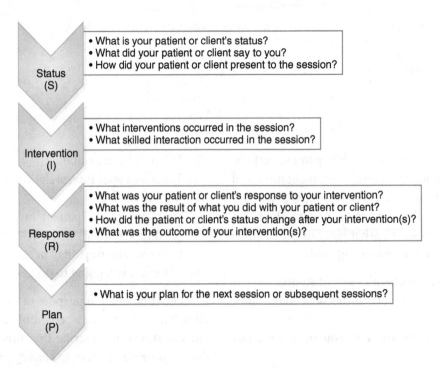

FIGURE 4-2 Use of SIRP for Creating a Daily Note.

your patient or client interprets his or her current condition or symptoms, how he or she responded to the events of the last session, or how he or she was able to implement home exercises, interventions, or modifications you prescribed at the last session. Be sure to only use quotation marks in this section to reflect exact value-added comments from your patient or client or caregiver. If your patient or client has no new information to report regarding his or her status, you may have to ask the patient or client, caregiver, or other members of the healthcare team further probing questions to identify relevant information. For example, you might ask if your patient or client is now able to perform an activity that previously was not possible. Alternatively, you may ask what activity limitations or participation restrictions remain that your patient or client cannot perform or achieve because of his or her current status. Rather than initiating the encounter with your patient or client by saying, "How are you doing today?" you might start by asking what he or she thought of a particular addition or adjustment to an intervention or perhaps his or her perception of his or her progress at the current point in the plan of care. In addition, reviewing the short- and long-term goals from your initial plan of care may lead to a conversation regarding your patient or client's current status, thus helping to generate the content of the status portion of the daily note. Consider the following example.

> Patient reports that his sleep was interrupted last night due to requiring assistance from nursing to transfer to the bedside commode × 3. Reports moderate fatigue this morning.

This content of the status section of the daily note relays that circumstances significant to the patient or client occurred since you last worked with him. This information should generate further conversation regarding your patient or client's ability to perform the transfer, the level of assistance needed, a comparison of prior ability with transfers, and the reason he required assistance three times in the middle of the night such as medication side effects, inappropriate fluid intake, or an undiagnosed medical problem. Gathering this information will assist you in your decision making for which interventions are required to meet your patient or client's needs in reducing this reported problem, thus setting up the framework for the remainder of your daily note. This detail will also allow another clinician not familiar with the patient or client

to generate a series of questions that could lead to ideas of how to initiate a treatment session without having to immediately probe further into prior documentation. Furthermore, this entry relays substance that indicates that continued care is necessary. Consider another example.

> Patient has no complaints.

It is reasonable that a clinical situation may exist where your patient or client is progressing as expected and that there is no new information to report. However, this documentation suggests that perhaps the patient or client no longer requires your skilled services. If this is truly the case, then discontinuing the episode of care is warranted. Consider another example.

> Mr. A reports that his shoulder pain is very limiting today and is a 6/10.

This content of the status section of the daily note relays a fairly superficial interpretation of one's status. While it may reflect what your patient or client said to you, it does not reveal a great deal of meaningful information that you can use to formulate how you might structure the session. In other words, the information reported here is simply data, rather than information recorded that would allow for further discussion that would lead to clinical decision making. Consider the following revision.

> Mr. A reports that his shoulder pain increased from zero at rest to a 6/10 after showering and getting dressed this morning.

This entry relays more detail that would allow you to further probe into the details of this situation. For example, you could determine the acuity and location of the pain, a comparison to a prior timeframe when the same activity was performed, or the manner in which the specific showering and dressing activities were performed. Furthermore, this note indicates that skilled care is warranted since basic activities of daily living increase pain. This information should assist you in constructing your session as well as the remainder of your daily note.

Intervention

The "intervention" section of the daily note details the actual events of the session. In this section, the interventions performed should be recorded. However, this section should be much more than a just a reference to the flow sheet or a list of the exercises and activities performed. Rather, this section should detail the skilled interaction you had with your patient or client. For example, the detail included in this section should reflect the interventions implemented based on your assessment of your patient or client's current status and your professional judgment of the patient or client's prior response to the interventions you prescribed. If you chose to write, "See flow sheet," it is important that the flow sheet reflect any exercise progression or other changes that you made to the interventions in that session. You could support this previous statement by indicating the detail of the activity you added to the flow sheet both in the flow sheet and in the daily note itself. For example, you could indicate that you added a particular exercise and the reason that exercise was added. Consider the following note.

> Added lateral overhead functional reaching task with 2# load to simulate retrieving item from shelf in shower. Dosed activity for motor control of the shoulder girdle per flow sheet.

If you determine that it is appropriate to perform interventions *exactly* as they were performed the session before without any modifications than it is important to indicate why changes were not made. This type of statement will support your clinical reasoning process for the decisions you made to keep the intervention the same rather than being interpreted by a third party as simply continuing the plan of care without skilled decision making. Therefore, this section should include any modifications made to the flow sheet or any interventions added within the session including details of an exercise's prescription, the level of assistance provided during an activity, education provided, or any addition to the home exercise program. Another component relevant to include in this section is the result of any tests and measures and outcome measures performed during the session. For example, assume that your patient or client indicates that he or she is having a much easier time getting up and down from a low seat such as the commode. You may decide to perform and record a Five Times Sit to Stand Test to determine if a clinically significant change in functional lower extremity strength has occurred. The numerical result of the outcome measure would be recorded in this section. Consider the following addition to the daily note in progress above.

> Practiced stand pivot transfers × 6 to/from the commode chair/hospital bed with an approach to the right and the left side of the bed. Provided education regarding fluid intake prior to sleep for the night. Five Times Sit to Stand = 19 seconds from 25-inch bed height.

This content of the daily note relays the exact activity performed in such a way that it could be reproduced by another member of your patient or client's healthcare team including the details of how the outcome measure was altered from its standard administration. Other details appropriate for this section of the daily note include your position relative to your patient or client, your patient or client's position, the presence of a caregiver or another healthcare provider, or your hand placement. You may also decide to talk with your patient or client's nurse to relay the details of your current session, and to find out further information regarding the events of the night before and the manner in which the transfers were actually performed. It is appropriate to include this detail in your note for future reference as well as to serve as the official record of what occurred in the session as follows:

> Practiced stand pivot transfers × 6 to/from the commode chair/hospital bed with an approach to the right and the left side of the bed. Spoke with nursing staff and determined that patient has been started on a diuretic medication, which may explain frequent assistance from nursing for toileting in the middle of the night.

This addition of the communication with other healthcare professionals to the content of the actual note can assist you in creating other components of the note as well as assist other consumers of the note to recognize a change in a patient or client's status and how it was managed.

Response

The "response" section of the daily note relays your interpretation of the acute reaction your patient or client had to the contents of the session. This section should include your professional judgment of your patient or client's response to the interventions you prescribed in real time using your observational skills. In other words, your judgment of your patient or client's performance is recorded in this section. Why certain improvements occurred or why certain deficits remain are relevant to include in this section. For example, you might consider including details regarding the types of cues or manual assistance your patient or client required to perform the desired intervention. Furthermore, you might record the details of what steps had to occur in order for your patient or client to perform an activity without pain or compensatory strategies. On the other hand, it would also be appropriate to record the details that prevented your patient or client from performing the activity using the desired approach. In addition, your interpretation of any outcome measures you collected during the session would be included in this section. For example, assume that your patient or client was able to perform the Five Times Sit to Stand Test in 11 seconds, which is a 12-second improvement from the performance on the initial examination. The interpretation that your patient or client has had a clinically significant improvement in lower extremity functional strength would be included here. A subsequent statement regarding the impairments in body functions and structures, activity limitations, and participation restrictions remaining that warrant skilled physical therapy intervention is then relevant. It is also relevant to include how your patient or client's status may have changed within the session based on the skilled intervention you provided during the session. For example, you may be working on developing lateral stepping balance reactions in your patient or client who has Parkinson's disease. It would be appropriate to include in this section of the note any improvement or lack of improvement in the ability to recover a loss of balance in response to repeated perturbations in a lateral direction. Consider the following addition to the daily note in progress above.

> Patient required contact guard assistance to prevent loss of balance during stand-pivot transfer to bedside commode; required verbal cues for right foot and right lower extremity placement during turn of transfer to the commode and again to the bed. Patient demonstrated improved lower extremity placement within the session requiring no verbal cues by end of session.

This content of the daily note relays your specific interactions with your patient or client based on his response to the intervention as it was being performed. The detail provided here completes the prescription of the transfer activity since the assistance level, type of cues

provided, and issues that prevented the transfer from being independent are included. Furthermore, it sets up the detail of the plan section of the note.

Plan

The "plan" section of the daily note should project what interventions or components of the plan of care should occur in a subsequent session. Simply relaying, "continue plan of care" does not reveal that a skilled decision-making process was employed to determine further movement through the established plan of care. This section should consider the content of the current session. For example, if your patient or client was not successful in achieving the appropriate upper extremity positioning for supraspinatus strengthening, then it would be appropriate to indicate in the plan to continue to perform motor control and proprioception interventions for the supraspinatus prior to initiating a strengthening dose. Incorporating this detail into the plan section of the note relays that you utilized skill in determining which portion of the plan of care to proceed with next. Consider the following addition to the daily note in progress above.

> Continue to practice stand-pivot transfers to/from commode chair for increased independence with toileting. Practice turns to facilitate improvements with stand-pivot transfers. Discuss fluid intake schedule with nursing and speech language pathologist and urinary frequency, possibly due to the addition of the diuretic medication, with physician.

This content of the daily note relays a skilled decision-making process and a proactive approach towards progressing your patient or client through the established plan of care.

The Flow Sheet

A critical component of the daily note is the flow sheet. Often a flow sheet format is used to list the interventions that were performed during a physical therapy session. A flow sheet could simply reflect the interventions performed in a list format, or it could take on a structure that has a clinical reasoning framework. Consider the following flow sheet.

Flow Sheet	Date:
Upper body ergometer	8 min
Standing rows	30# × 8
Lateral arm raises	4# × 8
Shoulder – external rotation	6# × 8
Shoulder – internal rotation	8# × 8
Biceps curls (eccentric)	5# × 20
Inferior glides (GH joint)	Grade III

Does this flow sheet have a clinical reasoning framework or is it simply a list of interventions? Do you think that the detail provided in this flow sheet is useful information? From the flow sheet above, you could assume that this patient or client may have performed a warm-up activity prior to initiating strengthening exercises at the shoulder. You might suspect the presence of a tendinopathy at the biceps based on the indication that the biceps curl is performed eccentrically. Lastly, you might infer that this patient or client has a capsular restriction at the glenohumeral (GH) joint based on the inclusion of grade III joint mobilizations. However, missing from this list is a framework for why these exercises might be included in the flow sheet. A clinical reasoning flow sheet (FIGURE 4-3) has an inherent structure from which decisions can be made and is not merely an inventory of interventions listed in the order in which they were performed. The medium for an interactive flow sheet such as this one is an electronic spreadsheet. Even if the documentation system with which you work is paper-based, a flow sheet could be created in a spreadsheet format and populated with blank spaces so that the appropriate interventions could be included. The first section of the clinical reasoning flow sheet shown in Figure 4-3 includes information that can serve as prompts or reminders regarding your patient or client's primary health condition, concurrent comorbid conditions, and any precautions or contraindications that may be relevant to his or her care. The subsequent sections begin with current procedural terminology (CPT) code headings such as manual therapy, therapeutic exercise, neuromuscular reeducation, and therapeutic activities. The flow sheet could be populated with any of the CPT codes you might use in that particular plan of care. Under each of the CPT code headings are a listing of the techniques you might use with your patient or client. For example, "soft tissue techniques" and "joint mobilizations" are listed under the CPT code heading "manual therapy." Additional rows could then be added under

Primary Health Condition
Comorbid Conditions
Precautions/Contraindications
Visit Count
Next Progress/Status Note Due
Outcome Measures to Track
Patient/Caregiver Education
Home Exercise Program

MANUAL THERAPY
Soft Tissue Techniques
    Deep tissue mobilization
Joint Oscillations
Joint Mobilizations
Neurodynamics

THERAPEUTIC EXERCISE/NEUROMUSCULAR RE-EDUCATION
Mobility/Symptom Relief/Tissue Health
Motor Control/Coordination
Endurance
Strengthening
Power

THERAPEUTIC ACTIVITIES
Functional Performance Training
Balance Activities
    Static
    Dynamic
    Center of Mass Perturbations
    Base of Support Perturbations
    Vestibular Training

FIGURE 4-3 Clinical Reasoning Flow Sheet.

the technique of "joint mobilizations" to include those interventions specific to that plan of care such as "grade III glenohumeral joint mobilizations." The CPT codes "therapeutic exercise" and "neuromuscular reeducation" are coupled in one row of the flow sheet to serve as a functional term for the purpose of listing a certain type of exercise under this heading. For example, an exercise listed under "mobility/symptom relief/tissue health" indicates that the exercise is being done with the goal of restoring tissue integrity and decreasing pain due to muscle guarding. Thus, the exercise dosing included in the adjacent cell should similarly reflect this goal. Likewise, an exercise listed under "strengthening" indicates that the exercise is being done with the goal of increasing force generating capacity and muscle mass. Therefore, the strengthening exercise should be listed with the appropriate exercise prescription. In addition to including a complete exercise prescription, the expanding cell within a spreadsheet format allows for further information such as the patient or client's position during the exercise and the cuing or level of assistance the patient or client required to complete the exercise. Organizing the flow sheet using CPT code descriptors as headings can then help you to ensure that your billing reflects your documentation of the interventions you actually delivered during your session.

Consider the flow sheet above that listed interventions for the shoulder. This flow sheet could be rewritten to look like the clinical reasoning flow sheet presented in **FIGURE 4-4**. From this flow sheet, you have access to multiple components of your plan of care in one location such as how many visits remain and when the next progress note is due. Similarly, you have a reminder of an outcome you would like to achieve by the end of the plan of care. The interventions are presented in the flow sheet in such a way that you are reminded about which exercises you decided to defer and which you have not yet considered. As you follow up with your patient or client at a subsequent session, you will be able to look at the flow sheet and use its contents as an adjunct to your clinical decision making as you draw meaning from what your patient or client is reporting about his or her current status, what interventions you would like to perform during the session,

Primary Health Condition	Supraspinatus tendinopathy; right
Comorbid Conditions	None
Precautions/Contraindications	None
Visit Count	3/12
Next Progress/Status Note Due	date
Outcome Measures to Track	Quick DASH; performance-based testing—overhead reach with 25# load
Patient/Caregiver Education	Sitting position while driving and when at the computer
Home Exercise Program (HEP)	See attached sheet; issued on date

MANUAL THERAPY
Soft Tissue Techniques
    Deep tissue mobilization
Joint Oscillations
Joint Mobilizations
    Inferior glenohumeral joint glides
Neurodynamics
	
	Grade III, supine, 5 min prior to motor control exercises

THERAPEUTIC EXERCISE/NEUROMUSCULAR RE-EDUCATION
Mobility/Symptom Relief/Tissue Health
    Wall slides
    Internal rotation standing at pulley
    External rotation standing at pulley
Motor Control/Coordination
    Lateral shoulder raises
    Lateral shoulder raises (eccentric)
Endurance
Strengthening
    Internal rotation standing pulley
    External rotation standing at pulley
    External rotation in side-lying position
Power
	
	Standing facing wall; in pain-free range, 30 × 2; also issue for HEP
	12# 3 × 25; 0 deg of abduction (towel under axilla)
	6# 3 × 25; 0 deg of abduction (towel under axilla)
	
	To 100 deg; standing at mirror, focus on scapulohumeral rhythm, 2 × 50
	From 100 deg; standing; therapist assist with concentric phase; 0# 3 × 12
	
	Deferred
	Deferred
	Deferred

THERAPEUTIC ACTIVITIES
Functional Performance Training
    Overhead reach shelf
    Lateral reach to shelf
Balance Activities
    Static
    Dynamic
    Center of Mass Perturbations
    Base of Support Perturbations
    Vestibular Training
	
	Deferred
	Deferred

FIGURE 4-4 Clinical Reasoning Flow Sheet – Shoulder.

your expectations of your patient or client's response to the interventions you prescribed, and your plans for future visits. Furthermore, you will be able to see what CPT codes are appropriate to bill based on the areas of the flow sheet you completed.

Federal Rules and Regulations

Since the daily note is a decision-driven rather than a data-driven document, the clinical practice setting in which you construct the note should not determine its contents. Some practice settings such home health agencies, skilled nursing facilities, inpatient rehabilitation facilities, or school-based settings utilize specialized forms or electronic health record templates to facilitate compliance with Medicare and Medicaid rules and regulations. Medicare's rules and regulations for documentation are considered the gold standard for payment and coverage policy and are typically replicated by other third-party payers.[12] However, documentation created in any setting where Medicare beneficiaries receive physical therapy care should still utilize the fundamental framework of relaying the patient or client's current **status**, describing the **interventions** completed during the interaction, conveying the patient or client's **response** to the interaction, and communicating the **plan** for the subsequent session. Medicare's guidelines that represent "reasonable and medically necessary documentation" reiterate the need to ensure that sound clinical decision making is at its root (**TABLE 4-4**).[13] Furthermore, the Jimmo v. Sebelius Settlement Agreement Program Manual Clarifications Fact Sheet[14] indicates that the justification of medically necessary skilled services should include that:

○ "The patient or client's condition has the potential to improve
○ The patient or client's condition is improving in response to therapy
○ Maximum improvement is yet to be attained
○ There is an expectation that the anticipated improvement is attainable in a reasonable and generally predictable period of time."[14]

These guidelines should not be considered as specialized instructions that should be applied only to Medicare beneficiaries. Rather, showing that you delivered "reasonable and medically necessary" skilled care should infiltrate every part of your documentation regardless of

TABLE 4-4   Medicare Guidelines for "Reasonable and Medically Necessary" Documentation of Therapy Services

Physical therapy services rendered must be:
Safe and effective.
Not experimental or investigational.
Appropriate in duration and frequency.
In accordance with the standards of practice for the patient/client's condition.
Provided in the appropriate setting to match the patient/client's medical needs and health condition(s).
Ordered and delivered by qualified personnel.
Appropriate to meet but not exceed the patient/client's medical needs.
At least as beneficial as an existing and available medically appropriate alternative.

Centers for Medicare & Medicaid Services. *Medicare Program Integrity Manual*, Chapter 13, 13.5.1- Reasonable and Necessary Provisions in LCDs (Rev. 473, Issued: 06-21-13, Effective: 01-15-13, Implementation: 01-15-13). Baltimore: Centers for Medicare & Medicaid Services. Available at: www.cms.gov/manuals/downloads/pim83c13.pdf.

the setting in which the therapy services are rendered, the entity providing the payment for services, or the consumer who will be using the documentation to make decisions.

Clinical Encounter Type

GROUP THERAPY

In constructing the daily note, the SIRP acronym not only applies in the context of a one-on-one clinical encounter, but it also applies to documenting group therapy, co-treatments, maintenance therapy, or prevention and wellness encounters. **Group therapy** is defined differently depending on the care setting in which it is delivered. The Centers for Medicare & Medicaid Services (CMS) define group therapy delivered in an outpatient setting as therapy provided simultaneously to at least two patients or clients who have similar or differing therapy needs as long as the therapist providing the group therapy gives constant attendance and provides skilled medically necessary services.[15] Group therapy in a skilled nursing environment is defined as therapy provided simultaneously to no more and no less than four patients or clients who are performing the same or similar activities.[16] CMS recommends that group therapy documentation, regardless of the specifics of the definition, should:

○ Reflect potential changes in the patient or client's medical condition.

○ Justify the plan of care.
○ Be properly tailored to the individualized goals of the patient or client.[16]

It may also be useful to include the number of patients or clients in the group therapy session. Consider the following daily note for one of your patients or clients who participated in group therapy with you and two other patients or clients.

> Mr. A reports that he was able to don his left shoe while sitting on his bed yesterday, which he was not previously able to do.
>
> See flow sheet for exercises completed during group session (six patients). Advanced intensity of seated knee extension strengthening exercise via wall pulley to 11# on the left .
>
> Mr. A demonstrates improved AROM at the left knee when donning shoes and when performing group sit-to-stand exercise from 18-inch height surface.
>
> Add step ups next session to continue to build lower extremity strength to facilitate Mr. A's ability to access the second floor of his home.

This daily note reflects a positive change in the Mr. A's status by relaying a new functional ability he has achieved. This note also justifies the plan of care by indicating an activity limitation that still exists. Finally, this note indicates that Mr. A's needs were addressed with skilled progression of the intervention. Including the ability of your patient or client to participate in the group session as well as indicating the value of the group session in comparison to the goals established in the plan of care will help you to relay that skilled care was provided for your patient or client involved in a group therapy intervention.

CO-TREATMENTS

The CMS defines **co-treatments** or team therapy as physical therapists or physical therapist assistants working together as a team to treat one or more patients or clients at the same time.[17] Other than indicating in your documentation that you worked with another member of the patient or client's healthcare team, the content of the daily note when you are involved in a co-treatment should be the same as documenting any other encounter and should include details relaying medical necessity as well as the skill utilized in the delivery of the service.

MAINTENANCE THERAPY

The CMS indicate that the goal of **maintenance therapy** should be to restore function; however it is also recognized that even in those situations where no functional improvement is expected, documentation should reflect that skilled therapy services are needed to prevent or slow a decline in the patient or client's current status.[14] You must be able to show however through your documentation that your patient or client's maintenance needs could not be addressed safely and effectively through the use of nonskilled personnel.[14] Consider the following example.

> Mrs. A reports that she has been able to implement the use of a nightlight to get to the bathroom at night without loss of balance consistently over the past 2 weeks.
>
> Added proximal upper extremity strengthening exercises to prevent loss of ability to use upper extremities to assist with dressing and toileting tasks.
>
> Mrs. A was unable to use a walker or other assistive device to support ambulation due to complete absence of functional grip strength bilaterally.
>
> Focus on strengthening biceps, triceps, and rotator cuff musculature bilaterally to compensate for loss of grip and to prevent deterioration of current abilities with dressing and toileting tasks.

This daily note indicates that you are providing skilled services with the goal of restoring abilities with functional tasks. Furthermore, this excerpt indicates that you are attempting to slow decline in this patient or client's current functional status by targeting a body region that is available to compensate for the lack of functional grip strength.

PREVENTION AND WELLNESS

Physical therapists and physical therapist assistants intervene to prevent impairments in body structures and functions, activity limitations, participation restrictions, and environmental barriers related to movement, functioning, and health.[18] Furthermore, providing physical therapy services to promote health, wellness, and fitness is considered within the scope of practice for physical therapy service providers.[19] Therefore, you must ensure that the documentation you generate on behalf of a patient or client engaged in **prevention and wellness** activities reflects that the service is medically necessary or is considered a service that can be provided only by a skilled professional. Consider the following scenario that occurs in an outpatient setting for your 48-year-old female patient or client for whom you have prescribed an exercise program to prevent a decline in bone mineral density.

> Mrs. A returns today with a completed exercise log that you issued 2 weeks ago. She reports that she no longer has muscle soreness across her shoulders and mid back and that her friends have noticed an improvement in her posture.
>
> Reviewed exercise program and progressed per sheet. Reassessed postural alignment. See status note.
>
> Improved scapular strength per reassessment.
>
> Perform progressed exercise program as indicated (see sheet) three times per week for 8 weeks. Client to return at the end of 8 weeks for further reassessment of strength gains. Exercise program to be reassessed and progressed as indicated at that time.

Providing follow-up physical therapy care for individual on a preventative fitness or wellness program is no different than the process you would implement for any other individual in whom you are providing skilled physical therapy services. Thus, the documentation that accompanies this type of encounter is also the same. For example, in the documentation example above the goal is for the patient or client to independently execute an exercise program to preserve bone health over a 2-week period. Just as in any other patient or client returning for a visit after 2 weeks, you reassess her status as well as her ability to carry out the plan you established together at the last session. This example assumes that a status or progress note was written and was attached to the daily note. The daily note above refers to the attached reassessment as well as to the progressed exercise program. Overall, the details of the reassessment should match the recommendations for the exercise progression and the plan for the future session indicating that skilled and medically necessary services were delivered.

WORKERS' COMPENSATION

While these same principles can be applied to the documentation for any patient or client regardless of the setting in which he or she received skilled physical therapy services, you may find it beneficial to include additional details in the daily notes of your **workers' compensation**

patients or clients to show that you are working towards the ultimate goal of returning your patient or client to work (**APPENDIX 4-A**).

Summary

Regardless of the type of session you document or the care setting in which you practice, reflect on the details of what you are writing in your daily note as you create its contents. **TABLE 4-5** provides reflective questions you can use to self-examine your daily note writing skills. Ask yourself, what value does this information add to this daily note? Does this information help relay the clinical situation? Does this information reflect the goals created at the initial examination? Does the information provided here build on prior daily notes? Does the detail provided here assist with developing a mental picture of the patient or client? In addition, be sure that when you document your professional opinion you are basing it on clear facts that are also evident in your documentation. Evaluating your own clinical skills in this way will undoubtedly demonstrate to you the quality of the information you include in your documentation. Furthermore, using the SIRP acronym to create the contents of your daily note can help you to plan not only the details of your current session, but also the progression of your plan of care. Remember, that the SIRP acronym is intended to help you populate the contents of the daily note. How you label each section of the note, SIRP or SOAP, is not relevant. In fact, many

TABLE 4-5 Guide to Daily Note Self-Reflection

Did I clearly relay my patient or client's status at this point in the plan of care?
Did I clearly relay the interventions completed during the session?
Did I clearly record my patient or client's response to the interventions completed?
Did I clearly record the plan for the subsequent session?
Does the information I included add value to this note?
Does the information I included reflect my observations of the patient or client before, during, and after the actual intervention?
Does the information I included indicate that skilled care was necessary?
Does the information I included supplement the content of the initial examination, re-examination documentation, or prior daily notes?
Does the information I included reflect the detail I would look for if I were reviewing this note?

BOX 4-1 The Electronic Health Record: Daily Note

Electronic health records (EHR) can be programmed to allow you to input the content of a daily note in a narrative format. However, there are also formats available that limit free-text input and provide pre-populated fields of text and drop-down menus from which you can create a sentence. It is important to recognize however, that eliminating the thought processes involved in creating the words of each included sentence could potentially decrease your understanding of how to infuse your daily note with relevant decision-driven content. CMS explicitly reports that phrases such as "Patient tolerated treatment well," "Continue with plan of care," and "Patient remains stable" are insufficient to establish the medical necessity of skilled services.[14] Be cautious that you are not incorporating short-cuts when documenting in an electronic system at the expense of your clinical reasoning. Other phrases to be cautious of include "See HEP" and "See flow sheet." These phases refer to additional documentation that lie outside of the structure of the daily note. Some electronic systems have built in flow sheet templates but others may not. If you are referring to documentation that you created utilizing alternative software such as a home exercise program, then it is important that you somehow link this information to your patient or client's record so that it can be easily referenced. Furthermore, it is important that your daily note, not just the flow sheet, explicitly indicates the progressions made and the skilled and medically necessary reasons that these occurred.

Another documentation pitfall is the use of abbreviations in a patient or client's health record. An EHR may facilitate the use of abbreviations due to software programming limits on available character spaces in any given data field. To save programming space in electronic systems, abbreviations might be used. Many organizations have created lists of approved abbreviations to be used in documentation to help standardize documentation across the system. While abbreviations have been widely used by many healthcare professionals regardless of the documentation medium, recognize that the APTA recommends that the use of abbreviations in a health record be minimized.[20]

Another common documentation mistake that occurs with the use of electronic systems is failure to sign and date a daily note in a timely manner. Many systems capture your signature one time electronically and then apply it along with a date and time to any subsequent note you write. However, there is often an additional step required of you after completing the content of your note to actually sign it. This action usually signifies that the note has been completed and that the charges you entered have been submitted to billing. Only then has the note been officially completed with the date, time, and your signature. It is important to note that while many systems record the time that your note was completed or signed, many systems do not capture the time during your session you spent on each intervention or the total treatment time of the encounter.

---

electronic systems specifically use the SOAP acronym as place holders for pre-populated fields and drop-down menus in the daily note template of an electronic health record (EHR). Ultimately, regardless of the acronym used, the fundamental framework of relaying the patient or client's current **status**, describing the **interventions** completed during the interaction, conveying the patient or client's **response** to the interaction, and communicating the **plan** for the subsequent session should be utilized for every patient or client encounter.

Discussion Questions

1. Listen to your clinical instructor or colleague greet a patient or client. Focus on the questions your colleague asked the patient or client.
   a. What are these questions?
   b. Create part of a daily note based on your observations.
   c. Compare this note to that of your clinical instructor or colleague.
2. Observe a physical therapy session between a patient or client and your clinical instructor or colleague. Focus on the outcomes measured and the interventions delivered.
   a. What are these measures and interventions?
   b. Create part of the daily note based on your observations.
   c. Compare this note with that of your clinical instructor or colleague.
3. Observe a physical therapy session between a patient or client and your clinical instructor or colleague. Focus on how the patient or client responded to the session

or how his or her status may have changed as a result of the intervention.

   a. What are these outcomes?
   b. How were they achieved?
   c. Create part of the daily note based on your observations.
   d. Compare this note with that of your clinical instructor or colleague.

4. Observe a physical therapy session between a patient or client and clinical instructor or your colleague. Focus on the plan for the next session.

   a. How did you know this plan?
   b. Create part of the daily note based on your observations.
   c. Compare this note with that of your clinical instructor or colleague.

5. Exchange a daily note with one of your clinical instructors or colleagues. Can you discern the clinical reasoning process from the contents of the note?

   a. What details of the note did you use to answer this question?

   b. Discuss your interpretation of this clinical reasoning process with the author of the note.
   c. Were you accurate in the detail you gleaned from the note? If not, what were the differences between your interpretation of the note and that of your clinical instructor or colleague?

6. After comparing notes with your clinical instructor or colleague in the question above, consider the guidelines presented in Table 4-5.

   a. Discuss the rationale for why each part of the note was included.
   b. Did your rationale differ from that of your clinical instructor or colleague?
   c. Did you identify any omissions from your note that you think should have been included?

7. Exchange flow sheets with one of your clinical instructors or colleagues. Does the flow sheet following a clinical reasoning format? Why or why not?

Case Study Questions

1. You are reviewing the health record of one of your clinical instructor's or colleague's patients or clients. You will be working with this patient or client this afternoon since your colleague went home sick. After reviewing the last daily note below, determine the issues you should potentially consider during your session with this patient or client. Identify the content of each component of the daily note. What are the potential relationships among the sections of this note? Also consider the flow sheet. What components of the flow sheet do you consider valuable? Why or why not?

> Patient states that she is feeling decreased stiffness in the left hip when standing from sitting to walk. She comments that she is very fearful to retrieve an object off the floor because she does not want to break her hip precautions.

> See flow sheet. Added item "retrieval from floor (used pencil and 3# cuff weight)."

> Pt required contact guard assistance when retrieving small object such as pencil from the floor due to decreased lateral stability in standing; however she was able to retrieve the 3# cuff weight with supervision only.

> Continue to practice retrieving items or varied sizes and shapes from the floor next session.

Primary health condition	L total hip arthroplasty date
Comorbid conditions	Osteoporosis
Precautions/contraindications	Hip – posterior approach
Visit count	5
Next progress note due	date
Outcome measures to track	Five Times Sit to Stand Test, Four Square Step Test, 10 Meter Walk Test, Single Limb Stance, Functional Gait Assessment
Patient or client/caregiver education	Updated home exercise program (attached) on date; practiced safe positioning while seated in shower chair to safely shave legs
MANUAL THERAPY	
THERAPEUTIC EXERCISE/ NEUROMUSCULAR REEDUCATION	
Mobility/symptom relief/tissue health	
Motor control/coordination	
Endurance	
Strengthening	
Sit to stand (17 in height)	11× in 30 sec; no UE A
Standing hip abduction	5# cuff 3 × 12 on L; 8# cuffs 3 × 12 on R; min UE A at counter (supervision)

Forward step ups (8 in step)	Lead with R 2 × 15 (1 UE A); lead with L 2 8 (2 UE A)
Power	

THERAPEUTIC ACTIVITIES

Functional Performance Training	
Item retrieval from floor	Pencil, 3# cuff weight; utilized one hand on nearby object for support; utilized extension of involved LE moving posterior as center of mass moved towards floor
Balance activities	
Static	
Single leg stance	On floor; no UE A; contact guard A; toes toward forwards or lateral target on floor 5 attempts R, L
Dynamic	
Lateral walking	4 × 25 feet stand-by A to contact guard A 3# cuffs B lower extremities
Backward walking	4 × 25 feet stand-by A to contact guard A 3# cuffs B lower extremities
March in place (eyes closed)	2 × 30 sec each (stand-by A)

2. **Consider the following daily note and flow sheet. Identify the content of each component of the daily note. What are the potential relationships among the sections of this note? What components of the flow sheet do you consider valuable? Why or why not?**

Patient states that he returned to rowing for 45 minutes on the ergometer at the gym 2 days ago and then rowed on the water for 45 minutes yesterday. He states that he has no pain currently and did not have any pain during rowing activities.

See flow sheet. Home exercise program reviewed—mid trapezius and lower trapezius targeted for motor control 3# dumbbells 3 × 30 each; daily

Normalized mobility of all thoracic spine segments and lower ribs via mobility testing; demonstrates proper form with all exercises including home exercise program; demonstrates understanding of importance of building strength of scapular musculature for rowing activity.

Continue home exercise program at this time as prescribed above for 1 week, patient to row with

rowing team without restrictions and contact clinic in 1 week to inform on progress with exercise. Will determine conclusion of the episode of care or furthering the plan of care at that time.

Primary health condition	Thoracic spine pain (facet joint dysfunction)
Visit count	4
Next progress note due	date
Outcome measures to track	Patient-Specific Functional Scale, pulling performance
Patient/caregiver education	Updated home exercise program (attached) on date

MANUAL THERAPY

Soft tissue techniques	
Deep tissue mobilization	(not performed this session) Positional release latissimus dorsi; L sidelying
Spine mobilizations	(not performed this session) T9–T11 (Grade III) (UPAs L)

NEUROMUSCULAR REEDUCATION/THERAPEUTIC EXERCISE

Mobility/symptom relief/tissue health	
All 4s (Thread the needle)	Reach to R with R then reach to L with L (follow movement with head) (elbow flexed) 20× per side; no hold
R sidelying over rolled pillow	L arm overhead (deep breathing; no hold) (3 min)
Motor control/coordination	
Standing trunk rotation	Pulley 40× each to R, L
Standing rows (unilateral)	Pulley 2 × 25 each to R, L
Seated rows	Pulley 50# 1 × 30; 1 × 15
Prone shoulder elevation (lower trapezius)	3 × 30 3# dbell B
Endurance	
Prone trunk extension	3 × 30 sec hold no weight
Strengthening	
Prone L shoulder extension	3# dbell 3 × 12; 3 sec hold
Power	
Serratus punch	Standing pulley; 30# quick contractions; extended elbow 3 × 12

References

1. American Physical Therapy Association (APTA). *Physical Therapy Documentation Reform.* Alexandria, VA: American Physical Therapy Association; June, 2013.

2. APTA. *Defensible Documentation: Improving Your Clinical Documentation: Reflecting Best Practice.* Alexandria, VA: American Physical Therapy Association; 2012.

3. APTA. *Defensible Documentation Elements.* Alexandria, VA: American Physical Therapy Association; 2012.

4. Weed LL. Medical records that guide and teach. *N Engl J Med.* 1968;278(11):593–600.

5. Cameron S. Learning to write case notes using the SOAP format. *J Couns Dev.* 2002;80:286–292.

6. Rubin A. Another way to enhance SOAP's usefulness [Letter]. *Acad Med.* 1998,73:445.

7. Donnelly, WJ. Why SOAP is bad for the medical record. *Arch Intern Med.* 1992;152:481–484.

8. Wainwright SF et al. Novice and experienced physical therapist clinicians: a comparison of how reflection is used to inform the clinical decision-making process. *Phys Ther.* 2010;90:75–88.

9. Heller M, Vea:40ch L. *Clinical Medical Assisting: A Professional, Field Smart Approach to the Workplace.* Clifton Park, NY: Delmar Cengage Learning, Inc; 2009:40..

10. Gensinger RA, Fowler J. ASOP: a new method and tools for capturing a clinical encounter. *Proc Annu Symp Comput Appl Med Care.* 1995:142–146.

11. APTA. *Defensible Documentation for Patient/Client Management.* Alexandria, VA: American Physical Therapy Association;. Available at http://www.apta.org/Documentation/DefensibleDocumentation/.

12. Daulong MR. Risk management: the spectrum of documentation – a resources guide to better ensure compliance. *PT in Motion,* November 2010. http://www.apta.org/PTinMotion/2010/09/RiskManagement/ Accessed June 29, 2014.

13. Centers for Medicare & Medicaid Services (CMS). *Medicare Program Integrity Manual,* Chapter 13, 13.5.1 – Reasonable and Necessary Provisions in LCDs, Rev. 473. Woodlawn, MD: Centers for Medicare & Medicaid Services; June 21, 2013 (Implementation: 01-15-13). Available at www.cms.gov/manuals/downloads/pim83c13.pdf. Accessed June 29, 2014.

14. CMS. *Jimmo v. Sebelius Settlement Agreement Program Manual Clarifications Fact Sheet,* Woodlawn, MD: Centers for Medicare & Medicaid Services; 2014. Available at http://www.cms.gov/Medicare/Medicare-Fee-for-Service-Payment/SNFPPS/Downloads/jimmo_fact_sheet2_022014_final.pdf. Accessed June 29, 2014.

15. CMS. *Medicare Carriers Manual* Part 3 – Claims Process. Transmittal 1753.. Woodlawn, MD: Centers for Medicare & Medicaid Services; May, 2002. Available at www.apta.org/Payment/Coding/OneonOneGroup/ Accessed June 29, 2014.

16. CMS. MDS 3.0 and RUG-IV, Updates and Training for FY 2012. Woodlawn, MD: Centers for Medicare & Medicaid Services; August 23, 2011. Available at www.cms.gov/Medicare/Medicare-Fee-for-Service-Payment/SNFPPS/downloads/mds30_rugiv_train_slides_081811.pdf. Accessed June 29, 2014.

17. CMS. 11 FAQs: Part B Billing Scenarios for PTs and OTs. Woodlawn, MD: Centers for Medicare & Medicaid Services; 2009. Available at www.cms.gov/Medicare/Billing/TherapyServices/Downloads/11_Part_B_Billing_Scenarios_for_PTs_and_OTs.pdf. Accessed June 30, 2014.

18. APTA. *Physical Therapists and Physical Therapist Assistants as Promotors and Advocates for Physical Activity/Exercise.* Alexandria, VA: American Physical Therapy Association; June 2008. [Previously titled: Promoting Physical Activity; June 2003] [Position].

19. APTA. *Physical Therapists' Role in Prevention, Wellness, Fitness, and Disease Management.* Alexandria, VA: American Physical Therapy Association; February, 2014 [Position].

20. APTA. *Defensible Documentation General Documentation Guidelines.* Alexandria, VA: American Physical Therapy Association; 2012.

Appendix 4-A Additional Daily Note Documentation for Workers' Compensation Patients or Clients

S:	○ Identify current status with job-related duties.
I:	○ Include job-specific interventions including any activities related to job demands. ○ Identify any barriers to recovery such as schedule and transportation conflicts or other contextual factors that could interfere with progress.
R:	○ Include response to and progress with job-related activities or an explanation for lack of progress.
P:	○ Identify progress made to date. ○ Identify rationale for continued plan of care. ○ Identify an action plan to address any contextual factors that are barriers to progress.

Data from the APTA's Defensible Documentation: Setting Specific Considerations in Documentation (2011).

CHAPTER 5

Documenting the Home Exercise Program

CHAPTER OBJECTIVES

1. Recognize that clinical reasoning assists in determining the content, delivery method, and documentation requirements for a home exercise program prescription.
2. Determine the components of a home exercise program and recognize where to document these components within the health record.
3. Recognize differing mechanisms of home exercise program delivery and how documentation of such programs might differ.
4. Establish a mechanism to efficiently update a home exercise program within the health record.

KEY TERMS

Home exercise program

Patient- or client-centered care

Introduction

The home exercise program is introduced in this chapter as an important adjunct to patient or client-centered care. The concept of the home exercise program as a unique product and service that is tailored to your individual patient or client's needs is relayed. A clinical reasoning process or framework is integral to creating a meaningful home exercise program for a patient or client and thus suggested criteria for the necessary characteristics of a home exercise program are presented. Lastly, the logistics of home exercise program delivery and documentation are offered.

Your patient or client is a consumer of the care you provide as a physical therapist or physical therapist assistant and may seek your services for a variety of reasons. Perhaps your patient or client was referred to you by another healthcare provider such as a physician or nurse practitioner after seeking an opinion from or having a routine visit with this professional. Perhaps your patient or client required pre- or postsurgical intervention. Perhaps your patient or client independently researched alternatives to surgical or pharmacologic management and decided to utilize your services as a means to achieve their health goals. Perhaps your patient or client is concerned about developing a certain health condition and is seeking your expertise on how to prevent it. Or perhaps your patient or client experienced a life-altering injury or event that makes receiving physical therapy services a non-negotiable necessity. Regardless of the reason your patient or client sits before you, they are a consumer of the services you provide.

Take moment to consider the last time you purchased a product or service. What factors influenced this purchase? Why did you ultimately choose to purchase this product or service? You likely generated a series of decisions that led to your purchase. For example, when purchasing a vehicle you might consider the quality of the vehicle or how that vehicle meets your needs and wants. You might consider how purchasing that vehicle may affect your car insurance rates or whether the vehicle is a new or used vehicle. You might consider the vehicle's seller such as a car dealership or an individual owner and whether there is a sale, special financing available for a loan, or a monetary gift that you are able to utilize in the purchase. You might consider your personal haggling skills in negotiating a deal. You might have a finite time frame in which to purchase this vehicle or you may have the time and resources to travel to a state that does not levy a sales tax on this type of purchase. Clearly, your expectations, preferences, resources, and personal circumstances play a role in your decision to purchase this product. Now consider purchasing a service for this vehicle such as an oil change and 75,000 mile inspection. You might have a mechanic whom you respect and trust to perform these services to your vehicle. You might rely on the recommendation of a friend or colleague, or you might turn to the media and advertising to locate a business with an effective marketing strategy who seemingly meets your needs. Again, your expectations, preferences, resources, and personal circumstances play a role in your decision to purchase this service.

In health care, the relationships between the consumer's expectations, preferences, resources, personal circumstances, and the product or service they seek are less clear. One key difference in shopping for a vehicle and shopping for a healthcare provider is that external criteria beyond the consumer's control influence the ultimate decision to choose that product or service. For example, the opportunity to implement a similar decision-making process as one that led to a vehicle purchase may not exist when investigating a healthcare provider. If your patient or client is insured, then a predetermined list of providers is available to them. Even though a patient or client may have the opportunity to seek care "out-of-network," the cost of this option may influence further decisions to pursue an alternative. In other words, you may have the expertise and reputation for providing exemplary care but because you are an out-of-network provider you are not considered. If your patient or client is uninsured, your patient or client may forego seeking your services due to a preconceived notion that such services are unaffordable for the uninsured. Furthermore, insurance or lack of insurance can be a source of stress or confusion surrounding the

understanding of one's coverage and personal responsibility in the form of co-pays or other out-of-pocket costs. Given the unpredictable nature of this environment, the details of which are often determined by administrative professionals before you even meet your patient or client, it is paramount that you as the provider recognize and are able to identify your patient or client's expectations and preferences and deliver a product or service that satisfies him or her as a consumer. Ultimately, it is your obligation to ensure that you meet the needs of your patients or clients once they set foot into your practice setting regardless of the factors that brought them there.

So what is the connection between knowing what the consumer wants and a home exercise program? Consider the **home exercise program** to be an example of a product *and* service that you provide as a physical therapist or a physical therapist assistant. Creating a home exercise program for your patient or client should be the ultimate example of delivering **patient- or client-centered care**, which indicates that you recognize your patient or client as an individual with unique needs affected by their health condition, impairments, activity limitations, participation restrictions, and contextual factors. "Patient- or client-centered" means providing care that is respectful of and responsive to individual patient or client preferences, needs, and values and ensuring that these values guide all clinical decisions.[1] Therefore, the home exercise program should not be added onto the end of an intervention session or plan of care as an afterthought, but instead integrated into the plan of care with a clear rationale for including its contents. It can be argued that a home exercise program is an integral part of the rehabilitation process for any patient or client, often representing the initiation of a lifestyle change for some and signifying the power to influence the chief complaint for others.[2] However, actually issuing the home exercise program to your patient or client is not the first step. Consider the following scenario.

Your patient or client is a 16-year-old junior in high school. He was referred to your outpatient physical therapy clinic by an orthopedic surgeon for shoulder pain. He is accompanied to the initial examination by his dad and reports that his shoulder pain started about 1 year ago when he was playing football. He states that he got low to make a tackle during a game and felt pain. He did not tell anyone about this pain because it seemed to have gotten better over time and he did not think that it was a big deal. However, he is now concerned because his shoulder hurts after his upper body conditioning workouts and when swimming. He states that football practice starts in 3 months and he wants to be ready to play. Your examination reveals what appear to be impairments, activity limitations, and participation restrictions associated with biceps tendinosis.

Do you think you should create a home exercise program for this patient or client? If so, when should it be established? At the initial encounter with the patient or client? At the first follow-up visit? On the last day of the episode of care? How would you determine if you should provide written instructions for the home exercise program or simply demonstrate what you expect your patient or client to do? How would you determine the contents of the home exercise program? How will you keep track of the contents of the home exercise program and whether or not your patient or client completes it as prescribed? How will you determine when to progress the home exercise program? How will you document all of this information? Before answering these questions, consider another scenario.

Your patient or client is a 32-year-old female who experienced a hemorrhage in the middle cerebral artery in the right temporal lobe in her brain. She was admitted to the inpatient rehabilitation hospital where you work over the weekend. The evaluating therapist indicates that this patient or client requires minimum assistance to roll in bed due to poor trunk control and poor strength. She also requires the maximum assistance of one person to perform a stand-pivot transfer due to poor trunk control, but also due to left-sided weakness and spatial orientation deficits. When you arrive to work on Monday, you see that this new patient or client was placed on your team.

Would you prescribe a home exercise program for this patient or client even though she is not at home? How would you ensure that other members of the multidisciplinary care team were aware of the home exercise program? Would you answer any of the questions posed after the above scenario differently? Why or why not? As you can see, many decisions are involved in creating, delivering, communicating, and documenting a home exercise program. Therefore, it is important to have an understanding of how your patient or client communicates and learns. It is equally important to understand the resources available to you for constructing the program as well as archiving the program not only for the purpose of it becoming a permanent part of your patient or client's health record, but also so that it can be referred to, retrieved, and refined as needed at some future time.

As you review the plan of care with your patient or client after conducting your initial examination, you likely mention the need to establish a HEP to ensure that gains made during the plan of care can be continued beyond the plan of care. Your patient or client then asks you, "What's the HEP?" What is your response? Of course, HEP is an abbreviation for "home exercise program," but how do you define the term *home exercise program*? As you reflect on your answer, consider the following criteria found in **TABLE 5-1** as the necessary characteristics of a home exercise program. In addition to maximizing your patient or client's adherence to the home exercise program you prescribe, it should be presented in simple, everyday language that is meaningful to your patient or client and tailored to suit their needs.[3] Consider the following two examples.

1. Perform sidelying hip abduction 3 × 12; 1 × daily.
2. Lie on your right side, right knee slightly bent. The left leg should be straight and in line with your body. Lift left leg about 1 inch and hold 5 seconds. If you can see your foot, direct your leg behind you slightly. Completely relax. Repeat 3 sets of 12; 1 time daily.

Which example above meets the criteria of "simple, everyday language"? While example "1" is concise it is not presented in layman's terms. Example "2," while more lengthy, relays how the activity should be performed and a specific compensation to be aware of when performing the activity.

TABLE 5-1 Characteristics of a Home Exercise Program

Characteristics of a Home Exercise Program
1. Effective
2. Efficient
3. Salient
4. Individualized
5. Brief
6. Explicit

Characteristics of a Home Exercise Program: Effective

A home exercise program should be *effective* in that it produces the results that your patient or client expects.[1] Therefore, it is appropriate to define your patient or client's expectations and establish goals for the home exercise program the same way you would establish goals for your plan of care.[3,4] Similarly, it is appropriate to determine how to measure progress towards these goals with the appropriate outcome measures. Revisit the football player in the above scenario. Assume that you have determined that this patient or client is experiencing secondary impingement at his biceps tendon due to instability at the glenohumeral joint likely caused by poor muscle performance of his scapular stabilizers and decreased glenohumeral joint capsule mobility. Since you are aware that he is symptomatic with his current conditioning workout it would be important to determine the contents of this workout. The details of the workout could be included in the evaluation section of the plan of care as below.

> John's health condition appears to be biceps tendinosis. His impairments include dysfunction in glenohumeral joint mobility as well as in muscle control, muscle performance, and muscle strength at the glenohumeral joint. His activity limitations include an inability to reach overhead and laterally with and without resistance, which restricts him from full participation in conditioning workouts required for his defensive lineman position on the football team. The contextual factors that affect this plan of care include the chronicity of the injury, current participation in conditioning workouts, and his eagerness to fully participate without limitation. Refer to the flow sheet for the current conditioning workout per patient or client's description and for a modified HEP designed to replace the conditioning workouts for 3 weeks. Will modify as necessary to control symptoms and promote tendon healing.

The contents of the current conditioning workout could be listed in a flow sheet format along with the contents of the home exercise prescription within the health record as shown in TABLE 5-2. It could also be an external document provided by the patient or client that you scanned into the health record. Alternatively, it could be a document that you created based on a verbal description or demonstration provided by the patient or client that you would also scan into the health record. Tracking your patient or client's current level of exercise or activity and the home exercise program as you have prescribed it in

TABLE 5-2 Intervention Flow Sheet

Date of Service	Date		
Visit Count	1 of 24		
Diagnosis	R shoulder biceps tendinosis		
Current Upper Body Conditioning Workout	Weight	Repetitions	Frequency
Push ups	20# weighted vest	50×	4 days per week
Pull ups	20# weighted vest	2 × 20	4 days per week
Dips	20# weighted vest	2 × 20	4 days per week
Bench press	120#	3 × 10	4 days per week
Bicep curls	20# db	3 × 10	4 days per week
Triceps extensions	80# pulley	3 × 10	4 days per week
Lat pull downs	70#	3 × 10	4 days per week
Pec flys	60#	3 × 10	4 days per week
Reverse flys	90#	3 × 10	4 days per week
Kayaking	--	1 hour	1 day per week
Swimming	--	1.0 mile	1 day per week
Running (sprints)	10# weighted vest	6 × 100 meters	3 days per week

(continued)

TABLE 5-2   Intervention Flow Sheet (*Continued*)

Home Exercise Program			
Eccentric load to biceps	Weight of arm	2 × 30	2 × daily
Prone scapular stabilization (120 deg elev)	2# db	3 × 8	Every other day
Prone scapular stabilization (90 deg abd)	3# db	3 × 8	Every other day
Shoulder ER (90°/90°)	Elastic band	2 × 30	2 × daily
Manual Therapy			
Joint mobilizations – inferior and posterior GHJ capsule	10 min		
Therapeutic Exercise – Tissue Healing/Symptom Reduction			
Eccentric load to biceps	3# db	1 × 15	
Therapeutic Exercise – Motor Control/Coordination			
Rhythmic stabilization – B UE on compliant surface	1 min × 8		
Therapeutic Exercise – Strength			
Lower trapezius (prone)	3# db	3 × 12	

HEP = home exercise program
GHJ = glenohumeral joint

TABLE 5-3   Example of Home Exercise Program Documentation

Exercise Description	Intensity	Frequency	Duration	Date Issued	Date Concluded
Active assisted shoulder elevation range of motion – face wall, with hand contacting wall, slide hand up wall in pain-free range, hold, return to start.	Weight of arm	2 × 30; 5 sec hold	3 × daily	4/20	4/27
Eccentric load to biceps – stand, hold dowel in both hands, curl, remove L hand and lower with R in controlled manner.	Weight of arm and dowel	2 × 30	2 × daily	4/25	--
Prone scapular stabilization (120 deg elevation) – lie on stomach on floor, face down, towel roll under forehead, rest arms by ears with elbows straight, retract shoulder blades, lift arms off floor; hold.	2# db	3 × 8; 5 sec hold	Every other day	4/25	--
Prone scapular stabilization (90 deg abduction) – same position as above, arms to side with elbows straight.	3# db	3 × 8; 5 sec hold	Every other day	4/25	5/10
Shoulder external rotation (90°/90°) – anchor band in door at eye level, stand, elbow in line with shoulder, forearm parallel to floor, rotate hand so fist is perpendicular to ceiling.	Elastic band	2 × 30; 2 sec hold	2 × daily	5/10	--

specific documents separate from the daily note, serves to remind you of the content and its progression. You could also indicate directly in the document you give to your patient or client if you reviewed, performed, progressed, added, or eliminated any of the home exercise program contents since it was initiated (**TABLE 5-3**).

Regardless of the format you utilize to house the home exercise program, consider it a mechanism to clearly communicate the details of the contents of the home exercise program as well as a means to relay your expectations in terms of home exercise program performance.

In the goals section of your plan of care, it would be relevant to incorporate goals about the home exercise program as below.

Short-term goal: In 3 weeks the patient or client will demonstrate the ability to perform HEP as issued at the initial visit without report of pain or limitation during or after exercise program.

Short-term goal: Incorporate strength dosing into HEP after patient or client is able to reach asymptomatically overhead at least 30× with 5# of resistance.

Long-term goal: Demonstrate the ability to perform advanced HEP including full participation in conditioning workouts without pain or limitation during or after workout.

The documentation above indicates where in the health record the actual home exercise program is located, how it compares with prior activity, when it was issued, how long the patient or client is to perform it before it is reassessed, and impairment-based (pain or limitation) or performance-based (overhead reach) tests and measures indicating if established goals have been met. When the patient or client's ability to perform the home exercise program is reassessed the goals should be updated to reflect progress. Anytime the home exercise program document is changed it should be saved to the health record or printed and scanned to the health record.

Characteristics of a Home Exercise Program: Efficient

Another necessary characteristic of a home exercise program is *efficiency* (Table 5-1). A home exercise program should be efficient in that it is well-organized and proficient. Consider that the home exercise program is the reiteration to your patient or client that you are dedicated to identifying what can be done to address his or her needs. Therefore, it is important to take the time to identify your patient or client's learning or communication style and create an appropriate program accordingly. For example, determine if your patient or client is a visual learner and requires demonstration or an opportunity to perform the exercise prior to the end of the session. Determine if your patient or client would prefer an illustration with written instructions in addition to actual practice, or if the written instruction would suffice. If you provide verbal instruction and demonstration, identify how you will record this intervention in your documentation. Consider the following scenario.

You determine after improving your patient or client's knee flexion range of motion with manual techniques that it is appropriate to prescribe an exercise for her to continue at home to maintain the range you have achieved to date. As she is putting on her shoes and gathering her things to leave, you verbally indicate that she is to perform deep squats to at least a 90-degree angle while holding onto her countertop or sink in the kitchen. You indicate verbally as you demonstrate that she is to hold each squat for 10 seconds, 10 times, 3 times per day until she returns 3 days later for her next session.

Since you did not provide a tangible picture or description to which you can refer, you must take the time to document in the session's daily note the exercise prescription which includes the description of the exercise, the frequency, intensity, and duration of the exercise, and some way of distinguishing that this activity is to be performed at home. Documentation of your verbal instruction in the scenario above might look like the following.

HEP: Patient to perform deep squats to at least a 90-degree angle at countertop or kitchen sink 10×, 10 sec hold, 3×day to improve active knee flexion range of motion. Patient indicated understanding of the demonstration and verbal instruction provided.

Even if your patient or client shows the ability to learn via verbal instruction, this method of giving verbal instruction lacks efficiency. Documenting in this way necessitates reviewing previous documentation to determine the contents of the home exercise program and when that particular part of the home exercise program was issued. Consider now that your patient or client has returned for a subsequent visit and complains of increased knee pain since the last session. It is possible that your patient or client misinterpreted your verbal instruction and performed the exercise in a way you did not intend. However, if you utilized a web-based software program featuring step-by-step instructions and pictures or a document you created yourself to manage your patient or client's home exercise program, you have a template that is separate from the daily note from which to work at a future time. The daily note for that same session would then have to refer to the attached home exercise program. You could quickly refer to this attached document and rectify any misinterpretation that may have occurred in the patient or client's execution of the exercise rather than relying on your written account of your verbal instruction and your assumption that your patient or client interpreted this verbal instruction and demonstration in the way you expected. This type of document could also be efficiently updated, printed, and handed to the patient or client in isolation of any other information from the health record. At a subsequent visit this document could be updated again, reprinted for the patient or client, and uploaded to the health record to document progression. The time you invest early in the plan of care to gather information regarding your patient or client's learning and communication style will help you to create an efficient program. In other words, you will not have wasted valuable time prescribing verbal or written instructions when your patient or client would have benefitted from demonstration or a picture.

Characteristics of a Home Exercise Program: Salient

In addition to effectiveness and efficiency, a home exercise program should be *salient* (Table 5-1). In other words, the home exercise program should hold significance or relevance to the patient or client. Research suggests that it is appropriate to identify the barriers, rather than what motivates an individual, to implement the home exercise program you prescribe.[2] One way to detect these barriers is by identifying relationships between the components of the World Health Organization (WHO) *International Classification of Functioning, Disability, and Health* (ICF) model. Recognizing the links between the health condition, impairments in body functions and structures, activity limitations, participation restrictions, and contextual factors will contribute to the overall success of your plan of care. Furthermore, identifying these relationships ultimately serves to facilitate thought processes and communications intended to reveal your patient or client's values, preferences, and activities or exercises he or she considers salient.

Consider your patient or client who suffered a hemorrhage and is in an inpatient rehabilitation facility in the scenario above. Assume that you have determined that the patient or client is demonstrating difficulty orienting herself to midline. This challenge is affecting her transfers and her ability to statically stand. She expresses frustration that she will not be able to stand and walk to get to the bathroom by herself if she is unable to balance. Her husband is present at one of your sessions and you establish that he is able to be an active participant in his wife's rehabilitation. **FIGURE 5-1** organizes her health

information using the ICF model framework so that relationships among components of the ICF model might be more readily identified.

Organizing this patient or client's health status and current level of functioning according to the ICF model framework may help you to decide how to utilize a home exercise program. For example, you could initiate a conversation with the patient or client based on the contextual factors that you identified as facilitators and barriers. You could discuss what specific activities she feels unable to complete or perform because of her current inability to walk. You could provide further education to her and her husband regarding the contribution of each of these impairments to the activity limitation of being unable to ambulate to the bathroom. This may lead you to educate your patient or client and her husband within a treatment session on an activity to help orient her to midline. You could then subsequently create a document electronically, such as that depicted in **TABLE 5-4**, print it, and hand it to the patient or client and her husband so that they have a tangible reference of what you have asked them to practice while not in a therapy session. This document could then be copied or printed and scanned to the permanent health record. Should a question arise about any detail of this activity from the patient or client, her husband, or other members of her healthcare team, there is a detailed account of the exercise prescribed.

Characteristics of a Home Exercise Program: Individualized

As mentioned above, you have several choices when creating a home exercise program for your patient or client. You can utilize a software program that provides diagrams and descriptions of selected exercises. You can create a typed or handwritten document or you can draw pictures of the activities or exercises you would like to prescribe. You can also verbally describe the activity or exercise to your patient or client and record the details of your education in the daily treatment note. Regardless of the method you chose to express the home exercise program and relay it to your patient or client, it is important that you ensure that you build it specifically for your patient or client so that it is *individualized*, another necessary characteristic of a home exercise program (Table 5-1). In other words,

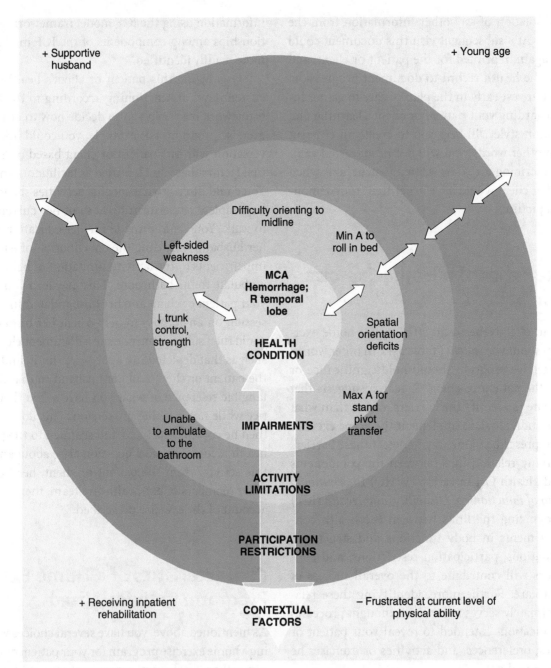

FIGURE 5-1 Circular Representation of the ICF Model – Patient with MCA Hemorrhage.

Data from Towards a Common Language for Functioning, Disability and Health (ICF). World Health Organization, 2002.

if you choose to use a predetermined set of exercises or a software-based or kit-based protocol ensure that you have determined that each exercise included is truly relevant for your patient or client. It is important to note that using the ICF model framework to organize the details of your patient or client's health status is in opposition to prescribing a predetermined set of exercises or using a protocol created for those with specific health conditions. Rather, the ICF model facilitates a high-level patient or client-centered reasoning process to identify salient and individualized activities to include in the home exercise program for your patient or client.

Characteristics of a Home Exercise Program: Brief

In addition to being effective, efficient, salient, and individualized, a home exercise program should also be *brief*. The literature supports prescribing a small amount of

TABLE 5-4 HEP Handout

HEP for: Patient or client's name	Issued on: date
_____ Rehabilitation Hospital	Therapist: _____

1. Sit at the edge of your bed in what you consider upright and erect posture with both feet firmly on the floor.

2. Your husband will sit directly in front of you in an armchair or large surface such as a couch.

3. Mirror the activities your husband performs with his leg, arm, and trunk. (These activities are to be done at the same time so that you can mirror your husband's movements.)
   a. Leg – Place the toes of your foot in front of the toes of your husband's foot on the floor. Try to mimic his movements as he moves his foot and leg to the side and back to midline. Repeat this movement 10 times on each side. Then repeat this movement without your husband to see if you can return to midline accurately.
   b. Arm – Place the palm of your hand on the palm of your husband's hand. Try to mimic his movements as he moves his hand and arm to his right and then back to midline; to his left and back to midline; up and back to midline; down and back to midline. Repeat this sequence 10 times in all directions. Then repeat this sequence without your husband to see if you can return to midline accurately.
   c. Trunk – Lean to the right onto the right elbow, pause 10 seconds, return to center. Then lean to the left onto the left elbow, pause 10 seconds, return to the center. Repeat to each side 10 times. Then attempt to perform the activity without your husband to see if you can accurately return to midline.

4. Repeat at least two times per day when you are not in a therapy session.

exercise and gradually increasing the amount if the individual shows adherence to this small amount.[5,6] You would then employ clinical reasoning to determine how many exercises constitute a "small amount of exercise." A brief home exercise program may be more successful in terms of adherence than a comprehensive program simply because a brief program is more convenient to accommodate. Therefore, it is important to identify what you and your patient or client consider the most important concerns based on the findings of the examination and build goals based on this information to create the home exercise program. It is also relevant to ask your patient or client how much time he or she is able to dedicate to performing a home exercise program. Consider the following scenario.

You are a home health physical therapist. You arrive at your patient or client's home to perform an initial examination. You are aware that she is 91 years old and was discharged from an inpatient rehabilitation facility after a 3-week length of stay. Four weeks ago she fell in her home and fractured her pelvis. She was admitted to acute care and stayed 1 week prior to transferring to inpatient rehabilitation. You plan on assessing her gait and balance with a 10-Meter Walk Test and a Berg Balance Test but as you progress through your examination you find that she is largely limited by pain at her right hip. You determine that she has significant muscle guarding at her hip musculature in addition to gluteus medius weakness bilaterally. You also determine that pain limits her bed mobility, transfers, and gait.

You may be tempted to simultaneously include items in her home exercise program that address her strength and balance deficits as well as exercises designed to decrease muscle guarding at her hip musculature, improve her transfers, her bed mobility skills, and her gait pattern. However, consider that the more complex or inconvenient a program, the less likely the patient or client will be able to adhere to it.[3,7] Rather than prescribe exercises to meet all of the goals you identify with your patient or client at once, it may be appropriate to prioritize these goals, adding new content to the home exercise program as each goal is managed. Therefore, it would be beneficial to create a document to guide you and serve as a reminder to you regarding the direction and the progression of the home exercise program. Such a document, as depicted in **TABLE 5-5**, can easily be retrieved and updated in the record.

Characteristics of a Home Exercise Program: Explicit

In addition to being effective, efficient, salient, individualized, and brief, a home exercise program should also be _explicit_. In other words, the home exercise program you prescribe should be unambiguous and overt in terms of detail so that there is little room for misinterpretation. It has been shown in the literature that providing clear instructions for home practice is positively correlated with patient or client satisfaction.[8] Thus, ensuring clear detail

TABLE 5-5 HEP Documentation

Goal	Exercise Description	Date Added
Decrease muscle guarding R hip adductors.		
Decrease muscle guarding at R hip internal rotators.		
Strengthen gluteus medius musculature.		
Improve bed mobility skills – rolling.		
Improve bed mobility skills – supine to sit.		
Improve transfers – sit to stand from low surface.		
Improve gait – stance time on R.		

will help to maximize the potential for optimal outcomes. Consider the following scenario.

> Your patient is 3 weeks status-post kyphoplasty procedure performed to support a spontaneous osteoporotic vertebral compression fracture at T5. He was admitted to the skilled nursing facility where you work after a hospital stay that was complicated with an infection at the surgical incision and a deep vein thrombosis in his left lower leg. You learn after meeting him that he is very deconditioned as a result of this hospital stay. At the conclusion of your examination, you ask him to sit at the edge of his bed two times per day and perform hip flexion (marches). You ask him to repeat 30 marches on each leg at least one time in the day. The next day when you see him you ask him about his marching exercise and he reports that he did not do it. You perform the activity with him again and ask him to repeat it one more time at the end of his afternoon before his evening meal. You see him later in the hall and ask him about the exercise. He reports again that he has not done it.

Prior to labeling your patient or client as noncompliant or nonadherent to your prescribed home exercise program, take the time to consider the barriers to your patient or client completing this task. Were your instructions explicit or did they lack clarity? Did you make an effort to ensure that your patient or client was able to learn the program? Are there physical impairments such as visual or hearing deficits that interfered with his performance? Does a cognitive impairment exist that you did not entirely examine? Do any cultural or personal beliefs exist as reasons your patient or client has not completed the activity you prescribed? Have you been ineffective in relaying the goals or the value of the home exercise program? Did you take the time to physically perform the home exercise program with your patient or client to enhance his ability to learn it and to allow for an opportunity for questions? Have you fully investigated your patient or client's ability to independently implement the program you have prescribed? Did you offer subsequent opportunities to learn the material? After all, learning is a required part of compliance.[6] Once you have explored potential barriers to home exercise program performance, revisit the contents of your original prescription and consider any alternatives.

Summary

It is a major responsibility of physical therapists and physical therapist assistants to prescribe, promote, and educate patients or clients on the importance and value of exercise as it relates to optimal function, wellness, and quality of life.[9] The home exercise program is one intervention within your plan of care and should be implemented, progressed, and documented as you would other interventions included in your plan of care. Similarly, it is your responsibility to continuously follow up with your patient or client regarding the home exercise program you prescribed. It will not be beneficial to issue a home exercise program if there is no mechanism in place to revisit and update the program. It will not be beneficial to establish goals for the home exercise program if the goals are not documented and progressed. Managing a home exercise program, including its documentation, involves several clinical decisions like any other decision you make during the course of implementing a plan of care to ensure that it includes the necessary characteristics of a home exercise program (Table 5-1).

Revisit the activity you prescribed your patient or client who suffered a middle cerebral artery hemorrhage in her temporal lobe to help orient herself to midline. Many objectives were met by creating and storing this home exercise program in the health record. First, you constructed a program around an actual activity limitation that you ascertained in your examination and took the time to practice during an intervention session increasing the possibility that the program is *effective* for improving this limitation. You provided a tangible, written or typed description of your expectations to the patient or client and her husband *after* performing the activity during treatment indicating that the program is *efficient*. You included the patient or client and her husband in the intervention plan by giving them a *salient* activity to practice. You customized the home exercise program making it *individualized* for your patient or client. You kept the program *brief* by including one primary activity within the home exercise program geared toward one specific goal identified during your examination. You created an *explicit* document you can easily refer to and update should you decide to progress or change this activity as well as a concrete account of the details and the dosing of the activity should questions arise from your patient or client or from other members of the care team. Because you have included these necessary elements of a home exercise program along with documentation to

---

> **BOX 5-1 The Electronic Health Record: The Home Exercise Program**
>
> Limitations may exist in an electronic health record regarding the user's ability to move backwards in time to a document that was previously created to update it. This is because the health record is a legal document and should not be edited without a specific reason using a specific process. Therefore, it may be necessary depending on the electronic system you are using to keep a separate record, perhaps on the hard drive of the computer on which you access the documentation system, to create materials for your patient or client's home exercise program. Like the flow sheet, it may be necessary to import the home exercise program into a document that will allow you to edit and save it or print and scan it to be uploaded to the health record after changes have been made.

support it, you likely relayed to your patient or client that you have considered her expectations and preferences in constructing and delivering a product and service that satisfies her as a consumer.

Discussion Questions

1. Consider a product that is important to you such as a computer, a pair of shoes, or a meal. What criteria do you look for in the product that would result in you purchasing that product? Now consider a service that is important to you such as getting a haircut, taking your clothes to the dry cleaner, eating out at a restaurant. What criteria do you look for in the service that would result in you purchasing that service? Now apply the criteria you developed to the creation, delivery, and documentation of a home exercise program. Are there any parallel criteria?

2. In your own words, create a definition of the term *home exercise program*.

3. When is the optimal time to prescribe a home exercise program for your patient or client? Why?

4. How will you determine your patient or client's learning and communication style?

5. How would you handle a situation in which your patient or client does not want to perform a home exercise program? What strategies would you use to persuade your patient or client to reconsider?

6. Your patient or client returns to your clinic for her first follow-up session since you performed her initial examination 1 week ago. At that time you asked her to perform the home exercise program as you had prescribed it once per day for 1 week. Upon her return you ask her if she has done the home exercise program over the course of the week. She replies that she did it twice over the course of the week. What is your response?

7. Use simple, everyday language to create a home exercise program for the patient or client in the scenario below.

   The patient or client is an 8-year-old girl who sustained a traumatic brain injury after falling off a swing at the playground. She has been in an inpatient rehabilitation setting for 9 days. Her Glasgow Coma Scale score at admission was 11. Currently, she has difficulty with gait and balance and is experiencing several episodes of loss of balance per day. These episodes are much more frequent in the afternoon and at night. She is usually able regain her balance when she is walking with her walker, but sometimes she catches her right foot on the ground and falls.

8. Use simple, everyday language to create a home exercise program for the patient or client in the scenario below.

   Your 82-year-old patient or client was admitted to the skilled nursing facility where you work after a 5-day acute hospital stay for a urinary tract infection. Her Berg Balance Score = 41/56 with most difficulty occurring with standing activities and her 6-Minute Walk Test = 359 feet with a rolling walker.

9. Obtain a home exercise program that you have created for one of your patients or clients. Critically analyze it for the necessary characteristics of a home exercise program as presented in Table 5-1. Does your program meet all of these requirements? Is there anything you would alter about this home exercise program based on your analysis? If so explain your changes.

10. Exchange home exercise programs with one of your peers. Repeat the activity described in #9 above.

Case Study Questions

1. Your patient or client is a 71-year-old man who comes to the outpatient clinic where you work with complaints of low back pain. He states that he has had episodes of low back pain over the course of the last 20 years, but this time he states that he knows the exact reason it flared up. He states that he and his wife have just moved into an assisted living community and that he has been moving furniture and packing boxes for the last 5–6 weeks. He states that one day nearly 2 weeks ago he could not stand after sitting in a chair for 30 minutes. He went to the emergency room and was released that day with pain medication and a referral to follow up with physical therapy. Currently, he has difficulty standing and walking after sitting for more than 10 minutes at a time. He is also unable to find a comfortable sleeping position. As you progress with your evaluation you note that you would like to see him in the clinic three times per week over the next 4 weeks in addition to building a home exercise program. He responds by telling you that in addition to the demands of moving he is the primary caregiver for his wife who has severe limitations due to Parkinson's disease. The results of your initial examination are as follows.
   - Anthropometric characteristics: BP rest = 131/78 mmHg; HR rest = 72 bpm; RR = 17 breaths/min
   - Assistive and adaptive devices: straight cane for household and community distance held in left hand to decrease pain on right
   - Environmental, home, and work barriers: volunteers at a local hospital as a courier for patient/client transport, cares for his wife who has Parkinson's disease (unable to assist wife with bed mobility tasks due to pain when bending)
   - Ergonomics and body mechanics: unable to bend to the floor from sitting or standing without pain to don shoes or retrieve items from floor
   - Gait, locomotion, and balance: 10MWT with straight cane = 1.16 m/s; utilizes wide base of support, decreased stance time on the right, decreased hip extension range of motion on the right at terminal stance, forward trunk flexion and left lateral lean
   - Joint integrity and mobility: hypomobility L2-S1; R sacroiliac joint
   - Muscle performance: poor ability to sustain contraction at right multifidus in prone via leg raise on left > 3 seconds; hip musculature 4/5 to 5/5 bilaterally however pain at central low back with resisted hip extension bilaterally
   - Pain: across low back; > on right; constant but worse with forward bend (putting on shoes and pants) and rotation (turning when driving); relieved by sitting on right buttock with legs crossed; lying on right side; no LE symptoms reported
   - Palpation: tender at L5-S1 spinous processes, right PSIS, erector spinae at thoracolumbar junction on right, at multifidus on right
   - Posture: decreased lumbar lordosis noted in standing
   - Range of motion: lumbar – decreased flexion 75% (little motion occurs at L3-4-5 spine segments)(pain on right); decreased extension 25% (pain on right); left rotation decreased 50% (moderate pain on right); + Quadrant Test; + sacroiliac joint Provocation Tests
   - Reflex integrity: L4 (patellar) and S1 (Achilles) – hyporeflexia = bilaterally; Babinski sign and clonus = negative bilaterally
   - Sensory integrity: intact and + to light touch and sharp/dull to lower extremities
   - Other: Oswestry Disability Index (ODI) = 60%

   a. Categorize this patient or client's health status using the ICF model framework.
   b. Create short-term and long-term goals based on the information above regarding the implementation of a home exercise program.
   c. Determine how you will measure and track progress of the home exercise program.
   d. Create a 30-minute treatment session using a flow sheet format. Be sure to distinguish between what

information is intended for the home exercise program.

e. Create a document that you will issue to the patient or client for him to take home to implement the home exercise program.

2. Your patient or client is an 86-year-old male who comes to your outpatient physical therapy clinic with complaints of poor balance despite his use of a straight cane when he walks and a history of three falls in the last 4 months. He reports that he lives with his wife of 60 years whom he cares for since she fell and fractured her hip last year. Upon completing his examination, you discover that he lacks protective sensation on the plantar surfaces of both feet and that he has inaccurate kinesthetic and proprioceptive awareness at his knees and ankles bilaterally. In addition, he has marked quadriceps, gluteus medius and gluteus maximus weakness.

a. Categorize this patient or client health status using the ICF model framework.

b. Create short-term and long-term goals based on the information above regarding the implementation of a home exercise program.

c. Determine how you will measure and track progress of the home exercise program.

d. Create a 30-minute treatment session using a flow sheet format. Be sure to distinguish between what information is intended for the home exercise program.

e. Create a document that you will issue to the patient or client for him to take home to implement the home exercise program.

3. Your patient or client is a 93-year-old man who was admitted to the skilled nursing facility where you work yesterday afternoon after a 7-day acute hospital stay with pneumonia. His past medical history is significant for coronary artery disease, hypertension, prostate cancer, hyperlipidemia, and osteoarthritis of bilateral knees and hips, hands, and spine. When you enter his room for the examination you find him awake in a semirecumbent position in his bed. The results of your initial examination with him are as follows.

○ Aerobic capacity and endurance: 2-Minute Walk Test = 32 feet (RPE = 16) with a four-wheeled rollator

○ Anthropometric characteristics: BP rest = 153/82 mmHg; HR rest = 78 bpm; RR rest = 25 breaths/minute; O_2 Sat% rest = 97%; BP activity = 181/94 mmHg; HR activity = 84 bpm; RR activity = 29 breaths/min

○ Assistive devices: four-wheeled rollator with seat, shower wheelchair

○ Peripheral nerve integrity and sensory integrity: intact and equal bilaterally to light touch and sharp/dull discrimination at bilateral upper extremities and lower extremities ; decreased kinesthesia at bilaterally knees and ankles; intact kinesthesia at bilateral hips

○ Gait, locomotion, and balance: unable to assess gait and standing balance after 2-Minute Walk Test due to poor endurance; sitting balance: static = independent; dynamic = required moderate assistance at edge of bed to avoid falling backward

○ Integumentary integrity: healing sacral wound at coccyx (size of a nickel); dressing in place at time of examination

○ Muscle performance: unable to perform test of functional lower extremity strength (Five Times Sit to Stand or Heel Rise Test); Manual Muscle Testing bilateral dorsiflexion = 4/5; quadriceps = 4/5 bilaterally; hamstrings 3/5 bilaterally; sitting tolerance = 1:07 sec then required supine rest due to fatigue

○ Pain: no pain reported

○ Posture: sits with forward head and rounded shoulders; stands with flexed knees (~10 degrees) and hips (~ 20 degrees) bilaterally; flexed trunk (~ 30 degrees)

a. Categorize this patient or client's health status using the ICF model framework.

b. Create short-term and long-term goals based on the information above regarding the implementation of a home exercise program.

c. Determine how you will measure and track progress of the home exercise program.

d. Create a 30-minute treatment session using a flow sheet format. Be sure to distinguish between what information is intended for the home exercise program.

e. Create a document that you will issue to the patient or client for him to take home to implement the home exercise program.

References

1. Jewell DV, Moore JD, and Goldstein MS. Delivering the physical therapy value proposition: a call to action. *Phys Ther*. 2013;93:104–114.

2. Forkan R, Pumper B, Smyth N, et al. Exercise adherence following physical therapy intervention in older adults with impaired balance. *Phys Ther*. 2006;86:401–410.

3. Bassett SF and Prapavessis H. Home-based physical therapy intervention with adherence enhancing strategies versus clinic-based management for patients with ankle sprains. *Phys Ther*. 2007;87:1132–1143.

4. Spink MJ, Fotoohabadi MR, Wee E, et al. Predictors of adherence to a multifaceted podiatry intervention for

the prevention of falls in older people. *BMC Geriatrics.* 2011;11:51–59

5. Hass R, Maloney S, Pausenberger E, et al. Clinical decision making in exercise prescription for fall prevention. *Phys Ther.* 2012;92:666–679.

6. Henry KD, Rosemond C, and Eckert LB. Effect of number of home exercises on compliance and performance in adults over 65 years of age. *Phys Ther.* 1999; 79:270–277.

7. American Geriatrics Society Expert Panel on the Care of Older Adults with Multimorbidity. Patient-centered care for older adults with multiple chronic conditions: a step-wise approach from the American Geriatrics Society. *JAGS.* 2012;1–12.

8. Hall A, Ferreira PH, Maher CG, et al. The influence of the therapist-patient relationship on treatment outcome in physical rehabilitation: a systematic review. *Phys Ther.* 2010;90:1099–1110.

9. American Physical Therapy Association. *Guide to Physical Therapist Practice.* Alexandria, VA: American Physical Therapy Association; 2001.

CHAPTER 6

Documenting Progress

1. Recognize the multiple terms used to describe a patient or client's progression through a plan of care including *progress notes/reports/summaries, re-examination notes/reports, re-assessment notes/reports,* and *status notes/reports.*

2. Implement a decision-making framework for determining when to document a patient or client's progress.

3. Implement a decision-making framework for developing the content of the re-examination note.

4. Demonstrate the ability to utilize a clinical reasoning process for creating the content of the re-examination note.

KEY TERMS

Clinical impression
Diagnosis
Evaluation
Goal achievement status

Outcome measures
Progress note, report, or summary
Re-examination
Tests and measures

Introduction

It is responsible clinical practice for you as a physical therapist to have knowledge of your patient or client's response to and progress with physical therapy interventions at any point during the plan of care. Thus, a decision-making process for 1) *when* during the plan of care to document progress and 2) the *format* in which to document progress is presented. The differences between a progress note and a re-examination note are relayed and a clinical decision-making algorithm for writing progress or re-examination notes is suggested. The components of a re-examination note are reinforced as well as the content of each of these components. Ways in which you can use other well-written components of your documentation to make clinical decisions regarding your patient or client's progress such as the evaluation or clinical impression of the initial examination, prior daily notes, or intervention flow sheets is relayed. The importance of your impression of your patient or client's goal achievement status and the content of the re-evaluation content within

the re-examination documentation is emphasized. Lastly, a guide to help you critically self-evaluate the content of the plan of care you have created on behalf of your patient or client is presented.

Defining Progress

How do you know if your patient or client is making progress with the plan of care you carefully created and documented at the initial examination? Reflect for a moment on the factors you consider when determining if your patient or client is making progress. Do you use your observational skills? Do you use tests and measures or outcome tools? Do you use the reported status your patient or client or caregiver shares? As a physical therapist, over time you hone your ability to synthesize all of this information to judge your patient or client's progress. But, which factors do you deem to be the most important in determining *when* you create a note that reflects your patient or client's progress through the plan of care? Consider the following scenario.

> You are an outpatient physical therapist working with a 32-year-old man who experienced a whiplash injury after a motor vehicle accident 10 days ago. He had his initial examination and 1 follow-up visit last week. He has now returned for his second follow-up visit.

Are you going to evaluate your patient or client's progress within his plan of care at this session? Will you create a re-examination note to document this progress? What will be the format of this note? Now consider this scenario.

> You are an outpatient physical therapist working with a 32-year-old man who experienced a whiplash injury after a motor vehicle accident 4 weeks ago. He has seen you for seven sessions and has now returned today for his eighth visit.

Are you going to evaluate your patient or client's progress within his plan of care at this session? Will you create a re-examination note to document this progress? What will be the format of this note? Did you use a different decision-making process for answering the questions in this scenario compared to the first scenario posed above?

A physical therapist or physical therapist assistant responsible for the delivery and implementation of a patient or client's plan of care should have knowledge of the patient or client's response to and progress with the physical therapy program at *each* visit regardless of the timeframe since the initial examination. Furthermore, when working with a patient or client, it is astute clinical practice to assess the need for an intervention prior to applying the intervention, to implement that intervention, and to then immediately reassess if that intervention had the desired effect during the session. While the effects of some interventions will not be known within the session, such as that of strength training, you can still assess your patient or client's response to the selected intervention and deem its appropriateness for inclusion in the plan of care at future sessions. The American Physical Therapy Association (APTA) affirms that documenting skilled care within each physical therapy session includes documenting observations before, during, and after an intervention as well as documenting the patient or client's response to the intervention.[1] Documenting the patient or client's

response to the interventions applied during the session will enhance your ability to determine your patient or client's progress. As indicated above, this ongoing reassessment process should occur at every session. However, there are two critical decisions surrounding your determination of the breadth and depth of the documentation of your patient or client's progress:

1. Determining *when* during the plan of care to document progress
2. Determining the *format* in which to document progress

Determining *when* to include details regarding your patient or client's progress and choosing the *format* in which to describe your patient or client's progress within the health record may in part depend on the definition of "progress." Multiple terms have been used to label a patient or client's progress within a health record including *progress note*, *progress report*, *progress summary*, *status report*, *reassessment note*, and *re-examination*. Some of these terms may have originated from electronic documentation systems or from terminology used by reimbursement entities. However, the APTA advocates for the use of two primary terms: progress note, report, or summary, and re-examination.

According to the APTA, a **progress note, report, or summary** is similar to a daily note but includes more detailed information regarding the patient or client's current status as compared to a previous time frame such as at the initial examination or the last re-examination.[1] Revisit the scenario above. When your patient or client returns for his second follow-up visit since the initial examination, you may decide to write increased detail in the "Intervention" (I) and "Response" (R) sections of your daily note to relay progress as indicated below.

> S: Patient reports that the intensity of his right-sided neck pain significantly decreased after last session for the rest of the afternoon. He notes that after about 6 hours, his pain returned, which limited his ability to find a comfortable position to sleep.
>
> I: See flow sheet. Cervical spine active right rotation range of motion = 60 degrees with pain at end range ipsilaterally (improved from 45 degrees with pain throughout entire available range at initial examination); extension = 45 degrees with pain at posterior head and on the right side of neck (improved from

20 degrees with pain into right upper extremity at initial examination); Deep Neck Flexor Endurance Test = 6 seconds (deferred at initial examination due to pain with concentric contraction of deep cervical flexors).

R: Patient demonstrates ability to perform overhead reaching tasks without pain due to improved active range of motion at cervical spine; also demonstrates improved recruitment of deep cervical flexors based on ability to tolerate Deep Neck Flexor Endurance Test. Able to lie in preferred sleeping position at end of session without neck or upper extremity pain.

P: Continue to improve cervical active right rotation and extension range of motion. Add motor control exercises for cervical flexors against gravity next session to improve postural stability during sitting activities at computer.

This note could be labeled as a progress note since detailed information is provided in the "Intervention" (I) section of the note that compares the patient or client's performance at this session to his performance at the initial examination. Even though this augmented documentation is occurring early in the plan of care, it is still considered a progress note because of the nature of the content. An equally acceptable daily note is below.

S: Patient reports that the intensity of his right-sided neck pain significantly decreased after last session for the rest of the afternoon. He notes that after about 6 hours, his pain returned, which limited his ability to find a comfortable position to sleep. Current right-sided neck pain = 4/10.

I: See flow sheet. Added active cervical supine rotation range of motion to the home exercise program to improve pain-free active cervical rotation; 2 × 30 repetitions to the right and left, 2 × per day.

R: Patient demonstrated the ability to perform added home exercise program without increase in pain. Able to achieve active cervical rotation in sitting to 65 degrees before onset of pain on right side of neck. No pain into right arm at any time during session. Able to achieve preferred sleeping position without pain at end of session.

P: Continue to improve cervical range of motion in pain-free range to allow for improved ability to look over shoulder when driving.

This daily note is comprehensive and relays relevant information regarding your patient or client's status, what interventions were completed, how he responded to the intervention, and what the plan is for the next visit. However, this daily note would not be labeled as a progress note because there is no overt comparison of the patient or client's current status to his status at a previous point in time during the plan of care. A further difference between the progress note and the daily note above is the detail provided in the "intervention" section of the note. In addition to activities indicated in the flow sheet, the "intervention" details the results of specific testing that was initially conducted at the initial examination and repeated in depth at a follow-up session. This is not to say that tests and measures and outcome measures collected at the initial examination could not be repeated at a follow-up session and included in a daily note. Rather, it is the depth and breadth of the re-testing that is performed *and* the comparison of the results to those obtained at a prior point in time to make a judgment of the patient or client's status that warrants the creation of a progress note. Creating a daily note at every session and foregoing the creation of a progress note throughout the plan of care would not sufficiently relay your patient or client's movement through the plan of care towards the goals established at the initial examination. Similarly, creating a progress note at every session may not be feasible as the patient or client may not make progress at the same rate at each visit. However, you should still be able to show that you are working toward a particular goal even when progress is not yet measurable. In addition, the requirement of both documentation formats, daily notes, and progress notes at some point during the plan of care may be indicated by the rules and regulations of the payer source or the setting in which you practice.

Regarding the patient or client example above, your note may take an alternative format from the daily note or the progress note when your patient or client returns for his eighth follow-up visit since the initial examination. In this case, you may decide that you should determine your patient or client's progress by performing a more comprehensive re-examination and documenting the findings in a re-examination note. According to the APTA, a **re-examination** is the process of performing selected tests and measures and outcome measures after the initial examination to evaluate progress and to modify or redirect interventions.[1] This is not to say that tests and measures and outcome measures could not be collected and used to determine progress during a time when a formal re-examination is not being conducted. For example, you could decide to re-administer a self-report outcome measure such as the QuickDASH to your client at the fourth visit to objectively gather your patient or client's perceptions of his status without conducting a formal re-examination or without creating any further detail in your daily note. Similarly, you could re-administer a performance-based test and measure such as the Deep Neck Flexor Endurance Test or a timed overhead reaching task with a prescribed amount of resistance to determine progress outside the context of a formal re-examination. In these examples, it is the comparison of the patient or client's current status to a previous status that earns the note the label of a progress note. A re-examination note would be created in lieu of a progress note or daily note when there is a need to re-examine every aspect of the plan of care including the goals established at the initial examination and to perform a re-evaluation to determine if any parts of the plan of care need to change.

Determining When to Document Progress

TIMING SINCE THE INITIAL EXAMINATION

Although the amount of time that has lapsed since the initial examination is an important factor to consider when documenting progress and determining in which format it should be documented, it is not the only factor you should consider in your clinical decision-making process for including your patient or client's progress within your documentation at any given session (TABLE 6-1). As discussed above, the time since the initial examination may trigger you to include progress within your documentation. For example, if you have written your plan of

TABLE 6-1 Factors to Consider in Determining When to Document Progress

1. Timing since the initial examination
2. Content of prior daily notes
3. Presence of new clinical findings
4. Unanticipated change in status
5. Clinical practice setting
6. Third-party payers

care for 4 weeks and you are ending the fourth week, you will likely decide to perform a formal re-examination to determine if you should continue the plan of care or conclude the plan of care with your patient or client.

CONTENT OF PRIOR DAILY NOTES

Another factor that may indicate the need for a progress note is the content of a previous daily note. Consider the following example of a note that was written by your colleague who worked with your patient or client during the weekend in an inpatient rehabilitation setting.

> S: Patient reports being very lethargic over the last 2 days due to inability to sleep because of increased right groin and right leg pain.
>
> I: See flow sheet. Modified weight-bearing exercise due to increased pain at groin when accepting weight on the right lower extremity.
>
> R: Patient was able to ambulate 3 × 15 feet with four-wheeled rolling walker. Patient demonstrated decreased ability to accept weight on right lower extremity during gait and during weight-shifting activities. Patient was not able to use a heel-toe step-through gait pattern. No increased lower extremity edema at ankles noted. No redness or tenderness to palpation noted at the right groin region.
>
> P: Continue to facilitate weight bearing for functional activities such as ambulation at least 50 feet to get to bathroom.

Because your colleague's documentation indicates a significant change in your patient or client's status in terms of his abilities, you will likely decide to comprehensively assess your patient or client to determine the reason for the poor performance with your colleague over the weekend. Based on your findings, you may decide to alter your plan of care to improve your patient or client's performance or you may decide to consult with the healthcare team to determine the next course of action. Your documentation should reflect the results of your reassessment and the outcome of your findings. Because there has been a marked change in your patient or client's activities and participation, a progress note would not likely include sufficient detail to relay a thorough investigation of the etiology of continued impairments in body functions and structures. Therefore, a re-examination note which includes an analysis of selected tests and measures and allows you to re-evaluate progress and modify or redirect interventions is warranted.

PRESENCE OF NEW CLINICAL FINDINGS

The presence of new clinical findings may also prompt you to include progress within your documentation. As in the scenario above, if new clinical findings become apparent during your interactions with your patient or client a progress note or re-examination note to document this new information is necessary. Consider the following scenario.

> You have been working with your older adult patient or client on improving her gait and balance for the last 2 weeks regarding the three falls she experienced over the last 6 months. Your impression after completing your examination 2 weeks ago is that she is deconditioned, weak, and has poor aerobic capacity after recovering from pneumonia. However, during the current session she indicates to you that she has been experiencing dizziness over the last day and a half.

Upon learning this new information, you will likely conduct further examination to determine the etiology of her dizziness and judge how to incorporate your findings into the plan of care. The details of this process should be recorded in your documentation. The depth of the relationships you identify among impairments in body functions and structures, activity limitations, participation restrictions, and contextual factors, in comparison to your original plan of care, will assist you in deciding if you create a progress note or a re-examination note.

UNANTICIPATED CHANGE IN STATUS

An unanticipated change in your patient or client's status is yet another factor that may prompt you to include progress or lack of progress within your documentation. Consider the following scenario.

> Over the last 4 weeks, you have been working with a 12-year-old boy who injured his knee when he landed awkwardly from a layup during a basketball game 5 weeks ago. The initial examination findings indicated that he suffered a sprain of his medial collateral ligament. However, due to persistent pain and lack of progression in the plan of care, you initiated communication with his physician to relay your findings and suggested that imaging may be indicated to rule

out a fracture. You subsequently learn that your patient or client suffered a tibial plateau fracture and has been put on a nonweight-bearing status for the next 6 weeks until further follow-up with his physician. After learning this information, you further communicate with the physician that you will modify the plan of care to account for this new change in status and to reflect the new goals of preventing disuse atrophy and maintaining core trunk and proximal leg strength since he plans on returning to competitive play.

The next time you see your patient or client, your documentation should not only reflect the communication you had with other healthcare providers on your patient or client's behalf, but it should also reflect this unanticipated change in status. Therefore, further reassessment and re-evaluation should occur and be recorded in the context of a re-examination note.

THIRD-PARTY PAYERS

Third-party payers may also dictate the presence of the content of documentation such as the progression of the plan of care. Payers such as Medicare, Medicaid, workers' compensation programs, and private insurance plans may have differing requirements for documenting progress based on the state or setting in which you practice. For example, a private healthcare preferred-provider plan may require you as an outpatient physical therapist to provide a progress or re-examination note after 25 visits. Therefore, it is feasible that during a 4-week, 12-visit plan of care for a patient or client with this third-party payer, that you are not required to create a formal progress or re-examination note in your documentation. Alternatively, Medicare requires that an outpatient physical therapist must document progress every tenth visit during a plan of care. APPENDIX 6-A details additional information to consider when documenting progress in your workers' compensation patients or clients. Therefore, not only must you be cognizant of the content of your re-examination or progress note as a physical therapist whose interest is to meet the goals established with your patient or client or caregiver in the plan of care, but you must also be aware of the rules and regulations that apply to your state and setting in which you are caring for your patient or client. Do varying requirements such as these then indicate that you only need to conduct a reassessment and note progress on those patient or client's whose payer source requires it?

No. Remember the progress note or re-examination note when written well is meant to guide you in further plan of care development. Consider the following note for an infant who has private insurance whom you are treating in an outpatient setting.

> S: Mother of child reports that child is attending to her left side given that she is now intermittently rolling to the left in response to a toy placed in her left visual field.
>
> I: See flow sheet.
>
> R: Child demonstrates steady progress towards goals.
>
> P: Continue to work towards goals as established at the initial plan of care.

It is important to recognize that simply indicating an improvement towards goals established at the initial the examination is an informal, nondescript comment that does not relay any meaningful detail about how you might continue to structure your interventions or what impairments in body functions and structures, activity limitations, or participation restrictions you might re-evaluate. The above note does not relay which aspects of the plan of care are progressing and which aspects of the plan of care continue to require your skilled oversight as a physical therapy professional.

Determining the Format for Documenting Progress

There are many factors to consider in determining when to document progress during the plan of care as discussed above and listed in Table 6-1. But how do you decide if a progress note or re-examination note is the most appropriate format to document factors such as the presence of new clinical findings or an unanticipated change in status especially when there are no other restrictions dictated by a payer source or the practice setting? Furthermore, is this the same reasoning process for deciding which format is the most appropriate when your plan of care is progressing the way in which you had intended? To help make this decision, consider the World Health Organization (WHO) *International Classification of Functioning, Disability, and Health* (ICF) framework in which you categorized your patient or client at the initial examination.

For example, you identified impairments in body functions and structures, activity limitations, participation restrictions, and contextual factors to help organize and create the details of your plan of care. Therefore, in the presence of additional information such as new clinical findings or an unexpected change regarding your patient or client's status consider the effect of this detail on your patient or client's activity limitations and participation restrictions (**FIGURE 6-1**). If the additional clinical information expands on or improves upon the activity limitations and participation restrictions that currently exist in the plan of care then consider creating a progress note using a daily note format by expanding on and reviewing the current plan of care. Alternatively, if the additional clinical information yields activity limitations and participation restrictions that are distinct and different from those present at the initial examination, then consider creating a re-examination note since this additional information requires a new and different clinical reasoning process than the one you employed when initial activity limitations and participation restrictions were identified within the original plan of care. Therefore, your decision

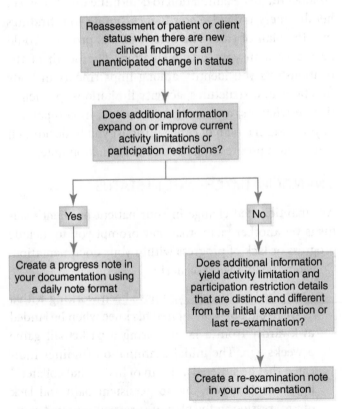

FIGURE 6-1 Algorithm for Writing Progress or Re-Examination Notes When There Are New Clinical Findings or an Unanticipated Change in Status.

to create a progress note using a daily note format or a re-examination note will depend on the level of ability defined by the activity limitations and participation restrictions you identify with verbal communication, skilled observation, and/or with specific tests and measures that indicate a change in your patient or client's ability status. Consider the following scenario.

> You have been working for 3 weeks in an outpatient setting with your patient or client who experienced a rotator cuff dysfunction after a traction injury sustained while walking his dog. His shoulder pain has been improving which has improved his ability to sit at his computer for work. However, your patient or client returns to a subsequent session with a complaint of neck pain.

You must decide if this neck pain expands on activity limitations and participation restrictions that you have already identified in your original plan of care or if it yields alternative activity limitations and participation restrictions than those present at the initial examination. You could decide to do this by asking him detailed questions regarding his neck pain, by using your observational skills of his movement patterns as you start your session, administering the Neck Disability Index, or some combination of these actions. If you then determine that his complaint of neck pain represents additional information that expands on current activity limitations and participation restrictions that you have already identified in your original plan of care, then you should continue your investigation of further impairments in body functions and structures and document these findings in a progress note using a daily note format (**FIGURE 6-2**). If, however, you determine that your patient or client's complaint of neck pain represents alternative activity limitations and participation restrictions than indicated at the initial examination, then you should continue your investigation of further impairments of body functions and structures and document your findings using a re-examination type of format (**FIGURE 6-3**).

Now revisit the scenario above and consider the following additional information.

> After 1 month of your plan of care, patient or client reports that he is doing well with his home exercise program and that he can manage his shoulder pain. After further discussion, you decide to re-test the elements of your plan of care and look at the progress he has made to date on the goals you established at the initial examination.

This scenario is ideal in that it indicates that the plan of care you have created for your patient or client has progressed as planned and that you now need to make a decision between continuing or concluding the episode of care. As you proceed through collecting data regarding your patient or client's current status compared to his status at the initial examination by reassessing the domains of the ICF model—body functions and structures, activity limitations, participation restrictions, and contextual factors—you will generate a judgment as to whether you should proceed with a re-examination or conclude the episode of care. Remember that many factors such as timing since the initial examination, content of prior daily notes, presence of new clinical findings, unanticipated changes in status, clinical practice settings, and third-party payers' influence when you will document your patient or client's progress. However, it is your patient or client's actual characteristics organized using the domains of the ICF model that also assist your decision to document progress or lack of progress using a progress note or a re-examination note format.

S: Patient/client reports that he rarely feels R shoulder pain but has R-sided neck pain (5/10) that seems to increase when he looks up or when he is working at his computer for his job as an accountant. He states that he also feels aching in his R arm (4/10) when he is not moving his neck or R arm.

I: R shoulder active range of motion: flexion = 160° (135° at initial exam); abduction = 150° (90° at initial exam); external rotation = 90° (85° at initial exam); internal rotation = 70° (70° at initial exam). Cervical active range of motion: R rotation = 45° (60° at initial exam); L rotation = 65° (55° at initial exam); R side bending = 5° (pain in lateral R upper arm, R side of neck); L side bending = 20° pulling on R side of neck; extension = 25° pain R posterior shoulder, R side of neck; flexion = 30° tight posterior neck. Provided education regarding sitting posture at computer (see flow sheet for details.)

R: R-sided neck pain 1/10 during cervical rotation after performing manual techniques per flow sheet to cervical spine. Patient/client demonstrated ability to assume appropriate positioning for prolonged sitting at his computer without increased pain by end of session.

P: Determine change in neck and R shoulder pain based on interventions performed today per flow sheet. Re-measure cervical spine active range of motion and review sitting position when patient is working at computer.

FIGURE 6-2 Progress Note Example After Identifying Additional Clinical Findings That Expands or Improves on Current Activity Limitations and Participation Restrictions Already Present in the Plan of Care.

Clinical Impression: Mr. A has made progress towards his goals as determined at the initial examination 3 weeks ago due to a right rotator cuff strain. However, he continues to display significant impairments in body functions and structures, activity limitations, and participation restrictions as indicated per the below reassessment.

Activity Limitations and Participation Restrictions:
○ Inability to sit at computer for > 10 minutes without neck and shoulder pain
○ Pain with reach to overhead shelf to retrieve or replace items (clothing in closet or overhead, washing hair, can in pantry, plate in cabinet) due to neck and shoulder pain

Peripheral Nerve Integrity: decreased light touch sensation in C6 dermatomal pattern R forearm and hand

Posture: moderate forward head and rounded shoulders

Palpation: hypertonicity and tenderness R anterior and middle scalenes; R levator scapula; R biceps tendon in bicipital groove

Pain: 6/10 R side of posterior neck and lateral aspect of R upper arm

Shoulder Active Range of Motion: R flexion = 175°, R abduction = 150°

Shoulder Passive Range of Motion: R flexion = 180°, R abduction = 165°; R external rotation = 50° at 90° abduction, IR = 70° at 90° abduction

Cervical Active Range of Motion: R rotation = 50° pain on R, L rotation = 75° pulling on R, extension = 30° pain on R side of neck and lateral aspect R upper extremity

Cervical Passive Range of Motion: R rotation = 55°, L rotation = 75°, extension = 35° pain on R side of neck and lateral aspect of R upper extremity

Muscle Performance: Craniocervical Flexion Test: activation score = 24 mmHg; R lower trapezius = 3/5; R middle trapezius = 3/5; R rhomboids = 4/5; R supraspinatus = 4/5; infraspinatus = 3/5; teres minor = 4/5, R biceps = 4/5

Special Tests: + ULTT (median nerve bias); + Spurling's Test; + Cervical Distraction Test; + pain with active shoulder ER

Other Outcome Tools: Neck Disability Index = 22/50

Goals Established at Initial Examination:
1. In 4 weeks, report the ability to walk dog on leash daily for at least 10 minutes without R shoulder pain. 50% MET
2. In 4 weeks, report the ability to perform overhead reaching for dressing and bathing tasks w/o R shoulder pain. 25% MET
3. In 4 weeks, improve pain as measured by the Numeric Pain Rating Scale by at least two points to indicate a meaningful improvement in R shoulder pain. 75% MET

Additional Goals:
1. In 4 weeks, demonstrate the ability to sit at computer for work for 30-minute bouts without limitation due to R shoulder or R-sided neck pain.
2. Improve activation score of deep cervical flexors via the craniocervical flexion test by at least 2 mmHg to indicate a clinically important change in motor control.
3. Improve Neck Disability Index score by at least seven points to indicate a clinically significant improvement in perceived neck disability.

Evaluation: Due to the impairments noted above in body functions and structures, activity limitations, and participation restrictions including decreased active range of motion, poor muscle performance, positive special tests, continued pain, decreased response to light touch sensation, and continued difficulty with sitting at computer for job tasks and reaching for basic activity of daily living tasks, Mr. A appears to have a C6 cervical radiculopathy in addition to continued rotator cuff pathology as indicated above. He has made some improvement with the current plan of care towards the goals established at the initial examination. He would continue to benefit from skilled physical therapy intervention two times per week for an additional 4 weeks to continue to work on initially established goals as well as additional goals created based on the reassessment above. Mr. A's prognosis is good based on progress indicated by the goals and his response to interventions per the flow sheet. A formal reassessment will be done in 4 weeks to determine further continuation of or discharge from this plan of care.

FIGURE 6-3 Re-Examination Note Example After Identifying Alternative Activity Limitations and Participation Restrictions from Those Present in Original Plan of Care.

Using Clinical Reasoning to Document Progress

Recall that the re-examination as defined by the APTA is created to evaluate progress and to modify or redirect the plan of care.[2] Thus, re-examination documentation should include all of the components necessary to make patient- or client-centered, evidence-based clinical judgments regarding your patient or client's progress with the plan of care. Therefore, the primary purpose of the re-examination is two-fold: 1) to ensure that a thorough reassessment of all of the components of the plan of care as delineated at the initial examination occurs; and 2) to ensure that any subsequent sessions where progress was indicated and assessed are revisited. It is during the re-examination when you decide if your plan of care should

TABLE 6-2   Components of the Re-Examination Note

1. Clinical impression or diagnosis
2. Objective reassessment of tests and measures and outcome tools
3. Goals status
4. Evaluation

continue as written or be modified in some way based on the response your patient or client has shown to date. It is important to recognize that you must include your clinical decision-making process and clinical rationale for your continued plan of care regardless of your decision to keep it the same or alter it in some way. Therefore, when determining the contents of your re-examination note (TABLE 6-2), think back to how you organized your documentation for your initial examination (FIGURE 6-4).

CONTENT OF RE-EXAMINATION COMPONENTS: CLINICAL IMPRESSION OR DIAGNOSIS

When creating your **clinical impression** or formulating your physical therapy **diagnosis**, you referred to your patient or client's past medical history, current history, and systems review. Remember to use the medical diagnosis or knowledge of a patient or client's health condition as another piece of data to formulate your clinical impression rather than the sole element that drives the plan of care. You then collated the results of your tests and measures to further refine your clinical impression or diagnosis of your patient or client's impairments in body functions and structures, activity limitations, and participation restrictions. This became the basis of your evaluation and allowed for subsequent identification of the prognosis, goals, and interventions as you finalized the plan of care. The APTA's *Guide to Physical Therapist Practice* defines the **evaluation** as a dynamic process in which the physical therapist makes clinical judgments based on data gathered during the examination.[3] Similarly, when creating your re-examination note it may be helpful to recapitulate your impression of the evaluation you created at the initial examination by first creating a synopsis of your patient or client's current status over the last one to two sessions based on his or her verbal report or subjective information such as the presence of pain or current activity limitations and participation restrictions (TABLE 6-3). From this data you can begin to build your clinical impression and determine how to proceed with your re-assessment. Consider

the following daily note for your patient or client in whom you have been working to improve the mechanics of the temporal mandibular joint.

> S: Patient reports that she is able to chew small pieces of meat such as steak and chicken with decreased left facial pain. She also states that she is able to sit at her computer for 10 minutes without experiencing increased neck or jaw pain on the left.
>
> I: See flow sheet. Added to home exercise program – Patient to perform mouth opening motor control exercises in front of the mirror 3 × 30 per day.
>
> R: Patient demonstrates an improved ability to open mouth symmetrically without deviation to the left when utilizing visual feedback.
>
> P: Perform re-examination next session.

As alluded to above, the last daily note can serve as the foundation for the re-examination note. In other words, you can use the subjective content from the last daily note regarding your patient or client's status as well as the evaluation from the initial examination as the basis for your current judgment of the clinical impression or diagnosis established in your initial examination documentation. Consider the evaluation from the initial examination of the patient or client in the above scenario.

> Ms. A is a 24-year-old female who demonstrates left-sided temporal mandibular joint disorder related to upper cervical spine dysfunction based on the findings from the above examination. Ms. A demonstrates impairments in body functions and structures that include muscle guarding of the left temporalis, masseter, and pterygoids; limited mouth aperture/opening, dyscoordination of the muscles of mastication, hypomobility of the atlanto-occipital joint, and C1 hypomobility. These impairments contribute to activity limitations and participation restrictions that include sleeping, chewing, and prolonged reading or typing in a sitting position. The contextual factors that impact Ms. A's plan of care include her young age, occupation as a veterinary assistant, and history of a motor vehicle accident with whiplash injury and concurrent left clavicular fracture 3 years ago. Ms. A would benefit from skilled physical therapy intervention 3 × week for 8 weeks to achieve the goals established above.

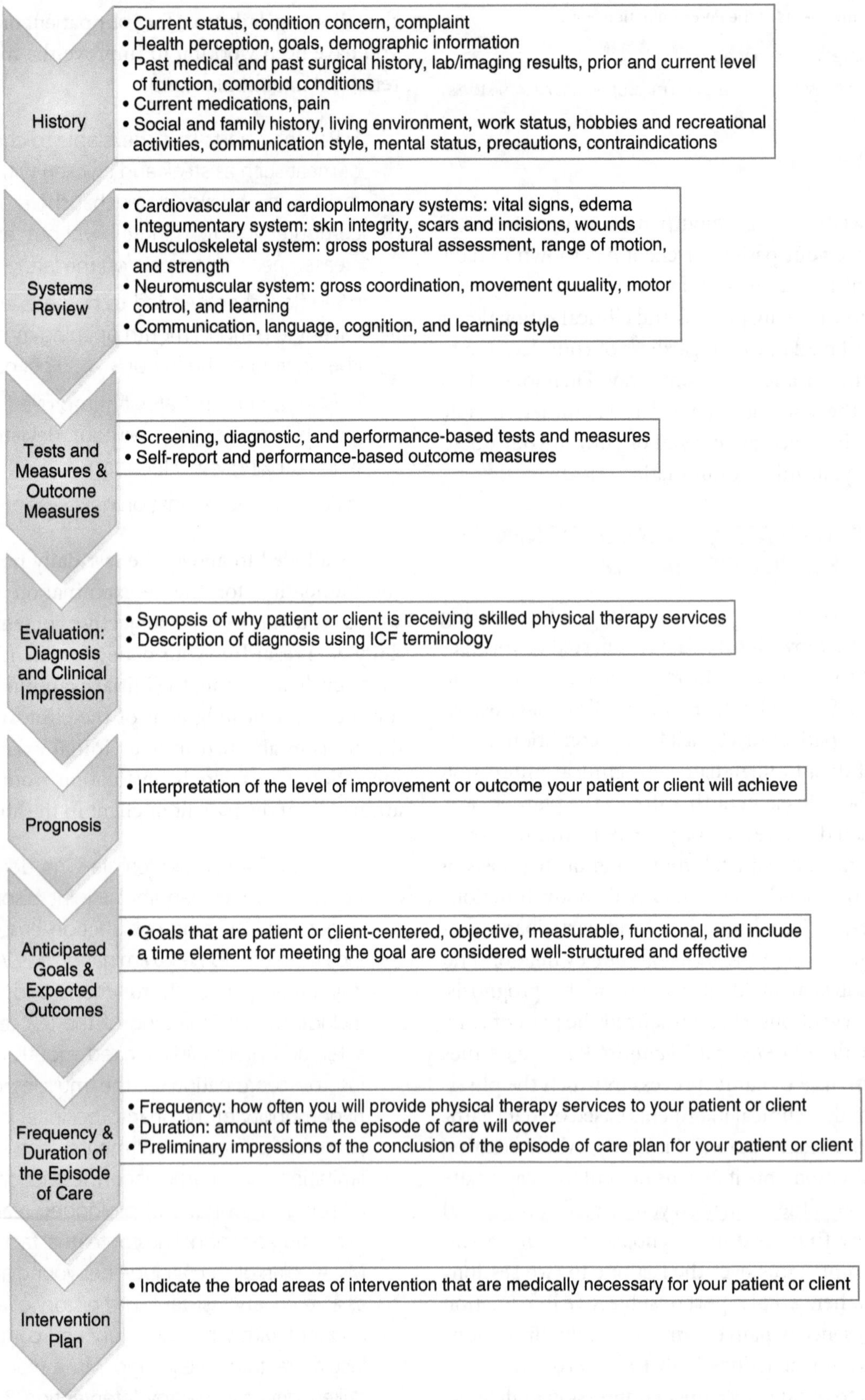

History
- Current status, condition concern, complaint
- Health perception, goals, demographic information
- Past medical and past surgical history, lab/imaging results, prior and current level of function, comorbid conditions
- Current medications, pain
- Social and family history, living environment, work status, hobbies and recreational activities, communication style, mental status, precautions, contraindications

Systems Review
- Cardiovascular and cardiopulmonary systems: vital signs, edema
- Integumentary system: skin integrity, scars and incisions, wounds
- Musculoskeletal system: gross postural assessment, range of motion, and strength
- Neuromuscular system: gross coordination, movement quuality, motor control, and learning
- Communication, language, cognition, and learning style

Tests and Measures & Outcome Measures
- Screening, diagnostic, and performance-based tests and measures
- Self-report and performance-based outcome measures

Evaluation: Diagnosis and Clinical Impression
- Synopsis of why patient or client is receiving skilled physical therapy services
- Description of diagnosis using ICF terminology

Prognosis
- Interpretation of the level of improvement or outcome your patient or client will achieve

Anticipated Goals & Expected Outcomes
- Goals that are patient or client-centered, objective, measurable, functional, and include a time element for meeting the goal are considered well-structured and effective

Frequency & Duration of the Episode of Care
- Frequency: how often you will provide physical therapy services to your patient or client
- Duration: amount of time the episode of care will cover
- Preliminary impressions of the conclusion of the episode of care plan for your patient or client

Intervention Plan
- Indicate the broad areas of intervention that are medically necessary for your patient or client

FIGURE 6-4 Review of Initial Examination Documentation Process.

TABLE 6-3   Content of Re-Examination Components

1. Clinical impression or diagnosis
   ○ Changes in patient or client status
   ○ Current activity limitations and participation restrictions
2. Objective reassessment of tests and measures, outcome tools
3. Goals status
   ○ Progress towards goals
   ○ Additional goals
4. Evaluation
   ○ Interpretation of tests and measures and outcome tools
   ○ Interpretation of goal achievement status
   ○ Prognostic status
   ○ Updated frequency and duration of the episode of care
   ○ Statement of why skilled intervention is recommended
   ○ Statement of plan to transition to next level of care

CONTENT OF RE-EXAMINATION COMPONENTS: OBJECTIVE REASSESSMENT OF TESTS AND MEASURES AND OUTCOME TOOLS

Reviewing the narrative of the information you created in the evaluation portion of your initial examination documentation to determine changes in your patient or client's current status will lead you to document the next part of the re-examination, the objective **test and measures** and **outcome measures**. In this section of the re-examination note, you are recording your patient or client's performance on the same measures you collected at the initial examination. It is important here to reassess each test and measure and outcome measure in the same manner it was originally performed so that an accurate interpretation of the test can lead to a meaningful judgment of your patient or client's progress. Your ability to use this information to make informed clinical decisions regarding your patient or client's progress will only be as valuable as data you chose to record. Consider the following clinical impression and accompanying documentation of tests, measures, and outcomes tools results.

Mr. B has made excellent progress towards his goals per the results of his re-examination indicated below. However, deficits in Mr. B's gait speed and balance continue to interfere with his ability to ambulate short distances with safety and without need for verbal cues.

○ Hip active range of motion = within functional limits
○ Gluteus medius strength = good bilaterally
○ Standing static balance = good

○ Static dynamic balance = fair
○ Five Times Sit to Stand Test = 28 seconds
○ Four Square Step Test = 31 seconds with straight cane

It is difficult to grasp if skilled intervention is still necessary for Mr. B based on the data presented above. For example, if hip active range of motion was recorded to be within functional limits and gluteus medius strength is scored as good bilaterally, then why do the performance-based measures above indicate compromised lower extremity functional strength and fall risk? Furthermore, why is there a need for an assistive device during the Four Square Step Test? Consider that the data you decide to document in your re-examination should continue to tell the story of your patient or client's journey through the plan of care and ultimately assist you with making meaningful decisions regarding future care based on the data you record. Consider an alternative to the above documentation.

Mr. B has made excellent progress towards his goals per the results of his re-examination indicated below. However, deficits in Mr. B's gait speed and balance continue to interfere with his ability to ambulate short distances with safety and without need for assistance to prevent lateral instability.

○ Hip active range of motion: right hip extension = 10 degrees, left = 15 degrees; right hip flexion = 95 degrees, left = 120 degrees
○ Gluteus medius strength = right = 3/5; left = 4/5
○ Standing static balance (Berg Balance Test) = 49/56
○ Static dynamic balance (Functional Gait Assessment) = 16/30
○ 10-Meter Walk Test = 0.93 m/s
○ Five Times Sit to Stand Test = 28 seconds
○ Four Square Step Test = 31 seconds with straight cane

The information indicated here provides greater detail that allows you to identify relationships not only between the listed impairments in body functions and structures, but also among the activity limitations and the listed impairments. For example, perhaps you question if your patient or client's limited active hip flexion range of motion on the right affected his performance on the Five Times Sit to Stand Test. Furthermore, perhaps you look specifically at the items on the Functional Gait Assessment to further judge your patient or client's decreased ability to safely ambulate without the need for physical assistance to prevent a loss of balance. The increased data reported in this section of the re-examination allows you to plan further reassessments and to more accurately determine your patient or client's progress within the plan of care.

Another tool that you can utilize when determining how to proceed with the tests and measures and outcome measures you would like to reassess during your re-examination is the intervention flow sheet you created at the time of the initial examination. One approach to the flow sheet is to organize it according to how you might progress your interventions over time. For example, rather than simply listing your interventions in the order in which they were performed during a session you might create categories for your interventions to reflect your clinical decision-making process such as symptom reduction exercises, motor control exercises, and strengthening exercises. This organization affords you the ability to look back over the flow sheet at previous sessions to see how you have progressed your exercise dosing for your patient or client over time. Also, included in this flow sheet is an indication of the outcome measures you collected at the initial examination and would like to re-collect at the time of the re-examination. Having this information available in your flow sheet can serve as a prompt to prepare for how you might structure a session in which a re-examination is to be performed. For example, rather than your patient or client starting on a particular intervention at the beginning of a session, you may decide to perform a certain outcome measure prior to the initiation of exercise for a result that is not influenced by fatigue or muscle activation. On the other hand, you may decide to allow for a period of exercise prior to collecting your outcome measures so that you can comment on your patient or client's ability to perform on the outcome measure despite a level of fatigue. Ultimately, organizing your flow sheet can help you structure the content and course of the tests and measures portion of your re-examination session.

CONTENT OF RE-EXAMINATION COMPONENTS: GOAL STATUS

The next section of the re-examination note is an indication of your patient or client's **goal achievement status** and includes your patient or client's progress towards the goals

you established at the initial examination as well as any additional goals you deem necessary to add (Table 6-3). In order to comment on goal progress, a reference to the goals as they were originally created in the initial examination documentation is warranted. This will allow for a direct comparison of goal achievement status. Whether or not the goals have been met, partially met, or not met should be clearly indicated to assist with the decision to continue to work towards the same goals as established at the initial examination, to alter these goals based on current progress, or to create new goals to reflect new findings recognized during the re-examination process. For example, you could choose a dichotomous, nominal scale of "MET" or "NOT MET" to record goal achievement status. Alternatively, you could choose a ratio scale to reflect partial goal achievement such as 0%, 25%, 50%, 75%, or 100% met. Consider the following goals from an initial examination that have been re-evaluated and labeled indicating goal status along the continuum of goal achievement.

1. In 1 week, patient or client will demonstrate ability to roll to right and left to facilitate independence moving from supine to sit at the edge of the bed. **GOAL NOT MET**

2. In 4 weeks, patient or client will report an improvement of right hip pain of at least 2 points as measured by the Numeric Pain Rating Scale to indicate a clinically meaningful change in right hip pain. **GOAL MET**

3. In 4 weeks, patient or client will improve on the 10-Meter Walk Test by at least 0.10 m/s to indicate meaningful improvement in functional mobility. **GOAL NOT MET**

4. In 6 weeks, patient or client will perform single-limb stance on a flat surface for 1 minute without loss of balance to improve lateral stability and dynamic balance. **GOAL NOT MET**

The goals above do not give enough information regarding which components of the plan of care have actually been beneficial or if your patient or client's potential for improvement continues to exist. Therefore, it will be challenging to create a meaningful narrative in the evaluation section of your re-examination note from the goals indicated above regarding your patient or client's progress. You might assume that some benefit to the patient or client is occurring since hip pain has decreased; however, this improvement could simply reflect natural healing over a 6-week time frame. The status of "NOT MET" for the other goals cannot be used to judge if the plan of care should continue as written or be altered due to lack of improvement. Now revisit these same goals that have been re-evaluated and labeled indicating goal status along the continuum of goal achievement using a more sensitive scale to indicate change.

1. In 1 week, patient or client will demonstrate ability to roll to right and left to facilitate independence moving from supine to sit at the edge of the bed. **GOAL 50% MET**

2. In 4 weeks, patient or client will report an improvement of right hip pain of at least 2 points as measured by the Numeric Pain Rating Scale to indicate a clinically meaningful change in right hip pain. **GOAL 100% MET**

3. In 4 weeks, patient or client will improve on the 10-Meter Walk Test by at least 0.10 m/s to indicate a meaningful improvement in gait speed and functional mobility. **GOAL 0% MET**

4. In 6 weeks, patient or client will perform single-limb stance on a flat surface for 1 minute without loss of balance to improve lateral stability and dynamic balance. **GOAL 25% MET**

The use of this more sensitive scale allows you to make further judgments regarding the current plan of care and to create a constructive narrative in the evaluation section of your re-examination documentation to further support your decision to alter or continue the plan of care. For example, for Goal #1 you may be able to conclude that your patient or client has achieved the ability to roll to at least one side but not the other since the documentation indicates that the goal has been 50% met. Similarly, Goal #4 indicates that the ability to single-limb stand can occur for at least a 15-second period since the documentation indicates that the ability to single-limb stand for one minute has been 25% met.

Meaningful goal interpretation cannot occur if goals are not well written. In other words, to be useful as an adjunct to your clinical decision making and appraisal of your patient or client's progress, goals should be written in an objective, functional, and measurable way. Consider the following example of goal documentation in a re-examination note.

Goal	Goal Achievement Status
In 4 weeks, patient or client will improve gait speed when ambulating short distances with safety and independence.	Goal Not Met
Improve static standing balance to decrease fall risk.	Goal 50% Met
Improve Five Times Sit to Stand Time to indicate increased lower extremity functional strength.	Goal Not Met
Demonstrate the ability to perform Four Square Step Test without a cane.	Goal 25% Met

Based on your patient or client's goal achievement as indicated above, is the continuation of the plan of care justified? Do you have an idea of how the percentage of goal achievement was determined? Do you have a sense of what interventions should continue based on the status of your patient or client's progress with the plan of care? Do you have a sense of why some goals were not achieved? Because the above goals lack tangible, objective data with which to gauge change, they are rendered meaningless to the evaluation portion of the re-examination note. Therefore, not only is it necessary to judge the level of goal achievement for each goal, it is also important to have an understanding of why each goal was or was not achieved. This understanding will allow you to determine if you need to extend these goals or set news ones. It may be beneficial to you to indicate in your re-examination note next to each goal why each goal was not achieved so that you have a visual reminder to carry this detail forward to your evaluation section of your plan of care. This addition to your clinical impression or evaluation of the plan of care section of your documentation will validate why skilled care is still necessary based on why previously set goals were not achieved and/or why new ones were set. Consider the following goals.

Goal	Goal Acheivement Status	Rationale
In 4 weeks, patient or client will improve on the 10-Meter Walk Test by at least 0.10 m/s to indicate a meaningful improvement in gait speed and functional mobility.	Goal Not Met	Patient or client continues to exhibit quadriceps and gluteus medius weakness.

Goal	Goal Acheivement Status	Rationale
In 6 weeks, patient or client will perform single-limb stance on a flat surface for 1 minute without loss of balance to improve lateral stability and dynamic balance.	Goal 50% Met	Patient or client able to perform single-limb stance for 30 seconds
Improve Five Times Sit to Stand time by 10 seconds to indicate increased LE functional strength.	Goal Not Met	Patient or client able to perform test in 22 sec; however with elevated surface and use of 1 UE to assist due to persistent knee pain.
Demonstrate the ability to perform Four Square Step Test in 20 seconds without a cane.	Goal 25% Met	Patient or client able to perform test in 35 seconds with straight cane and minimal assistance due to poor control of backwards step.

In addition to relaying why skilled care is still necessary, the format of the goals above enables you to accurately progress your interventions at your next session with your patient or client.

CONTENT OF RE-EXAMINATION COMPONENTS: EVALUATION

The last section of your re-examination note, the evaluation, is a narrative summary of your clinical impression of your patient or client's progress and recommendations for the plan of care. These recommendations are based on all of the information you have gathered during the reassessment process and includes a collation of an interpretation of the tests, measures, and outcomes collected, an interpretation of goal achievement status, prognostic status, updated intervention frequency and duration, a statement of why skilled intervention should continue, and a statement of the plan to transition to the next level of care (Table 6-3). Consider the evaluation documentation below based on the above scenario of Mr. B.

> Mr. B has made excellent progress with his plan of care as indicated in this re-examination. However the following deficits remain.
>
> ○ Impairments in body functions and structures include limited hip range of motion, poor gluteus medius muscle performance, impaired static

balance, impaired dynamic balance, slow walking speed, and fall risk.

> ○ Activity limitation and participation restrictions include inability to ambulate short distances (~75 feet) such as from bedroom to bathroom with safety and independence.

Mr. B has met three of five short-term goals and one of three long-term goals indicated in the above re-examination. The other goals being between 50% and 75% met indicate that Mr. B is benefitting from the current plan of care and will continue to make progress towards his goals to achieve independence and safety with household ambulation for the completion of basic activities of daily living such as getting to the bathroom, bathing, and dressing. Mr. B's prognosis is good based on the above progress indicated and his response to current interventions per attached flow sheet. Therefore, continue plan of care for two 30-minute sessions per day for an additional 3 weeks. Additional re-examination will occur at that time and continuation of plan of care or conclusion of the episode of care and discharge to home will be determined at that time.

The above evaluation is in a narrative format and highlights that despite improvement indicated by his goal achievement, deficits according to the ICF domains remain that continue to render him unsafe and at risk for falls during gait and other dynamic activities. A statement of Mr. B's prognosis, updated duration and frequency of interventions, and why skilled care continues to be necessary is concisely indicated and refers back to the re-examination note for corroborating details in the tests and measures collected and the comparison of goal achievement to those at the initial examination. Also consider, in the event that goals remain unmet, to indicate what elements of the plan of care contributed to the fact that these goals have not changed and to indicate an action plan for working towards them in the continued plan of care. Your action plan might include extending your previously set goals, which involves documenting clearly that physical therapy interventions aimed at reaching those goals are to continue as indicated in the above example.

Alternatively, your action plan might include setting new goals. These new goals should match any changes in your patient or client's body functions and structures, activity limitations, and participation restrictions. Additionally, if previously set goals that remain unmet are going to be dropped from the plan of care, an explanation of this change should be reflected in this section. Consider the following example of an evaluation that does not meet the above-recommended criteria.

> Mr. B has made excellent progress towards goals as indicated by improvement indicated in reassessment above. Mr. B's prognosis is good based on stated goals. Continue to work on unmet goals for an additional 2 × week for 3 × weeks.

This evaluation only superficially includes some of the content of the re-examination components recommended in Table 6-3. It is important to specifically reference the tests and measures and outcome tools that continue to indicate your patient or client's deficits, rather than to only refer the note's user to an alternative location in the note, as this data will support your claim for continued care. Additionally, the specific inclusion of your interpretation of the goal achievement status will support your prognosis as well as any continued frequency and duration of the plan of care. Furthermore, basing the need for continued care on the fact that some goals remain unmet is not a justification that skilled care is still necessary. Consider that this information could instead indicate that your patient or client has plateaued in the rehabilitation process and the unmet goals are a sign that further progress is not attainable.

Lastly, clarifying plans for transitions in care as well as indicating the structured plan for transition to the next level of care is also important detail to include in the evaluation component of a re-examination. This information shows that plans beyond long-term goal achievement such as terminating the episode of care has been considered in constructing the entire plan of care. Consider the following evaluation.

> Ms. C has made excellent progress as indicated in her re-examination performed today. She has met all of her goals except for returning to playing a full softball game at first base on her softball team. Ms. C has been issued an updated comprehensive overhand throwing and shoulder-strengthening home exercise program based on her above improvements. She will continue this program on her own every other day for the next 4 weeks in addition to playing first base in one to two softball games per week. Ms. C will return for one follow-up visit in 4 weeks to ensure ability to continue

with her role as first baseman on her softball team and to update her exercise program.

Now consider this evaluation.

> Mr. D has made slow but steady progress with his plan of care as indicated by his ability to meet his goals established at the initial examination. Due to his ability to tolerate sitting upright in his wheelchair while maintaining a steady blood pressure and heart rate, Mr. D will be transferred to an inpatient rehabilitation facility in 2 days. Will continue to work towards progressing transfers from a squat-pivot method to a stand-pivot method until his day of discharge.

Both of the evaluation examples above clearly indicate the next level of care and what is to occur between the present time and the actual termination of the episode of care.

Reflection for Documenting Progress

The re-examination process and creating the subsequent re-examination documentation can be viewed as a critical self-check on the plan of care you have created on behalf of your patient or client. Use your re-examination documentation to critically evaluate your ability to hone your communication skills for determining your patient or client's current status, write short- and long-term goals, interpret outcome measure results, measure goal achievement status, determine prognosis, define frequency and duration of intervention planning, and create succinct and meaningful summaries of all the information gathered in the re-examination process. Use the questions listed in **TABLE 6-4** to guide you through this self-assessment process. Challenge yourself to answer these questions in the context of your re-examination documentation. This process will consistently lead to a clear re-examination note that supports your intentions.

Summary

Determining your patient or client's progress within a plan of care requires you to integrate information you collect about your patient or client from the initial examination and from subsequent physical therapy sessions

TABLE 6-4   Questions for Critical Self-Assessment of Re-Examination Documentation

1. How well did your patient or client achieve the goals you created at the initial examination?

2. Are your skilled services still required and on what details are you basing this information?

3. Have you ensured that you are performing the interventions indicated by the CPT codes under which you have billed?

4. Have you indicated which areas of the plan of care have not yet been achieved by providing an interpretation of the goal achievement status?

5. Have you relayed prognostic status?

6. Have you clearly indicated plans for transitioning the plan of care from the current setting to an alternative setting (home, other healthcare facility)?

7. Have you updated the frequency and duration for the episode of care?

BOX 6-1 The Electronic Health Record: Documenting Progress

An electronic health system can allow you to create a template for the re-examination note that mirrors the content of the initial examination thus affording you efficiency and saving you valuable time. In some electronic systems, selecting the re-examination template will populate the note with the same tests and measures and outcome tools you collected at the initial examination, the results of these items at the time of the initial examination, and other details of the plan of care such as the frequency and duration of care and the short- and long-term goals. Information provided in an organized and predictable template can help you structure your re-examination note in real time as suggested in Table 6-3 without having to toggle back and forth between your current note and your initial examination documentation.

throughout the plan of care. Capturing progress during this time in a well-written progress or re-examination note requires careful organization of all of the information gathered throughout the plan of care. One could argue that if you do not create documentation that would assist you in making future decisions on your patient or client's behalf or in creating future meaningful documentation within your patient or client's plan of care, then you have wasted your valuable time and resources creating mediocre documentation. Recall that a progress note is written when additional clinical information expands on or improves upon the activity limitations and participation restrictions that currently exist in the plan of care. Alternatively, a re-examination note is written when additional clinical information yields activity limitations and participation restrictions that are distinct and different from those present at the initial examination. Therefore, organizing your thoughts about your patient or client's progress around relationships you can identify among the domains of the ICF model will assist you in ensuring that your plan of care circles back to the primary patient- or client-centered goals of resolving or minimizing impairments in body functions and structures, activity limitations, and participation restrictions that initially indicated the need for skilled physical therapy services.

Consider however that some electronic systems may have content of the re-examination note such as an area

for the clinical impression, objective reassessment of tests and measures and outcome tools, and goal status at different locations within the electronic record. In other words, a re-examination template may simply be a drop-down menu of tests and measures from which you select the ones you want to re-examine on your patient or client. The goals may also be featured in data fields that are partially populated and are designed for you to fill in patient- or client-specific information. Furthermore, other components of the evaluation, such as the frequency and duration of the episode of care, may be housed in a location that indicates the insurance benefits for your patient or client so that this information can be easily considered when making your recommendations. When creating your re-examination documentation you would have to remember to go back to this location in the electronic record to update this component of the evaluation. Overall, be aware that the electronic health record may eliminate a narrative option for the clinical impression and evaluation content of your re-examination note. Be sure that pre-populated data fields or drop-down menus do not disrupt the integration information into your re-examination note.

Discussion Questions

1. What is the purpose of the progress report or re-examination note?
2. What is the difference between a progress note and a re-examination note? Give a clinical example of when you would create a progress note. Give a clinical example of when you would create a re-examination note.
3. What factors do you consider when you are determining your patient or client's progress within the plan of care?
4. What factors do you consider when determining the timing of:
   a. A progress note within the plan of care?
   b. A re-examination note within the plan of care?
5. Review the health record of one of your clinical instructor's or your colleague's patients or clients. Can you distinguish daily notes from progress notes? Can you distinguish progress notes from re-examination notes? What details differentiate these entries into the health record?
6. Exchange re-examination notes with one of your clinical instructors or your colleagues. Identify the components of the re-examination note as indicated in **TABLE 6-2**. Label the components of the:
   a. Clinical impression or diagnosis
   b. Objective reassessment of tests and measures and outcomes tools
   c. Goals status
   d. Evaluation
7. Identify an initial examination note among your documentation. Create a re-examination note based on the review of your initial examination documentation.

8. Based on the last one to two daily notes you have created for one of your patients or clients, can you identify activity limitations and participation restriction details that allows you to determine your patients or client's current clinical status?
9. Ask your clinical instructor or your colleague to review the plan of care of one of your patients or clients. Then ask your clinical instructor or colleague to describe your patient or client's current status. Is your clinical instructor or colleague's report of your patient or client accurate? If so, identify what information was present to allow for this accurate description. If not, what data was missing and where in the plan of care should it have been included?
10. Identify the evaluation you created in the initial examination documentation of a plan of care you created. Is the information in this evaluation useful to you for creating the initial content of a re-examination note? If so, what components are present that are useful? If not, what components are missing that would assist you in your ability to begin your re-assessment note?
11. Identify the tests and measures and outcome tools in an initial examination you created. Have you created meaningful documentation that would enable you to use this information in a re-examination note? Why or why not?
12. Identify the short- and long-term goals in an initial examination you created. Are these goals functional, objective, and measureable such that you could judge your patient or client's progress with the plan of care in a meaningful way? Why or why not?

Case Study Questions

1. Would you classify this note as a daily note or a progress note? Provide the rationale for your choice.

   Patient or client returns today with her exercise log, which indicates that she has lost 5 pounds over the last 4 weeks.

   Reviewed HEP and provided progression per sheet. BP rest = 152/88 mmHg, HR rest = 89 bpm (BP rest = 142/82 mmHg, HR rest = 80 bpm 4 weeks ago); 6-Minute Walk Test = 582 feet; RPE = 15 (412 feet; RPE = 17 4 weeks ago); 30-Second Chair Stand = 9 times (7 times 4 weeks ago)

   Improving resting vital signs due to improved aerobic fitness and lower extremity strength.

   Patient or client to continue her exercise program for the next 3 weeks at which time patient or client will return for further progression of exercise program.

2. Would you classify this note as a daily note or a progress note? Provide the rationale for your choice.

   Mr. E reports that his left hip is sore but feels more weak than painful. He notes that he continues to get tired quickly when he is walking what he considers very short distances in his home.

   Added gastrocnemius strengthening on leg press after performing Heel Rise Test: right = 3/5, left = 2/5; hip flexor strength: right = 4/5, left = 3/5

Mr. E demonstrates poor control of left lower extremity at terminal stance during gait with straight cane or rolling walker over 50-foot distance.

Continue to improve gastrocnemius strength to improve push off at terminal stance. Add hip flexion strengthening to facilitate lower extremity clearance during gait.

3. Transform the following goals into those that would allow you to accurately judge the patient or client's level of achievement at a certain point in time.
   a. In 4 weeks, demonstrate improved stance time on right during gait to decrease tendency to catch left toe on rug.
   b. Improve quadriceps strength to a 4/5 bilaterally.
   c. By 12 weeks, report improved tolerance to job duties.
   d. Improve standing tolerance for increased independence with basic activities of daily living.

4. Create the evaluation component of your re-examination note based on the following information.

   Mrs. F has made excellent progress after her R total knee arthroplasty 4 weeks ago towards her goals as indicated by the re-examination results below (results from initial examination are in parenthesis).

   ○ Patient-Specific Functional Scale:
     ○ Unable to drive = 0 (0)
     ○ Difficulty ascending stairs (4) into home (no device) = 4 (0)
     ○ Unable to get on and off the floor to play with grandchildren = 0 (0)
   ○ LE fatigue after walking far distance such as across parking lot into the grocery store (no device) = 6 (0)
   ○ Nonpitting edema at joint line: right = 54 cm (57 cm), left = 48 cm (49 cm)
   ○ Incision: Healing, closed and dry; minimal scabbing in place at distal inferior end of incision (surgical bandage still in place)
   ○ Knee flexion AROM: right = 102 degrees (67 degrees); left = 131 degrees (129 degrees)
   ○ Knee extension AROM: right = –4 degrees (–10 degrees); left = 0 degrees (0 degrees)
   ○ Patellar mobility = decreased superior-inferior glides (not assessed due to surgical bandage covering incision)
   ○ Timed Up and Go = 21 sec with no assistive device (18 sec with rolling walker)
   ○ 10-Minute Walk Test = 0.91 m/s no assistive device (self-selected speed) (0.86 with rolling walker)
   ○ Five Times Sit to Stand Test = 19 sec; 18 in chair height (23 sec; 21 in chair height)
   ○ Gluteus medius strength: right = 3/5 (2/5); left = 4/5 (4/5)

References

1. American Physical Therapy Association (APTA). *Defensible Documentation: Components of Documentation within the Patient/Client Management Model.* Alexandria, VA: American Physical Therapy Association; last updated March 8, 2012. Available at: www.apta.org/Documentation/DefensibleDocumentation/. Accessed on July 15, 2014.
2. APTA. *Defensible Documentation Elements.* Alexandria, VA: American Physical Therapy Association; last updated March 8, 2012. Available at: www.apta.org/Documentation/DefensibleDocumentation/. Accessed on July 15, 2014.
3. APTA. *Guide to Physical Therapist Practice* 3.0. Alexandria, VA: American Physical Therapy Association; 2014. Available at: guidetoptpractice.apta.org/. Accessed on July 15, 2014.

Appendix 6-A Considerations for Documenting Progress for Workers' Compensation Patients/Clients

Progress Notes	Re-Examination Notes
Include specific work abilities including modifications and compensations.	Ensure that current abilities with job duties and job-related tasks are explicit in order to compare to prior performance.
Identify any barriers to recovery such as scheduling, transportation, or other contextual factors.	Identify any changes and additions in interventions to address remaining limitations for successful performance of job duties for return to work.
Include communications with case manager, physician, and employer regarding progress and ultimate return to work.	
Ensure that action plans to address identified barriers with time lines are clearly indicated.	

Data from the APTA's Defensible Documentation: Setting Specific Considerations in Documentation (2011).

CHAPTER 7

Conclusion of the Episode of Care

CHAPTER OBJECTIVES

1. Recognize the components of a conclusion of the episode of care summary.
2. Recognize how the content of the episode of care summary can differ depending on:
   a. The care setting.
   b. The clinical scenario.
3. Demonstrate the ability to create a detailed conclusion of the episode of care summary.
4. Utilize a clinical reasoning framework for creating a conclusion of the episode of care summary.

KEY TERMS

Algorithm

Conclusion of the episode of care

Introduction

The conclusion of the episode of care summary represents the closure of the episode of care. Therefore, it is important to have a solid understanding of the components of the conclusion of the episode of care summary along with the content of each component to formulate the foundation of the conclusion of the episode of care documentation. Therefore, this information is presented followed by varied clinical scenarios that represent the ways in which you might document the conclusion of the episode of care summary. The ability to plan the details of the conclusion of the episode of care at the time of the initial examination is a skill that develops with clinical expertise and exposure to certain practice settings. Therefore, a clinical reasoning algorithm for determining your patient or client's readiness for the conclusion of the episode of care is suggested.

The Purpose of the Conclusion of the Episode of Care Summary

At the 69th Annual Session of the House of Delegates in Salt Lake City, Utah in June 2013, the term "discharge/discontinuation of intervention" was replaced by "conclusion of episode of care" and the term "discharge summary" was replaced by "episode of care summary."[1] The expectation is that this terminology be incorporated into all relevant American Physical Therapy Association (APTA) publications, documents, and communications on a scheduled revisions cycle.[2] The term "conclusion of the episode of care" is somewhat of a misnomer in that planning for the end of the episode of care with your patient or client starts immediately upon initiating that episode of care. Even though the creation of the conclusion of the episode of care documentation occurs at the termination of the episode of care, the content of this document requires data collected from the first encounter with your patient or client. Consider the following scenario.

You work in an outpatient physical therapy setting and are reviewing your schedule for tomorrow. You see that your first patient or client is a 70-year-old man with a referral from his orthopedic surgeon for physical therapy 6 weeks after a distal biceps tendon repair.

Based on this review alone, you might be thinking about how this person could present to physical therapy. Will he be wearing an elbow brace? Will he have started actively moving his elbow? Will he have concurrent wrist or shoulder pain? Does he have any comorbid conditions that may affect his healing? How does his age affect his healing? What injury did he experience that warranted a surgical intervention? How long after the injury did he have surgery? What phase of healing has he achieved 6 weeks after a tendon repair? Even with the limited information presented in the scenario above, you can start to develop your thoughts about what impairments in body functions and structures, activity limitations, participation restrictions, and contextual factors might exist, how these components might be objectively measured, and how they then might be resolved with physical therapy interventions. You can judge which outcome measures to utilize and from which domains (e.g., self-report, performance-based) based on if the measure has been deemed reliable and valid in an individual such as your patient or client. Similarly, you can judge which interventions to implement based on if these interventions have been deemed efficacious in an individual such as your patient or client. As you conduct your initial examination, including the history, systems review, and tests and measures and outcome measures, answers to these preliminary questions develop and further impressions about the episode of care, including the prognosis, goals, intervention plan, duration and frequency of care, and conclusion of the episode of care plan, are formulated.

According to the *Guide to Physical Therapist Practice*, the term "**conclusion of the episode of care**" is intended to indicate that a single episode of care has ended when the anticipated goals and expected outcomes have been met.[3] However, the patient or client's status and clinical rationale regarding why an episode of care is concluding when anticipated goals and expected outcome have not been must also be documented. Thus, a conclusion of the episode of care summary should also be created when:

○ The patient or client's declines to continue.
○ Continuation is not feasible due to medical, psychosocial, or financial barriers.
○ The physical therapist determines that the patient or client will no longer benefit from physical therapy services.[5]

Ultimately, it is important that you plan for successful achievement of the goals and outcomes you create for your patient or client from the inception and throughout the entire episode of care.

Components of the Conclusion of the Episode of Care Summary

According to the American Physical Therapy Association, the episode of care summary includes all of the elements found in **TABLE 7-1**.

CURRENT STATUS

The patient or client's physical or functional status is typically determined at the final visit via a reassessment of the progress made towards the goals established at the initial examination. Based on your observations of the patient or client's performance with physical therapy interventions, the subjective report of signs and symptoms, and the results of your tests and measures, you determine the need to terminate or continue the plan of care. At the completion of your testing, it is then appropriate to indicate your clinical impression of the patient or client's current physical or functional status just as you do during the evaluation process at the initial examination. Consider the results from the re-examination shown in **TABLE 7-2**.

The outcomes assessed in this scenario indicate that impairments in body functions and structures present at the initial examination have improved with the exception of deficits that remain in upper extremity strength as indicated by biceps and supinator manual muscle testing and performance-based testing. Furthermore, your reassessment of the QuickDASH and the Patient-Specific Functional Scale (PSFS) indicates that your patient or client

TABLE 7-1   Elements of an Episode of Care Summary

Current physical or functional status
Criteria/justification for termination of physical therapy services in that setting
Degree of goals/outcomes achieved
Reasons for goals/outcomes not being achieved
Plans related to the patient or client's continuing care such as:
Home exercise program
Referrals for additional services
Recommendations for follow-up physical therapy care
Family and caregiver training
Equipment provided

Adapted from: 1. GUIDELINES: PHYSICAL THERAPY DOCUMENTATION OF PATIENT/CLIENT MANAGEMENT BOD G03-05-16-41. 2. http://www.apta.org/Documentation/DefensibleDocumentation/ Accessed on 7/21/2013.

TABLE 7-2   Outcomes Data – Patient/Client Status Post (s/p) Distal Biceps Tendon Repair

Test and Measure/ Outcome Tool	Result Initial Examination	Result (4 week Re-Examination) (10 weeks s/p surgery)	Result (8 week Re-Examination) (14 weeks s/p surgery)
AROM Wrist Flexion	65°	75°	80°
AROM Wrist Extension	45°	65°	70°
AROM Elbow Flexion	110°	135°	145°
AROM Elbow Extension	−25°	−5°	−2°
AROM Forearm Supination	45°	70°	80°
MMT: Biceps	Deferred	3/5	4/5
MMT: Supinator	Deferred	3/5	4/5
MMT: Triceps	Deferred	4/5	5/5
MMT: Flexor Digitorum Superficialis	4/5	4/5	5/5
MMT: Flexor Digitorum Profundus	3/5	4/5	5/5
MMT: Extensor Carpi Radialis	3/5	4/5	5/5
MMT: Extensor Carpi Ulnaris	4/5	4/5	5/5
MMT: Extensor Digitorum	3/5	4/5	5/5
Grip Strength	65#	96#	120#
Joint Mobility			
Proximal radioulnar joint	Normal mobility	Normal mobility	Normal mobility
Humeralulnar joint	Normal mobility	Normal mobility	Normal mobility
Performance-Based Tests			
Lift and carry ≤ 5# in L hand	Deferred	Able 5 × w/ 4#; 10 × w/ 3#	Able 2 × 10 w/ 5#
Retrieve and replace 8# object on/off overhead shelf	Deferred	Able 10 × w/ 2#	Able 10 × w/ 5#; 1× w/ 8#
Modified push ups (knees on ground)	Deferred	Able to assume all-fours position	× 4
Pull ups (20% of body weight = 42#)	Deferred	Deferred	× 3
Quick DASH (symptom/disability score)	61.4%	30%	0%
Patient-Specific Functional Scale (Total Score)	1.80/10	6.40/10	10/10
Opening jars/containers	2/10	5/10	10/10
Brushing teeth	4/10	10/10	10/10
Washing hair	3/10	6/10	10/10
Driving manual transmission	0/10	7/10	10/10
Pick up/hold 2-year-old grandchild	0/10	4/10	10/10

has returned to desired activities and is able to participate in them without limitation. Your clinical impression of your patient or client's progress could be documented in your evaluation as below.

Mr. X has benefitted from skilled physical therapy intervention to date and is able to continue to improve remaining upper extremity strength deficits on his own via a home exercise program (attached) as indicated via performance-testing conducted today. He has regained full ability and participation in activities according to the PSFS and QuickDASH. He has met all established goals except for the ability to return to his previous exercise program, which included upper body resistance training. He has executed some of the activities of his previous exercise routine, however not at the pre-injury intensity level. At this time, he demonstrates safe execution of the home exercise program designed to continue to build upper extremity strength. Discontinue current episode of care at this time.

Criteria/Justification for Termination

The above documentation for Mr. X illustrates that you have determined, based on objective data from your reassessment, that it is appropriate to conclude the episode of care for your patient or client. By relaying the results of your re-examination and formulating your clinical impression via your evaluation, you have indicated your professional judgment of your patient or client's current physical and functional status. You have also indicated that skilled physical therapy care is no longer necessary for your patient or client to work towards the remaining unmet goal of returning to his previous exercise program. By defining the plan for addressing the impairments in body functions and structures, activity limitations, and participation restrictions that remain, you have relayed the criteria or justification for termination from the outpatient physical therapy plan of care, which is another important element of the conclusion of the episode of care summary (Table 7-1).

Degree of Outcomes/Goals Achievement

Another appropriate section to include in the conclusion of the episode of care documentation is an indication of the degree to which your patient or client's outcomes or goals were achieved (Table 7-1). If you are to make a judgment regarding the extent to which goals were met, the actual goals established at the start of care and any goals established during a subsequent re-examination should be listed and included as part of the conclusion of the episode of care summary. The degree of goal achievement can be indicated by a ratio scale (TABLE 7-3) or by a categorical or ordinal scale such as "goal met" or "goal unmet" or goal "fully," "partially," or "not met," respectively. Delineating the degree of goal achievement in the conclusion of the episode of care documentation will permit you to indicate reasons why some goals or outcomes may not have been met. In the scenario above, your patient or client did not meet the long-term goal relating to regaining full functional upper extremity strength. It

TABLE 7-3   Measurement of Goal Achievement in the Conclusion of the Episode of Care Summary

Goal Term	Goal	Achievement (4 Week Reassessment)	Achievement (8 Week Reassessment)
Short	In 3 weeks (9 weeks post-op), patient or client's will demonstrate full active ROM of the L elbow and forearm to allow for improved mobility for dressing, grooming, and feeding tasks.	~ 90% met	~ 95% met
Short	In 4 weeks (11 weeks post-op) patient or client's will demonstrate the ability to carry objects at least 5# in L hand to allow for improved ability with household tasks such as putting objects (dishes) away in cabinets.	~ 70% met	100% met
Long	In 7 weeks (13 weeks post-op), patient or client's will demonstrate the ability to retrieve and replace 8# object on overhead shelf to assist with household tasks such as retrieving a gallon of milk from the refrigerator.	~ 25% met	100% met
Long	In 8 weeks (14 weeks post-op), patient or client's will demonstrate the ability to assume an all-fours position on the floor to ensure ability to access and retrieve items from floor-level cabinets.	~50% met	100% met
Long	In 8 weeks (14 weeks post-op) patient or client's will demonstrate the ability to push or pull at least a 50# load to ensure ability to perform tasks such household chores and to resume pre-injury workout routine.	0% met	~85% met
Long	In 8 weeks (14 weeks post-op) patient or client's will improve the Patient-Specific Functional Scale average score by three points demonstrating meaningful and clinically significant improvement in function.	100% met	100% met
Long	In 8 weeks (14 weeks post-op), patient or client's will improve QuickDASH symptom/disability score by 10 points demonstrating meaningful and clinically significant improvement in function.	100% met	100% met
Long	In 8 weeks (14 weeks post-op), patient or client's will be independent with a self-directed home exercise program aimed at regaining upper extremity strength.	~50% met	100% met

is appropriate to speculate on why this goal was deemed as not fully met to reaffirm your decision to implement the conclusion of the episode of care plan despite falling short of meeting this goal. The conclusion of the episode of care documentation in the scenario above states that a clinically significant improvement in activity limitations and participation restrictions was indicated by the self-report and performance-based outcome measures used. Therefore, it is pertinent to relay the plan for those goals that have not been met by the end of the plan of care and indicate that continued progress can be achieved with a self-directed home exercise program designed for continued strength building.

PLAN RELATED TO CONTINUING CARE

Plans related to the patient or client's continuing care are appropriate details to include in the conclusion of the episode of care documentation. In the scenario above, continuing care includes implementing a self-directed home exercise program. Additionally, it is relevant to include a description or list of any equipment provided to the patient or client to aid with implementing the conclusion of the episode of care plan such as a tub bench, a rolling walker, the home exercise program document itself, or resistance bands, for example. Lastly, alternative plans may include referrals for additional services or recommendations for continued physical therapy care in a different setting.

Content Specific to the Care Setting

The content of the conclusion of the episode of care summary should include information as indicated in Table 7-1 regardless of the clinical setting or clinical scenario. However, the format of this documentation may vary and additional content may exist specific to the clinical setting or clinical scenario that is pertinent to include in the conclusion of the episode of care summary.

Assume that your patient or client from the scenario above had comorbid conditions or complications after the distal biceps tendon repair that warranted a hospitalization. A conclusion of the episode of care summary containing all the recommended elements (Table 7-1) after a 2-week inpatient rehabilitation facility stay might appear as indicated in **FIGURE 7-1**. The patient or client's current physical or functional status is relayed via the Functional Independence Measure (FIM) scores. The "Assessment" and "Plan" sections of the summary indicate the justification for the termination of physical therapy services in the inpatient rehabilitation setting. The degree of goal achievement is clearly stated in the "Activity" and "Additional PT Goals" sections, as is an indication for goals 4–6 not being met. Lastly, the conclusion of the episode of care recommendations section indicates that a home exercise program has been prescribed and issued, a list of durable medical equipment has been recommended, and a referral for additional home health physical therapy services has been suggested. Additional information that is specific to the conclusion of the episode of care summary in an inpatient rehabilitation facility could include length of stay, the reason for hospital admission, and a summary of the procedures or interventions delivered during the length of stay.

Now assume that after 4 weeks of home health physical therapy, the conclusion of the episode of care summary recommends that your patient or client continue with outpatient therapy. This conclusion of the episode of care summary might appear as indicated in **FIGURE 7-2**. The patient or client's physical and functional status, justification for termination of physical therapy services in the home care setting, the degree of goal achievement, reasons for some goals not being met, and plans related to continued care are clearly indicated but appear with alternative headings than those presented in Table 7-1.

Now assume that your patient or client was attending outpatient physical therapy as in the scenario above, but requires assistance from a family member or a caregiver to safely execute the home exercise program you provided due to some other barrier to independent performance such as a gait and balance disorder or cognitive impairment. Documentation to reflect this assistance might appear in the conclusion of the episode of care summary from the outpatient setting as indicated below.

> Mr. X demonstrated the ability to safely execute the home exercise program as issued today (handout) with intermittent verbal cues for appropriate body position and alignment. Because of his impaired memory, his wife has agreed to deliver verbal reminders and provide tactile cues as needed during daily home exercise program performance. She demonstrated the ability to effectively assist with the home exercise program during today's session.

Xxxx Rehabilitation

Physical Therapy Conclusion of the Episode of Care Summary

Patient Name; DOB: Xxxxx Xxxxx; xx/xx/xxxx   **Physician:** Xxxx Xxxxx

Health Record #: 123456   **Admission Date:** 07/31/2013   **Room #:** Xxx

Length of Stay: 07/31/2013 to 08/16/2013   **Units of Service during Length of Stay:** Xxx

Reason for Hospital Admission: R distal biceps tendon repair on 7-25-2013. Patient or client suffered a myocardial infarction (MI) with subsequent quadruple coronary artery bypass graft surgery (CABG) surgery on 7-26-2013.

Intervention Targets: therapeutic exercise; home exercise program, durable medical equipment recommendations; functional training (bed mobility; transfers).

Summary of Rehabilitation Stay: patient or client was admitted to facility on 7-31-2013 from acute hospital with a diagnosis of acute MI with subsequent quadruple CABG 2 days s/p R distal biceps tendon repair. Patient or client was seen for an initial examination on 7-31-2013 and received PT and OT services until discharge from hospital on 8-16-2013.

Past Medical History: primary condition: CAD with acute MI; CABG. Secondary condition: R distal biceps tendon repair; atrial fibrillation. See health record for further details.

Precautions: safety/observation of chest precautions during transfers, bed mobility, dressing, grooming and bathing tasks; avoid heavy exertion, limit shoulder ROM and thoracic extension.

Contraindications: None.

Patient or Client's Goals for PT: Improve stamina, regain use of R arm.

Impairments in Body Functions and Structure:

Cognition – awake, alert, and oriented to person, place, time, and event.

Strength – Five Time Sit to Stand = 26 sec (41 sec initial); see OT Discharge Summary for other UE strength measurements; Grip strength: R = 35#; L = 74# (R = 16#; L = 65# initial).

Endurance – 6-Minute Walk Test (6MWT) = 472 feet; rest breaks as needed (no device) (368 ft w/ 4-wheeled rolling walker initial).

ROM – AROM of B LE allow for functional mobility; L UE allows for assistance with sit-to-stand transfers and bed mobility.

Posture – mild forward head; rounded shoulders; continues to wear hinged elbow brace on R UE locked in 45 deg of flexion during most waking hours and to sleep.

Integument – healed sternotomy incision at anterior chest; healed chest tube incision at L upper quadrant; heeled saphaneous vein incision L LE from proximal medial malleolus to mid inner thigh; healed incision 1 inch distal to R cubital fossa.

Edema – mild pitting edema at R medial forearm ~ 4 inches distal to olecranon.

Sensation – decreased to LT in a stocking-in-glove distribution at the R forearm (volar surface) from incision to proximal radioulnar joint; intact B LE.

Tone – hypertonicity noted in R forearm flexors.

Gait: 10-Meter Walk Test (10MWT) = 0.91 m/s (no device); slow speed with intermittent rest breaks after 125 feet (0.82 m/s initial).

Fall Risk: Functional Gait Assessment (FGA) = 23/30 (14/30 initial).

Balance: Berg Balance Scale (BBS) = 48/56 (39/56 initial).

Pain (avg. in last week): 6/10 volar surface of R forearm; 3/10 dorsal surface of R wrist; 5/10 posterior aspect of R shoulder.

FIGURE 7-1 Conclusion of the Episode of Care Summary from an Inpatient Rehabilitation Facility.

Activity Limitations:

FIM	IE	Current	LTG	STATUS	DATE
Rolling R	NA	NA	NA	NA	8/16/2013
Rolling L	MOD A	I	SUP	Met	8/10/2013
Sit-to-Supine	MAX A	I	I	Met	8/13/2013
Supine-to-Sit	TOTAL	MOD I	MOD I	Met	8/13/2013
W/C to Bed					
Stand-pivot	MOD A	SUP	SUP	Met	8/10/2013
Toilet Transfer					
Stand-pivot	MAX A	SUP	SUP	Met	8/10/2013
Tub/Shower	MAX A	MOD I	SUP	Met	8/16/2013
Car	NA	MOD I	MOD I	Met	8/16/2013
W/C Set Up	MOD A	I	I	Met	8/10/2013
W/C Propulsion	TOTAL	I	I	Met	8/10/2013
Sitting Balance	MIN A	I	I	Met	8/4/2013
Standing Balance	MOD A	SUP	SUP	Met	8/16/2013
Sit-to-Stand	MAX A	SUP	SUP	Met	8/7/2013
Ambulation	MIN A	SUP	SUP	Met	8/16/2013

Ambulation Distance – See tests above.
Ambulation Device   None.

Curbs (8 inches)	NA	SUP	SUP	Met	8/16/2013
Steps (4 inches)	NA	SUP	SUP	Met	8/16/2013

Additional PT Goals:

1. Improve grip strength at R UE to within 50% of L UE grip for ADLs.   GOAL MET
2. Improve FGA Score to at least a 22/30 to indicate a decreased likelihood of falls.   GOAL MET
3. Improve BBS at least 8 points to indicate a clinically significant improvement in balance.   GOAL MET
4. Improve 6MWT distance by at least 50 meters indicating a clinically significant increase in cardiovascular endurance for ADLs.   GOAL NOT MET*
5. Improve 10MWT by at least 0.13 m/s indicating a clinically significant increase in gait speed for ADLs.   GOAL NOT MET*
6. Improve Five Times Sit to Stand time to ≤ 15 seconds indicating a clinically significant increase in LE strength for ADLs.   GOAL NOT MET*

*goals partially met

Conclusion of Episode of Care Recommendations: Ambulate as primary means of mobility; recommend tub bench (owns), grab bars (installed); home exercise program provided (attached).

Assessment: Patient or client has demonstrated increased functional skills during inpatient LOS.

Plan: Conclude episode of care to home from inpatient rehabilitation physical therapy services based on current level of function and level of family/caregiver support; requested referral issued by physician for home health physical therapy services for UE ROM, strength, and function, and falls risk assessment.

Date: 08/16/2013

Therapist: Xxxxxx Xxxxxxx

FIGURE 7-1

XXXXX Home Health Services, Inc.

Conclusion of the Episode of Care Summary: Physical Therapy

Patient Name: Xxxxxx Xxxxx   **Health Record Number:** 123456

Date: 09/09/2013

Start of Care Date: 08/19/2013   **Last Visit Date:** 09/09/2013

Reason for Conclusion of the Episode of Care: Mr. X has made excellent progress toward improving his gait speed, aerobic endurance, and overall functional ability with bed mobility and transfers. He continues to demonstrate deficits with his UE and LE strength, R elbow ROM, and fall risk. Mr. X has met goals established at the initial examination as indicated below and is able to continue towards unmet goals with more intense outpatient physical therapy services.

Continued Services Recommended: outpatient physical therapy services are recommended to improve UE strength and function and to decrease fall risk.

Current Physical/Functional Status:

- Transfers = Independent
- Bed Mobility = Independent except rolling to R and side lying on the R due to pain that persists at R elbow and forearm
- AROM UE = All allows for full function with transfers and bed mobility except R elbow = 3 to 129 degrees
- MMT UE = Grossly 4+ to 5/5 L UE; R biceps = 3/5; R triceps = 4-/5; R supinator = 4/5; R wrist flexors = 4/5; R wrist extensors = 3+/5; R shoulder flexors and abductors = 4/5
- Gait = Timed Up and Go = 18 sec (initial = 24 sec) (no device); 10MWT = 1.07m/s (initial = 0.90m/s); 6MWT = 608 feet
- LE Functional Strength = Five Times Sit to Stand = 22 sec (initial = 29 sec)
- Fall Risk = Mini-BEST Test = 18/28 (initial = 14/28)
- Pain (avg. in last week) = 7/10 volar surface of R forearm; 3/10 dorsal surface of R wrist; 3/10 posterior aspect of R shoulder

Goals/Outcomes:

1. Demonstrate the ability to perform supine-to-sit transfer with safety and independence to allow for bedside commode chair transfer in the middle of the night.   GOAL MET
2. Demonstrate the ability to perform tub/shower transfer with safety and modified independence (use of grab bars, seat).   GOAL MET
3. Demonstrate the ability to ambulate household distances without shortness of breath or need for sitting break indicating improved aerobic capacity and endurance.   GOAL MET
4. Demonstrate improved elbow AROM to allow patient/client to independently don/doff shirt and jacket.   GOAL MET
5. Demonstrate improved elbow AROM to allow patient/client to independently wash and groom hair.   GOAL NOT MET
6. Demonstrate improved UE strength to allow for patient/client to retrieve at least a 3# item from eye-level shelf.   GOAL NOT MET
7. Improve Mini-BEST Test score to 22/28 to indicate an improvement towards a decreased fall risk.   GOAL NOT MET
8. Improve Five Times Sit to Stand time to ≤ 15 seconds indicating a clinically significant increase in LE strength for ADLs.   GOAL NOT MET
9. Improve 10MWT by at least 0.13 m/s indicating a clinically significant increase in gait speed for ADLs.   GOAL MET

Conclusion of the Episode of Care Instructions to Patient/Family: Recommend continued performance of daily HEP as prescribed (attached) until outpatient physical therapy services start.

Notification of Conclusion of the Episode of Care to Referring Physician:

☐ Yes   ☐ No   Reason:

PT Signature: Xxxxxxx Xxxxx

FIGURE 7-2 Home Health Conclusion of the Episode of Care Summary.

Content Specific to the Clinical Scenario

In addition to the necessary elements of the conclusion of the episode of care documentation as recommended by the APTA, other essential components include the patient or client's identifying information such as a name and a health record number on each page of the health record, as well as the name of the physical therapist who created the document. Aside from this general information, scenarios exist that warrant additional details in the conclusion of the episode of care planning and documentation. You may have patients or clients whose conclusion to the plan of care is less straightforward than the patient or client who makes specific progress with intervention and is able to continue with a self-directed home exercise program. As you proceed through creating your plan of care, you may realize that it can be challenging to accurately envision the execution of the actual discharge plan at the time of the initial examination. According to the *Guide for Physical Therapist Practice*, creating the plan of care includes not only developing goals and expected outcomes, recommending an anticipated level of improvement or recovery, and proposing an estimate of the duration and frequency interventions, but also generating the anticipated conclusion of the episode of care plans. As the plan of care progresses and reassessment or re-examination occurs, it is important to determine if the anticipated goals and expected outcomes have been met. If this criterion has been met, then the conclusion of the episode of care, as indicated for Mr. X above, is warranted. If goals and expected outcomes have not been met, then a decision about the continuation of the plan of care must be made and supporting documentation indicated. If you conclude an episode of care for a patient or client when goals and expected outcomes have not been met, then a rationale for the decision to conclude the episode of care for the patient or client must be included in the conclusion of the episode of care summary. Consider the following scenario.

> Your patient or client is a 39-year-old female with complaints of right heel pain. She states that this pain started about 1 year ago after she participated in a 5K walk that was part of a fundraising event. She reports that her worst pain was attempting to walk after getting out of bed upon waking in the morning. She indicated that she experienced similar left heel pain about

6 months ago after a 5K event. You discussed the possibility of orthotics to improve her foot mechanics based on your findings at the examination. She indicated at that time that she likes to wear different shoes so she is not interested in orthotics. After eight visits with no change in symptoms, you reintroduce the use of orthotics. She reiterates that she will not likely wear them. You indicate that you are referring her to her physician for further care given the lack of progress towards the goals and expected outcomes by the end of the established plan of care.

In the scenario above, you may decide to keep the health record open to determine a further plan of care based on future discussions with the patient or client and the referring physician. Alternatively, you may deem it appropriate to write a conclusion of the episode of care summary as indicated below.

> Ms. R received physical therapy services two times per week for 4 weeks for impairments in body functions and structures, activity limitations, and participation restrictions due to right heel pain. After eight visits, Ms. R reports that significant pain and dysfunction persists per the re-examination conducted today (attached). Interventions included manual therapy, therapeutic exercise, ultrasound, ice packs, and a home exercise program aimed at symptom management. Due to minimal progress towards the goals established at the initial examination, follow-up medical care is recommended to determine further intervention. The patient has not previously used orthotics or a prescribed anti-inflammatory medication and has indicated that she prefers not to utilize these interventions. Ms. R indicated today that she will continue with her home exercise program as it provides temporary relief of pain, until she is able to make a follow-up appointment with her physician. Conclude current physical therapy episode of care at this time.

The current physical or functional status is relayed via the re-examination performed at the conclusion of the episode of care visit since this is the mechanism that will allow you to determine progress towards the goals and expected outcomes created at the initial examination. Similarly, the justification for the termination of the plan of care is also gleaned from the re-examination data. Details of what interventions were implemented and those the patient or client has not yet tried are noted, which may give some insight as to potential future plans related to continued care.

Alternative clinical scenarios may exist such that you do not have an opportunity to determine if the patient or client's goals and expected outcomes have been met or not. Consider that your patient or client does not return for any follow-up visits after the initial examination. The conclusion of the episode of care summary in this situation could appear as follows.

> Mrs. A was initially examined on 10/23/2014 for low back pain. A plan of care was established at that time; however she did not return for any follow-up visits. A voicemail was left for her on 11/3/2014 and again on 11/10/2014. Conclude the episode of care at this time since attempts at contacting Mrs. A were not successful.

It is a professional courtesy to attempt to contact an individual who has not attended a missed appointment to determine the reason for the absence and to resolve any barriers that may exist to the patient or client attending physical therapy. It is then appropriate to document the outcome of the attempted communication in the conclusion of the episode of care summary.

Clinical Reasoning to Determine Conclusion of the Episode of Care Readiness

The ability to accurately define each necessary component for the conclusion of the episode of care summary at the time of the initial examination is a skill that develops over time as you gain experience self-reflecting on the clinical decisions you make. **FIGURE 7-3** depicts an **algorithm** intended to assist you with the clinical decision of determining if your patient or client is approaching conclusion of the episode of care readiness as you progress through the plan of care created at the initial examination. The algorithm indicates that a pertinent initial question when determining the appropriate timing for concluding an established plan of care is, "Do functional deficits persist?" If the answer is "no," as in the case of Mr. X above, then the algorithm asks, "Is the patient or

client set with appropriate home exercise program or self-management strategies?" If the answer is "yes," then it is appropriate to conclude the physical therapy plan of care. If the answer is "no," then an additional time for the plan of care is warranted to establish the home exercise program and subsequently conclude the plan of care. As you progress through the plan of care, if functional deficits persist then the algorithm indicates a follow-up question, "Are deficits likely to change with skilled intervention?" If the answer to this question is "no," then the algorithm directs you to issue a home exercise or self-management program and prepare the patient or client for concluding the plan of care. If you determine that your patient or client's deficits are likely to change with your intervention, then an appropriate follow-up question is, "Are your skills required to make the change?" If the answer is "no," then again you are to consider the delivery of a home exercise or self-management program and subsequent conclusion of the plan of care. If you determine that your skills are required to make further progress towards the anticipated goals and expected outcomes, then an appropriate follow-up question is, "Does the patient or client wish to continue?" If the answer is "no," then the appropriate course is to prescribe a home exercise or self-management program and conclude the plan of care. If your patient or client does wish to continue with the plan of care, then an appropriate follow-up question is, "Do financial resources exist to continue needed services?" If the answer to this question is "yes," then the plan of care should continue towards the goals and expected outcomes as established at the initial examination or as updated at a subsequent re-examination. If the answer is "no," then an appropriate follow-up question is to determine if your patient or client is willing to pay out-of-pocket for the recommended services. If your patient or client is able to self-pay, then care should continue until you and your patient or client are satisfied with the outcomes of the plan of care. If your patient or client is unable or unwilling to self-pay, then the algorithm directs you to pursue alternative reimbursement options such as charity funding, for example. If alternative funding options do not exist then the algorithm directs you to prescribe the appropriate home exercise or self-management strategies and subsequently conclude the plan of care.

Consider that you are working with a patient or client who continues to display functional deficits; however

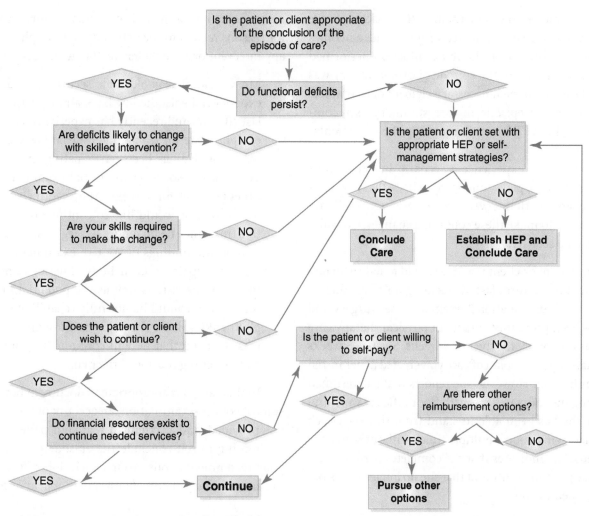

FIGURE 7-3 Conclusion of Episode of Care Algorithm.
Created by and used with permission from Raine Osborne.

these deficits are unlikely to change with physical therapy intervention such as in the scenario below.

Your patient or client is a 66-year-old male with right shoulder pain. He has been diagnosed with a supraspinatus tear and a labral tear. His physician has recommended physical therapy to address the existing impairments, activity limitations, and participation restrictions before discussing surgical management. After 8 weeks, your patient or client's function has minimally improved due to persisting pain and disability.

Your conclusion of the episode of care summary is as follows.

Mr. A has made slow and minimal progress towards regaining his function and abilities with skilled physical therapy intervention due to the presence of a full-thickness rotator cuff tear with labral involvement at the right shoulder. The attached re-examination indicates that significant functional deficits persist including the inability to complete dressing and grooming tasks as well as activities required for participation in his job as an accountant. He has been educated regarding a sleeping position that minimizes pain and sleep disruption, as well as a home exercise program designed to maintain current available shoulder active range of motion. Conclude current plan of care at this time with referral to the physician for consultation regarding further management of right shoulder pain.

It is assumed in the conclusion of the episode of care summary above that the degree of goals and outcomes achieved are indicated in the re-examination performed when the conclusion of the episode of care summary was created. Otherwise, each necessary element of a complete conclusion of the episode of care summary as recommended by the APTA is represented in the documentation above.

You may also experience a scenario in which your patient or client displays functional deficits that may continue to change with intervention; however your skills are not necessary to make these continued changes. Consider the following scenario.

> Your patient or client is a 55-year-old female who had a total knee arthroplasty 5 weeks ago. You conducted her initial examination 2 weeks after her surgery and have been providing outpatient physical therapy care 3 days per week for the last 3 weeks. She has 3 weeks remaining in the plan of care you created at her initial examination. However, she reports that she resumed taking the stairs to her fourth floor office at work and that she has been able to stand from the low couch in her living room multiple times without using her hands. She indicates that she completes her home exercise program daily and that she no longer needs her pain medication.

In this case, it is appropriate to verify your patient or client's abilities against the goals and expected outcomes established at the initial examination and provide an updated and comprehensive home exercise program. Your conclusion of the episode of care documentation may appear as follows.

> Mrs. B has met all of her established goals and expected outcomes as indicated by the attached re-examination. She demonstrates the ability to safely perform and implement a home exercise program (attached) dosed to allow for continued independent strength building. Conclude current plan of care at this time.

It is also likely that you experience a situation where, according to your judgment, significant functional deficits persist. However, your patient or client does not wish to continue with the plan of care for reasons related to personal or environmental contextual factors rather than for reasons related to the actual delivery of physical therapy interventions. Consider the following scenario.

> Mr. C is a 40-year-old male security guard. He has experienced episodic low back and leg pain over the last 10 years and recently has experienced an episode of right posterior leg pain and distal lower extremity weakness. He has been participating in the plan of care you developed at the initial examination three times per week for 3 weeks. At his tenth visit he relays to you that he would like to continue on his own at this time since he no longer has leg pain. You educate him on the findings of your re-examination regarding the impairments in body functions and structures that persist, as well as the potential for future recurrences should he not fully rehabilitate. He simply thanks you for the help you have given him and reassures you that he will continue his core and leg strengthening routine at the gym.

In this case, it is appropriate to document both the results of your re-examination, an account of the education you provided, and a statement that your patient or client is choosing to self-conclude the episode of care against your recommendations. Your conclusion of the episode of care summary documentation may appear as follows.

> Mr. C has made progress to date towards the goals and expected outcomes established at the initial examination. However, it is Mr. C's desire at this time to terminate his plan of care 3 weeks early in favor of continuing on his own at his gym. According to a re-examination conducted at today's visit (attached), significant impairments in body functions and structures remain including his distal lower extremity weakness, restricted lumbar range of motion, lumbar instability, and poor motor control. Mr. C has been educated regarding the deficits that remain and that the goals and outcomes established at the initial examination have not yet been met. He expresses understanding and reports that he knows which activities to continue at the gym to build strength. A gym/home exercise program with education regarding safe lifting and bending mechanics was recommended per the attached document. Conclude current plan of care at this time.

Plans of care may also terminate for reasons unrelated to the actual delivery of physical therapy interventions including insurance or financial limitations. Consider the following scenario.

D is a 14-year-old female high school basketball athlete who had an anterior cruciate ligament reconstruction 4 weeks ago. She has been coming to outpatient physical therapy two times per week for the last 3 weeks and is making steady progress towards improving her knee range of motion, her gait mechanics without her crutches, and the activation of her quadriceps musculature. Your patient or client's mother informs you at the seventh visit that she will no longer have insurance coverage and that her daughter will be unable to continue with physical therapy. After discussing alternative payment options, your patient or client's mother determines that her daughter will not be able to continue.

In this case, in addition to documenting your patient or client's current physical and functional status with a re-examination, the degree of goal achievement to date, and any education provided, it is important to indicate what avenues have been explored in an effort to continue care for your patient or client. Your conclusion of the episode of care summary documentation may appear as follows.

D is making steady progress towards the goals and expected outcomes established at the initial plan of care; however she is unable to continue physical therapy due to the fact that her mother no longer has insurance coverage. Her mother has also indicated that she is unable to pay the discounted self-pay rate. Therefore, the patient or client has been given a progressive home exercise program as issued today (attached) designed to build strength over the next 3 months. The patient or client and her mother demonstrate understanding of how to progress this exercise program and have agreed to check in with her surgeon in 1 week for the scheduled follow-up appointment. The patient or client's mother has also agreed to return to a physical therapist with her daughter for a progression of the exercise program and for a re-examination of her daughter's knee prior to the start of basketball season so that future injury can be avoided. Conclude current plan of care at this time.

Summary

A conclusion of the episode of care summary represents the closure of the plan of care. The initiation of the plan of care is the appropriate time for a physical therapist to plan for the patient or client's conclusion of care and to be thinking about any potential referrals to alternative healthcare providers. A complete and informative conclusion of the episode of care summary should include all of the elements detailed in Table 7-1 regardless of the document's format, which varies depending on the care delivery setting or the electronic tools used to generate components of an electronic health record. Overall, the content of the conclusion of the episode of care documentation should be driven by your clinical reasoning process as the physical therapist finalizing the plan of care. In other words, the content of the conclusion of the episode of care summary should not be determined by a third-party payer or the type of setting in which the patient or client received physical therapy care. There are unique documentation requirements that exist, however, of which you should be aware as a physical therapy professional. The Outcome and Assessment Information Set (OASIS) is a group of data elements that formulates the basis for documentation in a home health setting required by Centers for Medicare and Medicare Services for certified home health agencies. **Appendix 7-A** includes the content that would be added to the conclusion of the episode of care documentation for a patient or client filing a claim under worker's compensation. Realize however, that regardless of the setting or third-party payer, the basic structure and content of documentation that supports reasonable and medically necessary physical therapy services is the same.

Adopting a systematic approach to creating the conclusion of the episode of care summary document should assist you with becoming more proficient at accurately determining the details of the conclusion of the episode of care summary content at its inception at the initial examination. The APTA *Guide to Physical Therapist Practice* indicates that the primary criterion for a patient or client's conclusion of the episode of care is the achievement of the anticipated goals and expected outcomes. The content of a conclusion of the episode of care summary should therefore highlight if the goals and outcomes occurred as you hypothesized, with a rationale explaining any shortcomings of your predictions.

> **BOX 7-1 The Electronic Health Record: The Conclusion of the Episode of Care Summary**
>
> One important goal of an electronic health record is to improve efficiency and facilitate real-time documentation. Real-time documentation, also known as documenting at the point-of-service, refers to the idea that you complete your documentation during your encounter with your patient or client rather than wait until the end of the morning or the end of the afternoon to complete all of your documentation for the day. Additionally, it may be tempting to delay the creation of the conclusion of the episode of care documentation since the patient or client's episode of care is over and they will not be immediately returning to your clinical setting. Consider, however, that there may be other consumers of your documentation such as a third-party payer or a case manager waiting for your documentation to be complete so that they can make decisions based on it on behalf of your patient or client. Consider also that you could be contacted by the patient or client who wants to take your documentation to a new healthcare provider to relay what they achieved in physical therapy.
>
> Documenting in real time as the service is being rendered will help you to record accurately the actual events that occurred at the patient or client's final visit. Documenting the conclusion of the episode of care in a timely manner can also help you to gain insight to your ability to prescribe a plan of care for your patient or client and how your patient or client was actually able to carry out the conclusion of the episode of care with your assistance. In the electronic health record, it is likely that the initial examination and the re-examination you create will carry over specific content to populate data fields in your conclusion of the episode of care summary. Therefore, the quality with which you create those early documents at the beginning of the episode of care will have a direct impact on the quality of the conclusion of the episode of care summary.

Discussion Questions

1. In your own words, what is the purpose of the conclusion of the episode of care summary?
2. When you write a conclusion of the episode of care summary, who is the intended audience? What is the take-home message you expect the note's user to get from the conclusion of the episode of care documentation you create?
3. Identify a conclusion of the episode of care summary that you have written and examine it according to the following criteria.
   a. Have you included a statement of the patient or client's current physical or functional status?
   b. Have you indicated the criteria for the termination of physical therapy services in that setting?
   c. Have you indicated the degree of goals or outcomes achievement?
   d. Have you included reasons that goals or outcomes were not achieved?
   e. Have you indicated plans for the continuation of care?
4. Repeat the exercise above with a conclusion of the episode of care summary created by one of your peers, colleagues, or clinical instructors. Give your feedback regarding the content of the conclusion of the episode of care summary.

Case Study Questions

1. You have been working with your patient or client for 12 visits. At the 10th visit at the end of last week, you completed a re-examination and determined that your patient or client would continue to benefit from skilled physical therapy care. Over these last 2 visits you mutually agree that the patient or client will continue with a home exercise program and that it is time to conclude the episode of care. The re-examination that you completed 2 visits ago is below. Create an episode of care summary from this information.

Clinical Impression: Mr. A has made progress towards his goals as determined at the initial examination 4 weeks ago due to a right rotator cuff strain. However, he continues to display significant impairments in body functions and structures, activity limitations, and participation restrictions as indicated per the below reassessment.

Activity Limitations and Participation Restrictions:

○ Inability to sit at computer for > 10 minutes without neck and shoulder pain

○ Pain with reach to overhead shelf to retrieve or replace items (clothing in closet or overhead, washing hair, can in pantry, plate in cabinet) due to neck and shoulder pain

Posture: Moderate forward head and rounded shoulders

Palpation: Hypertonicity and tenderness right anterior and middle scalenes; right levator scapula, right upper trapezius

Pain: 4/10 right side of posterior neck and lateral aspect of right upper arm

Shoulder Active Range of Motion: right flexion = 175°, right abduction = 150°

Shoulder Passive Range of Motion: right flexion = 180°, right abduction = 175°; right external rotation = 80° at 90° abduction, internal rotation = 85° at 90° abduction

Cervical Active Range of Motion: right rotation = 75° pain on right; left rotation = 60° pulling on right, extension = 40° pain on right side of neck

Cervical Passive Range of Motion: right rotation = 80°, left rotation = 75°, extension = 45° no pain in any plane

Muscle Performance: Craniocervical Flexion Test: Activation Score = 24 mmHg;

right lower trapezius = 3/5; right middle trapezius = 4/5; right rhomboids = 5/5; right supraspinatus = 4/5; right infraspinatus = 3/5; right teres minor = 4/5, right biceps = 4/5

Special Tests: - Upper Limb Tension Test (median nerve bias); - Spurling's Test; - Cervical Distraction Test; - pain with active shoulder external rotation

Other Outcome Tools: Neck Disability Index = 24%

Goals Established at Initial Examination:

1) In 4 weeks, report the ability to walk dog on leash daily for at least 10 minutes without right shoulder pain. 75% MET

2) In 4 weeks, report the ability to perform overhead reaching for dressing and bathing tasks without right shoulder pain. 50% MET

3) In 4 weeks, improve pain as measured by the Numeric Pain Rating Scale by at least 2 points to indicate a meaningful improvement in right shoulder pain. 100% MET

Additional Goals:

1) In 4 weeks, demonstrate the ability to sit at computer for work for 30-minute bouts without limitation due to right shoulder or right sided neck pain.

2) Improve activation score of deep cervical flexors via the craniocervical flexion test by at least 2 mmHg to indicate a clinically important change in motor control.

3) Improve Neck Disability Index score by at least 10% to indicate a clinically significant improvement in perceived neck disability.

Evaluation: Due to the impairments noted above in body functions and structures, activity limitations, and participation restrictions including decreased active range of motion, poor muscle performance, and continued difficulty with sitting at computer for job tasks and reaching for basic activity of daily living tasks, Mr. A has neck pain that appears to be due to muscle guarding and hypertonicty of cervical musculature. He has made some improvement with the current plan of care towards the goals established at the initial examination. He would continue to benefit from skilled physical therapy intervention 2 times per week for an additional 4 weeks to continue to work on initially established goals as well as additional goals created based on the reassessment above. Mr. A's prognosis is good based on progress indicated by the goals and his response to interventions per the flow sheet. A formal reassessment will be done in 4 weeks determine further continuation of or discharge from this plan of care.

2. Imagine a scenario where your patient or client does not return to physical therapy after the initial examination. You see that the patient or client had four appointments scheduled after the initial examination but did not return. You call your patient or client to follow up regarding her status and she shares with you that she had to go out of town for a family emergency. Your patient or client reports that her pain is much better with the intervention you provided at the initial examination and that she gets relief from the home exercise program you prescribed. She indicates that she is unsure when she will be able to return to physical therapy and you mutually agree that the plan of care will be concluded at this time. Create a conclusion of the episode of care summary based on the information you learned.

3. Mrs. A is your patient or client in an inpatient rehabilitation facility. She was admitted to your facility 1 week ago after experiencing a concussion related to a fall. You were informed by the patient or client's case manager that she was suddenly admitted to an acute care facility the night before due to respiratory distress. Create a conclusion of the episode of care summary based on this information.

4. During the evaluation after conducting the initial examination for your patient or client you educate him about your findings regarding the etiology of his vertigo. You explain that you can perform an intervention and prescribe a home exercise program for him to follow for 1 week at which time you would like him to return for a reassessment of his symptoms. He agrees. The next week you receive a message from your front office administrator thanking you for your work. Your patient or client's symptoms have resolved and since he has a $50 copay he is not going to return. Create a conclusion of care summary based on this information.

5. You work in an outpatient physical therapy center. You are reviewing your patient or client's health records and see that one of your patient or client's has not been to therapy in 2 weeks. You give her a call and learn that she thought that she had her final visit. The documentation indicates that she was seen for her last three visits by the physical therapist assistant and to continue the plan of care. Further discussion reveals that the patient or client does not wish to return to therapy at this time since she is managing well with her home exercise program. Create a conclusion of the episode of care summary based on this information.

6. You work in a skilled nursing facility. You learn that your patient or client was transferred over the weekend to an acute care facility for cardiac surgery. How can you integrate this information into a conclusion of the episode of care summary?

7. Mrs. Y is an 83-year-old sedentary female with a history of falls due to gait and balance deficits. She has myasthenia gravis diagnosed 7 years ago. She experienced a fall resulting in a hip fracture that was treated with an open reduction internal fixation approximately 3 months ago. She had a 3-week inpatient rehabilitation stay, a 6-week skilled nursing facility stay, and has been receiving home health physical therapy services for the last 4 weeks. According to your re-examination she has not fully met all of the goals and expected outcomes that you established together at her initial examination. It is your impression based on your re-examination that she has made progress with skilled physical therapy intervention to date, but that significant deficits remain. You recommend that she continue with home health physical therapy services to make additional gains towards these remaining deficits. She relays to you however that she is not interested in continuing with therapy since she has plenty of family support to help her with her daily activities. Write a conclusion of the episode of care summary to reflect this information.

8. Your patient or client is a 29-year-old female cosmetologist. She came to your outpatient clinic 6 weeks ago with complaints of right wrist and elbow pain after she reached out to catch a box of hair styling products that slipped off a shelf as she was reaching for it while at work 7 weeks ago. According to your re-examination, she has met all of the goals established at the initial examination including the ability to manage scissors and hold items such as a curling iron and a blow dryer without wrist and elbow pain. She indicates that she has not yet returned to work at the full-time status she held prior to her injury 7 weeks ago. She states that she has spoken with her employer who has agreed to allow your patient or client full return to work as a cosmetologist based on your recommendations. What information is important for you to include in her conclusion of the episode of care summary? Write documentation to reflect this information.

References

1. American Physical Therapy Association (APTA). *Standards of Practice for Physical Therapy*, RC 17-13. Salt Lake City, UT: House of Delegates of the American Physical Therapy Association; June 2013. Available at www.apta.org/HOD/. Accessed on July 7, 2014.

2. APTA. *Integration of Episode/Conclusion of Care Terminology*, RC 18-13. Salt Lake City, UT: House of Delegates of the American Physical Therapy Association; June 2013. Available at www.apta.org/HOD/. Accessed on July 7, 2014.

3. APTA. *Guide to Physical Therapist Practice* 3.0. Alexandria, VA: American Physical Therapy Association; 2014. Available at guidetoptpractice.apta.org/. Accessed on July 7, 2014.

4. APTA. *Guidelines: Physical Therapy Documentation of Patient/Client Management*. Alexandria, VA: American Physical Therapy Association; March 2005. Available at www.apta.org/Documentation/DefensibleDocumentation/. Accessed on July 21, 2013.

5. American Physical Therapy Association (APTA). *Guide to Physical Therapist Practice*, 2nd ed. Alexandria, VA: American Physical Therapy Association; 2001:49/S41.

Appendix 7-A Recommended Content for the Conclusion of the Episode of Care for Workers' Compensation Patients or Clients

Criteria for termination from the physical therapy plan of care
  ○ Return to work details such as previous job or new position with alternative job requirements

Current physical and functional status

Degree of goals/outcomes achieved
  ○ Ability to perform required job duties
  ○ Education provided for future injury prevention

Summary of any communications with patient or client's physician, case manager, adjuster, or employer

Documentation of the necessity for further clinical evaluation such as an advanced return to work program or Functional Capacity Examination

Data from the APTA's Defensible Documentation: Setting Specific Considerations in Documentation (2011).

SECTION III

Critical Issues in Physical Therapy Documentation

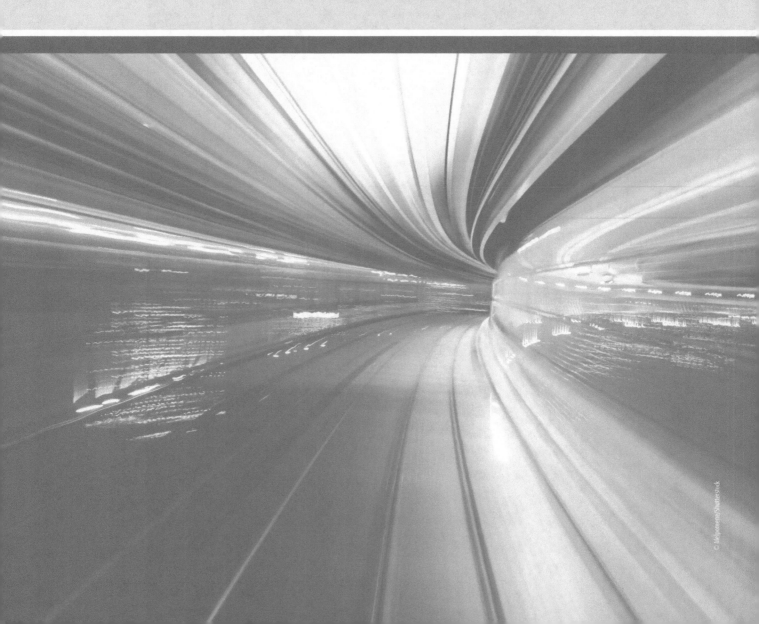

CHAPTER 8

Principles of Measurement in Documentation

Raine Osborne PT, DPT, OCS, FAAOMPT

CHAPTER OBJECTIVES

1. Review basic concepts related to the principles of measurement.
2. Describe the relevance of the principles of measurement to clinical practice and documentation.
3. Identify a framework for considering principles of measurement within clinical practice and documentation.

4. Provide examples and suggestions for integration of the principles of measurement into clinical practice and documentation.

KEY TERMS

Reliability
Responsiveness

Validity

Introduction

Applying the principles of measurement in clinical practice is a skill that is important to providing comprehensive, quality physical therapy care to your patients or clients. Therefore, it is important to possess an understanding of how to incorporate these principles into your documentation. This chapter defines the key principles of reliability, validity, and responsiveness of tests and measures and outcome tools and further develops a framework for how to incorporate this information into your documentation. Specifically, a framework for including this information in your clinical decision making and documentation that is structured around your knowledge of test selection, test performance, and test interpretation is presented.

Measurement is a concept very familiar to physical therapy professionals. The ability to select, perform, and interpret tests and measures is a principle fundamental to physical therapy education and clinical practice.[1,2] Unfortunately, the degree of knowledge and skill required to

effectively apply these principles is currently not well reflected in the documentation of physical therapy services. A recent motion passed by the APTA House of Delegates specifically directs the APTA to "...pursue documentation standards that focus primarily on clinical reasoning and decision-making in the provision of physical therapist services."[3] This represents an important paradigm shift from recording technical skills to demonstrating professional knowledge and expertise. In other words, the APTA's position represents an evolution from simply recording *what* you do within a given encounter with a patient or client to providing a rationale for *why* you are doing it. This paradigm shift in thinking and documentation is essential to the continued provision of best care to patients or clients and to demonstrate the necessity and value of our services to payers and healthcare policy makers. In order to demonstrate necessity and value, you need to provide evidence of sound decision making that leads to effective interventions resulting in meaningful outcomes. Sound decision making requires the collection and analysis of quality information. Recognizing how you can apply the principles of measurement clinically to ensure that you are collecting the best possible information, interpreting the information appropriately, and documenting this process in a manner that demonstrates your skill, knowledge, and value as a healthcare professional is essential to creating successful documentation. Consider the following scenario.

In reviewing your schedule for the day you notice a patient or client you have not previously treated is scheduled with you for a follow-up visit. The patient or client was previously seen by a therapist new to your facility. You are not familiar with the patient or client or the primary therapist, who is not working today. Appropriately, you open the patient or client's record to review the plan of care. You identify that the patient or client is 3 weeks status post right total knee arthroplasty, the prognosis is good, and the intervention frequency prescribed is three sessions per week to improve lower extremity strength and knee range of motion. Interventions include therapeutic exercise, manual therapy, neuromuscular re-education, therapeutic activities, and cryotherapy. Next you review the previous daily notes to gain an understanding of the specific interventions applied to date, the patient or client's response to these interventions, and overall progress with the plan of care. You see that the patient or client has only attended two physical therapy sessions since the initial examination. The daily notes are as follows.

VISIT 1

S: No change since examination.

I: See flow sheet for details.

R: Tolerated treatment well.

P: Continue plan of care.

FLOW SHEET

Intervention	Details
Bike	10 min
Quad sets	3 × 10
Hamstring curl	3 × 10 5 lbs
Straight leg raise	3 × 10
Knee flexion stretches	3 × 30 sec
Knee extension stretches	3 × 30 sec
Ice pack	To right knee 20 min

VISIT 2

S: No increase in pain after last session.

I: See flow sheet for details.

R: Tolerated treatment well.

P: Continue plan of care.

FLOW SHEET

Intervention	Details
Bike	10 min
Quad sets	3 × 10
Hamstring curl	3 × 10 5 lbs
Straight leg raise	3 × 10
Knee flexion stretches	3 × 30 sec
Knee extension stretches	3 × 30 sec
Ice pack	To right knee 20 min

After reading the scenario above, hopefully you have more questions than answers. If you do, then you realize that in order to make sound clinical decisions about your plan for today's session there is a lot more information you need. One series of questions you might ask is:

1. What was the amount of range of motion present in the knee joint at the initial examination?
2. What is the current range of motion of the knee joint?
3. What effect did the first two sessions have on range of motion of the knee joint?

In order to answer question number 1 you would look at the objective data from the initial examination. On review, you find the following.

Movement	Active ROM/Passive ROM
Right knee flexion	85 degrees/90 degrees
Left knee flexion	130 degrees/135 degrees
Right knee extension	–15 degrees
Left knee extension	5 degrees

What value does this information provide to your clinical decision making? You can obviously identify that there is a difference between the range of motion values for the left knee and the right knee. But, do these values represent a true difference between the right and the left knee? Do the values represent an answer to the clinical question you are asking? Indeed, you can speculate based on your knowledge and clinical experience that the differences in knee range of motion provided above are clinically significant. But how clinically significant are these values? What if the impairment in body functions and structures was a 1 cm difference in girth measurements, or a 3+/5 versus a 4–/5 difference in manual muscle testing rather than a 45-degree difference in knee flexion range of motion? In order to adequately interpret objective values you need to know some basic information about how the measurements were performed and the psychometric properties of the chosen method. For example, to interpret the clinical significance of a knee range of motion measurement, you need to know the instrument utilized to measure the range, the level of skill the primary therapist had when performing the measurement, and the position of the patient or client during the measurement. This information will provide valuable information related to the reliability and validity of the measurement.

The **reliability** of a measurement describes how confident a clinician can be that the values obtained from the measurement are free from error and would be the same if tested multiple times.[4] The **validity** of a measurement describes the clinician's confidence that the measurement is truly measuring what it is intended to measure (p.77).[4] If you were to measure the knee range of motion again and found a 10-degree increase in knee flexion range of motion and a 3-degree increase in knee extension range of motion, would this reflect a true change in the amount of range of motion in the patient or client's knee? To answer this question, not only do you need to know if you measured the range using the same instrument with the patient or client in the same position as the original measurement, but you also need to know something about the responsiveness of the measurement. The **responsiveness** of a measurement describes the amount of change in value necessary to be confident that a change has truly occurred (p.112).[4] Thus, knowing that a goniometer has a measurement error of 5 degrees allows you to judge that knee range of motion improved to a level that is deemed clinically significant and that knee extension range of motion did not. As a clinician, understanding the extent to which each of these measurement principles is present in the objective measure being considered is essential to sound clinical decision making. Furthermore, the ability to document the levels of reliability, validity, and responsiveness of tests and measures and how you interpreted

the results will likely be an increasingly important part of how physical therapy professionals demonstrate the level of care and resources required to achieve cost-effective healthcare outcomes.

To successfully incorporate data that will enhance your clinical decision making into your documentation requires knowledge of test selection, test performance, and test interpretation. Test selection includes knowing the important attributes inherent to a measure when using them to inform your clinical decision making. Test performance refers to the actual procedures utilized when executing the test such as the positions of the patient or client and the tester, the materials used to implement the measurement, the setting in which the test is conducted, and the population on whom the test is being used. Lastly, test interpretation links test selection and test performance to evidence-based decision making.

Test Selection

Volumes of textbooks, journal articles, and instructional manuals have been published or distributed describing tests and measures for all types of health conditions, impairments in body functions and structures, activity limitations, and participation restrictions related to the examination of various patient or client populations in various clinical settings. Many of these tests and measures were developed by experienced clinicians utilizing knowledge gained through many years of training and practice and passed along both formally and informally through mentoring, teaching, or publication. Historically, the selection of the "best" test or measure for any given attribute was based on the opinion of recognized expert clinicians. In 1992, Guyatt and colleagues[5] coined the term "evidence-based medicine" and heralded the shift toward more objective forms of clinical decision making (p.1).[6] Current professional practice expectations described in the *Normative Model of Physical Therapist Professional Education*[1] include the use of evidence-based practice (EBP), which has led to an increasing body of literature investigating the psychometric properties of tests and measures and the development of new tests and measures that are better able to inform clinical decision making.

Recognizing the psychometric properties of a test or measure refers to your ability to identify the characteristics of a test that can be analyzed to discern how well it measures a particular attribute. As a clinician, you are expected to select tests and measures based on the best available evidence to inform your decision making regarding diagnosis, prognosis, intervention planning, and outcomes assessment. Improved decision making through EBP is expected to result in improved health outcomes.[7] Additionally, having the knowledge and understanding of the relative strengths and weakness of various tests and measures and how to select the most appropriate tests and measures relative to the complexities of real-world clinical environments and patient or client contextual factors demonstrates your professional skill and value as a physical therapy professional. The ability to document the clinical decision making behind test selection may be necessary to justify the need for physical therapy services to third-party payers, to collaborate with other healthcare professionals, and to defend decision making in lawsuits.

The individual who selects tests or measures to be used affects the clinical decision-making process as well as documentation. Since test selection influences decisions related to diagnosis, prognosis, intervention planning, and outcomes assessment, the person who selects the tests and measures to be used carries a level of responsibility. This degree of responsibility highlights the importance of a thorough understanding of EBP, continued active participation in post-professional development, and regular review of current literature related to specific area(s) of practice. You as a physical therapy professional are well positioned to select which tests and measures will most appropriately support the plan of care you developed with your patient or client. It will be important for you as a physical therapist or physical therapist assistant to work together to ensure that the measures used are in fact the optimal choices for the patient or client. In some practice environments, a management team may select one or more of the tests and measures that are applied to all patients or clients or to those patients or clients with certain conditions. This may be done for different reasons including establishing standards of practice, tracking data for quality assurance, collecting data to demonstrate outcomes, or conducting scientific research. In these situations, you should ensure that you understand the reasoning for the selection, how to perform the tests or measures properly, how the selection will impact your clinical decision making, and if any additional tests or measures are needed to supplement the information

obtained from the standard tests and measures chosen. There are also instances where larger institutions, such as third-party payers or governmental agencies, select a set of tests and measures that are incentivized or required from a payment or regulatory standpoint. One example of this is the Physician Quality Reporting System (PQRS) developed by the Centers for Medicare & Medicaid Services.[8] These programs are generally developed to collect large amounts data that can be utilized to describe or track various aspects of health or health care in large populations, and then to create policy or programs to effect a desired change. Ultimately however, it is you who continues to hold responsibility for the care of your patient or client.

Whether you are an individual selecting tests and measures for your patient or client or you are part of a group charged with selecting tests and measures for a clinic, organization, or population, there are several factors that you should consider in the selection process (TABLE 8-1). Appropriate test selection requires an understanding of the intended purpose of the test or measure, the known reliability and validity of the test or measure, the population to which the results of the test or measure can be generalized, and the likelihood of being able to reproduce the test or measure in the intended clinical setting. Consider the following scenario.

> You are working in an outpatient clinic and you are examining a 35-year-old female with low back, buttocks, and posterior thigh pain. The patient or client reports that the pain began after missing a step coming down a ladder. She now reports pain rolling over in bed, with sit to stand transfers, when walking fast, and going up and down stairs.

As you plan your clinical examination, you must decide which tests and measures to perform. First, consider what clinical questions you have related to this patient or client. In the scenario above, you may be asking if your

TABLE 8-1 Factors to Consider When Selecting Tests/Measures/Outcome Tools

1. What is the intended purpose of the test?
2. Is the test reliable?
3. Is the test valid?
4. In what populations was the test evaluated?
5. In what settings was the test evaluated?

patient or client's pain is related to the lumbar spine or sacroiliac joint. This question would help you determine the patient or client's diagnosis. Diagnostic tests and measures are those that accurately differentiate between the presence and absence of a certain condition or attribute (p.619).[4] Therefore, diagnostic tests should demonstrate high levels of reliability and validity. Reliability is the extent that a measurement is consistent and free from error (p.77).[4] When determining reliability, consider the standard error of measurement (SEM), or the degree of variability expected in the values obtained from a given test assuming the testing procedure remains constant (p.608).[4] For example, you may decide to use a Straight Leg Raise Test to determine the presence of a lumbar radiculopathy. It is important to know if the Straight Leg Raise Test has been established as a reliable test in a young adult female population for use in an outpatient setting regardless if the test was performed by you initially or by a different clinician.

Reliability is a prerequisite to establishing validity. Put another way, a test that demonstrates poor reliability cannot be valid (p.97).[4] Validity then assures that a test actually measures what it is intended to measure (p.77).[4] There are various statistical methods used to determine reliability and validity. Some of the more common methods for reporting the reliability of a test or measure include the reliability coefficient (r), interclass correlation coefficient (ICC), or the kappa statistic (κ). The validity of a diagnostic test can be described in terms of the sensitivity and specificity, predictive values, or likelihood ratios. More complete descriptions of these methods can be found in other texts.[4]

In the scenario above, a diagnostic question is posed regarding the presence of pathology in the lumbar spine versus the sacroiliac joint (SIJ). Based on this question you may choose to include pain provocation tests for the SIJ as part of your examination. Many such tests exist to examine the SIJ. How do you select the tests to perform? How many tests are necessary? Current literature suggests that a cluster of five SIJ pain provocation tests—SIJ distraction, SIJ compression, thigh thrust, Gaenslen's Test, and Patrick's Sign—is useful in determining the presence or absence of pain originating from the SIJ. Individually, these tests have demonstrated variable reliability. However, when performed as a cluster, the reliability has been shown to be acceptable [weighted kappa 0.70 (95% CI = 0.45 – 0.95)].[9] The same is true regarding the validity of these tests. Individually, SIJ provocation tests are insufficient to make diagnostic determinations. When performed as a cluster, however, three or more positive tests represent a positive likelihood ratio (LR+) of 4.02, and fewer than three positive tests represent a negative likelihood ratio (LR–) of 0.19.[10] A LR+ of 4.02 represents a small to moderate shift in the probability that pain related to the SIJ is present. A LR– of 0.19 represents a moderate shift in the probability that pain related to the SIJ is not present (p.628).[4] The final level of confidence in the presence or absence of SIJ pain would be based on how likely it was that SIJ pain was present before performing the test. This degree of diagnostic accuracy would provide you with useful information to answer your clinical question as to the origin of your patient or client's pain.

Understanding the reliability and validity of potential tests and measures is only a first step in making an appropriate selection. The next step is to consider the characteristics of the population used in the reliability and validity studies and how similar this population is to your patient or client. The cluster of SIJ pain provocation tests described above was studied in a population of patients or clients from the Netherlands between the ages of 18 and 80 who were referred to a pain clinic with chronic low back pain below L5, over the posterior aspect of one SIJ, with or without leg pain. None of the patients or clients were pregnant, had a leg-length discrepancy of more than 2 cm, osteoporosis, osteoarthritis of the hip with clinical symptoms, radicular pain, or neurologic signs of radiculopathy.[10] If you practice in the United States does this limit your ability to generalize the results of this study done in the Netherlands to your patients or clients? What if your patient or client is pregnant or has hip osteoarthritis? What if your patient or client is in a skilled nursing setting? Does your patient or client have a characteristic that may interfere with the performance or interpretation of the test? Are there other tests that are more specific to the characteristics of your patient or client? These are all important questions to consider when selecting the most appropriate diagnostic tests to apply to your patients or clients.

The final step in selecting a test is to consider the reproducibility of the test in your specific practice setting. Does the test require special equipment that is not available to you? Does the test require a certain set of skills that you currently do not possess? Is the time required to perform the test prohibitive in relation to the value of the information obtained? Remember, a good diagnostic test is only as good as your ability to perform the test reliably and accurately in the clinical setting.

DOCUMENTING TEST SELECTION

Documenting your clinical decision making related to test selection may simply appear as a listing of the tests and measures you performed. It is important that you use terminology that is consistent with the literature supporting the use of your selected tests or measures. Therefore, if the user of your note such as your colleague or an auditor is unfamiliar with the test or measure they will be able to go to the literature for relevant information. Unfortunately, tests and measures have many abbreviations and acronyms that may not be used consistently. Material such as the APTA *Guide to Physical Therapists Practice*[2] has been implemented to address the consistency and universal understanding of nomenclature. Furthermore, the APTA emphasizes that the use of abbreviations in healthcare documentation be minimized.[11] As electronic documentation systems become more sophisticated there may be an opportunity to create direct links between the listed tests and measures and information related to the description, psychometric properties, and interpretation guidelines for each test and measure.

A strategy to capture the intended purpose of a test or measure is to organize your documentation into categories that reflect the context in which the test results should be interpreted. For example, you may have a section in your documentation labeled "Screening Tests and Measures" with subcategories for the particular attribute being screened (FIGURE 8-1), or "Health Condition Tests and Measures" with subcategories for the specific conditions (FIGURE 8-2). Inherently, tests and measures that have better sensitivity or negative likelihood ratios will be utilized as screening tests and those that have better specificity or positive likelihood ratios will be utilized diagnostically.[12] The simple act of documenting these tests in the appropriate category demonstrates your understanding as a clinician of the properties of the tests and the diagnostic process. Tests and measures designed to collect data related to impairments in body functions and structures can be labeled as such with subcategories to reflect the body functions and structures that are being examined (FIGURE 8-3). Another relevant category for documenting test selection is "Outcome Measures." Subcategories may include items such as various functional measures, quality of life measures, or pain measures (FIGURE 8-4).

When you select a test or measure, you should be able to produce relevant evidence supporting your selection if asked. For example, when collaborating with colleagues or other health professionals, you should be able to provide additional information regarding the level of evidence currently available related to the selected tests or measures and be able to discuss your clinical reasoning process that led to your selection. Similarly, when clinic or organization management selects a set of tests and measures for use by clinicians within that organization, the rationale, selection process, description of the standard procedure for performing the tests or measures, and relevant data related to test interpretation should be reflected in the policy and procedures manual for the clinic or organization. Documentation of this information will provide you as well as others such as your colleagues, payers, regulators, or legal professionals with the necessary information to understand the rationale behind the selection and the intended purpose of the information collected. It is also important for large entities such as governmental agencies and third-party payers to document and make easily available information related to selection, performance, and interpretation of tests or measures they require or recommend be included in the clinical care of patients or clients. It is important that everyone involved

Attribute or Condition Screened	Tests or Measures	Result
Deep vein thrombosis	Wells Criteria Score	0/8
Shoulder pathology	Neer Test	Negative
Pain catastrophizing	Pain Catastrophizing Scale	4/52

FIGURE 8-1 Screen-Based Tests and Measures.

Health Condition	Tests or Measures	Result
ACL rupture	Lachman Test	Positive
Cervical radiculopathy	Ipsilateral Rotation < 60°	Positive
	Spurling's Test	Positive
	Distraction Test	Positive
	Upper Limb Tension Test	Positive

FIGURE 8-2 Health Condition-Based Tests and Measures.

Function or Structure	Tests or Measures		Result	
Postural alignment	Visual observation		Increased knee flexion and decreased weight-bearing on right lower extremity	
			Left	Right
	AROM	Knee flexion	130°	95°
		Knee extension	0°	−10°
	PROM	Knee flexion	140°	100°
		Knee extension	0°	−5°
Joint mobility		Tibiofemoral anterior glide	Normal	Normal
		Tibiofemoral posterior glide	Normal	Hypomobile
	Passive Accessory Motion	Patellofemoral medial glide	Normal	Normal
		Patellofemoral lateral glide	Normal	Normal
		Patellofemoral inferior glide	Normal	Hypomobile
		Patellofemoral superior glide	Normal	Hypomobile
	Light Touch Sensation		Normal	Normal
	Pin Prick Sensation		Normal	Normal
			Left	**Right**
	Myotome Testing	L1-2 (hip flexion)	5/5	5/5
		L3 (knee extension)	5/5	5/5
		L4 (ankle dorsiflexion)	5/5	5/5
Peripheral nerve integrity		L5 (great toe extension)	5/5	5/5
		S1 (ankle plantar flexion)	5/5	5/5
		S2 (hamstring flexion)	5/5	5/5
	Deep Tendon Reflexes	L4 (patellar tendon)	2+	2+
		L5 (ext. digitorum brevis)	2+	2+
		S1 (Achilles)	2+	2+

FIGURE 8-3 Impairment-Based Tests and Measures.

Category	Tests or Measures	Result
Self-report measures	Lower Extremity Functional Scale	45/80
	Patient-Specific Functional Scale	Avg. 6/10
Performance-based measures	Five Times Sit to Stand	17 sec
	10-Meter Walk Test	0.64 m/sec
	Timed Up and Go	12 sec
	Functional Gait Assessment	20/30
Pain	Worst pain (last 7 days)	8/10
	Least pain (last 7 days)	2/10
	Current pain	4/10

FIGURE 8-4 Outcome-Based Tests and Measures.

in a patient or client's care share a common understanding of the relevant information surrounding the selected test so that informed decision making can occur on the patient or client's behalf.

Test Performance

Test performance refers to the details for administering the test or the conditions under which the test was delivered. This includes factors such as the tester's expertise, the equipment or instrumentation used to administer the test, the time of day the test was administered, the setting in which the test was given, or the characteristics of the individual who was given the test. Any detail that has the potential to influence the results of the test should also be considered to influence a test's performance. Consider the following scenario.

You work in a skilled nursing facility and have a team conference today regarding a patient or client who has received physical therapy for the last 6 weeks. You know the conversation will focus on planning for the conclusion of the episode of care. Your patient or client is an 89-year-old female who underwent an open reduction internal fixation of the right femur 10 weeks ago secondary to a fall. She has several co-morbidities and very poor functional mobility. You have to decide if she is making progress with her lower extremity muscle performance and her ability to perform chair to bed transfers. The physical therapist who initially examined the patient selected the Five Times Sit to Stand Test (FTSST) as a performance-based measure of lower extremity functional strength and ability. At the initial examination, the therapist documented that the patient or client was unable to perform even one repetition of sit-to-stand. At 2 weeks, the FTSST was reassessed by a different clinician and the documented result of the test was 23 seconds. At 4 weeks a third clinician administered the test and documented that the patient or client was only able to complete two repetitions in 35 seconds. Looking at this data, you recognize an abnormal pattern in the values.

OUTCOME MEASURES

Category	Tests or Measures	Initial Exam	2 weeks	4 weeks
Performance-Based Functional Measures	Five Times Sit to Stand Test	Unable to complete 1 repetition	23 sec	2 reps in 35 sec

The differences in the values recorded in the scenario above are likely related to differences in how the test was performed. For example, the evaluating therapist may have administered the test using a standard height chair without allowing the patient or client to utilize her arms for assistance. The second clinician may have administered the test from sitting on the edge of an adjustable mat table and allowed use of the upper extremities for assistance, and the third clinician may have instructed the patient or client to rise from the edge of the hospital bed without allowing the use of upper extremity assistance. Without knowing how the test was performed previously, how will you decide the procedure for performing the test today? Furthermore, how will you compare the results of the test today with the previous results?

The scenario above illustrates the importance of documenting not only which test is performed but also how it was performed. Even when the test or measure is very

common and a general acceptance of the proper procedure for performing the test exists, there are frequently factors that require the clinician to change the performance of the test or measure or alter it from its standard protocol. For example, a patient or client may not tolerate the typical testing position or may require alterations to the setup of the test due to a secondary health condition or additional impairments in body functions and structures. When documenting test performance it is useful to utilize the phrases "standard procedure" and "modified procedure" to relay any alterations you may have made from the way the test was intended to be performed. It is generally understood in clinical practice that a test is performed in the manner in which it was validated. Therefore, a standard procedure is one that has been previously described and tested in the literature and has been accepted as the usual method for performing a test or measure. A modified procedure is one where some change has been made to the standard procedure, which may or may not have been tested for reliability or validity in the literature. For example, an accepted standard position for measuring passive knee range of motion is in supine. If your patient or client is unable to assume a supine position and you opt to measure knee range of motion in sitting you should document that the value was obtained with the patient or client in sitting. There are also instances where a specific modification is needed to accommodate a unique situation. For example, you may wish to assess your patient or client's ability to achieve the prone position; however, they have a percutaneous endoscopic gastrostomy (PEG) tube that limits the ability to achieve prone. Therefore, your judgment and subsequent documentation regarding your patient or client's performance on this task will need to reflect the presence of the PEG tube.

As stated above, a standard procedure is one that has been previously described and accepted as the usual procedure for performing a test or measure. Consider your daily practice in reference to this definition. Do you have standard procedures for each test and measure you perform? Most clinicians likely have a typical method for performing the tests and measures they most frequently utilize. However, it is also likely that these procedures are not available such that someone reading their documentation could access the description in order to understand how the test or measure was performed. Furthermore, clinicians may accept their particular methodology as the usual procedure for a test or measure when it may actually represent a procedure that is utilized by a very small minority of clinicians. This is not to say the clinician should change the procedure he or she typically utilizes. Rather, a description of the procedure utilized should be available to other users of the documentation to better understand and reproduce the procedure as needed. The process for selecting the standard procedure should be based on a thorough review of the literature as well as on the current knowledge and skills of the clinicians who will perform them. Clinicians selecting the procedure for performing the test or measure should be able to produce relevant evidence from a thorough literature review to support the decision (TABLE 8-2). For example, a clinician who is questioned about the procedure for performing the test or measure as part of a utilization review or legal case should be able to answer the questions posed in Table 8-2 and provide the literature supporting the rationale. Not all tests or measures have been empirically investigated to the same degree, however. In situations where there is ambiguity or a lack of evidence in the literature, the clinician should be able to identify the gaps in the available data and describe the clinical rationale for the chosen procedure. For example, in describing the procedure for performing a timed tandem stance test, a question may arise regarding allowing

a patient or client upper extremity assistance to achieve the starting position before the timing begins. There may be literature that supports allowing upper extremity assistance as well as alternative literature indicating that upper extremity assistance to achieve the starting position alters the construct that the test is intended to measure.

Clinics or rehabilitation departments where there is a great degree of variability between who performs the initial examination and who performs the re-examination would likely benefit from establishing standard and alternative procedures that are accessible in a written or electronic format. The rationale for the decision, along with a detailed description of the standard and alternative procedures, should be documented and placed in a location that can easily be accessed by all clinicians. The clinic or department management should ensure that all clinicians understand each procedure and are proficient in performing it in a reliable manner. When these steps have been taken, clinicians can make informed evidence-based decisions utilizing the results of tests or measures performed by other clinicians.

DOCUMENTING TEST PERFORMANCE

Documenting test performance is simplified when standard procedures are utilized. The clinician may choose to include a sentence in the plan of care stating that standard procedures were utilized for all tests and measures unless otherwise noted. If the description of standard and alternative procedures is located somewhere such as a policy and procedures manual, an additional sentence indicating that tests and measures utilized in the examination are described in the policy and procedures manual for the clinic can also be included. If an alternative procedure was utilized then the clinician should make note in the documentation which alternative procedure was performed. For example, assume that instead of measuring passive knee flexion range of motion in supine, you opted to collect this data with your patient or client in prone due to poor tolerance to lying supine. In this scenario the clinician should state in the documentation "measured in prone" adjacent to the recorded range of motion data. The prone procedure should be listed and described as an alternative procedure in the manual describing standard and alternative procedures for tests and measures utilized in your clinic. Documentation of an unconventional method for performing a test or measure also requires a description of the modifications somewhere in

TABLE 8-2   Guidelines for Investigating the Psychometric Characteristics of a Test or Measure

Clinical Questions
1. What procedure was used when determining the reliability and validity of the test or measure?
2. If reliability and validity data exist for multiple procedures related to a test or measure, which one has the best properties?
3. To what populations can you generalize the results of the test or measure if multiple procedures exist for performing a test or measure?
4. In what setting or settings was the procedure for the test and measure investigated?
5. Do the populations of patients or clients identified in your investigation of the test or measure compare to the patients or clients you serve?
6. Did the clinicians or researchers in the study receive any special training for performing the particular procedure?
7. What were the characteristics of the clinicians or researchers performing the test or measure in the literature you reviewed?
8. Was special instrumentation used to investigate the properties of the test or measure?
9. Are the reliability and validity properties of the test or measure consistent across multiple studies?

the patient or client's health record. For example, assume your patient or client is performing a Five Times Sit to Stand Test but was unable to perform the test from a standard height chair without the use of the upper extremities for assistance. If you decide to utilize an elevated chair and allow the use of upper extremities for assistance you should include the height of the chair and the level of assistance allowed when recording the time for the patient or client to complete the test. This additional description of the test performance will allow you and any clinician who follows up with your patient or client to immediately understand how the test was performed and reproduce the testing procedure if necessary. This documentation also allows you to judge progress if your patient or client is able to perform the test from a standard height chair at subsequent testing sessions. The clinician does not have to describe the components of the testing procedure that are consistent with the standard procedure, only those aspects that deviate from standard procedure description.

In the event that the test or measure is uniquely designed for a particular patient or client, a more detailed description would be required in your documentation. For example, assume your patient or client works for the postal service and has shoulder range of motion limitation and pain while sorting mail into a series of boxes on the wall. You may decide to measure the length of time your patient or client can perform a simulated task in the clinic holding a 1-pound weight before the onset of symptoms. In your documentation, you would note that the test involves measuring the "length of time before pain or postural compensation onset at the shoulder when reaching from waist height to a series of four targets on the wall at arm's length in a 2 foot × 2 foot square starting at shoulder height to 6 inches above eye level while holding a 1-pound weight." This description provides enough detailed information for any clinician to accurately reproduce this test at a later date so that a reasonable determination of progress with the activity can be made.

Test Interpretation

Test interpretation refers to the meaning or value assigned to the results of a test or measure. The interpretation of a diagnostic test is represented by the degree to which your confidence in the presence or absence of particular condition shifts based on a positive or negative test result.

For outcome measurements such as range of motion, the Timed Up and Go, or the Oswestry Disability Index, for example, your interpretation is related to the significance of any change identified in the measurement. In order to make this determination, you need to know how the measurement was initially performed as well as how much variability in the measurement you can expect even when no change actually occurred. Consider the following scenario.

You are a clinician working in a home healthcare setting. For the last 4 weeks you have been working with an 89-year-old man who returned home following a 6-week hospital stay secondary to congestive heart failure and subsequent complications. He continues to display significant weakness and mobility limitations. You are re-examining him to determine his progress during your plan of care. At the initial examination you selected the Timed Up and Go (TUG) Test due to its ability to identify mobility limitations in this population.[13,14] As you prepare to reassess your patient or client's performance on the test you realize there are several details about the testing procedure of which you are unsure. The patient or client has some rooms that have hard floor surfaces and some rooms that have thick carpeting. You do not remember in which room you performed the TUG at the initial exam. The patient or client is able to walk without an assistive device, but generally he uses a straight cane when walking room to room in his home. You are unsure if the cane was used for the TUG during the initial exam. There are many chairs in the patient or client's home as well and you do not remember which chair you used initially.

The inability to answer these questions prior to performing the test will greatly affect your interpretation of the results. To illustrate this point, first assume that you decide to have the patient or client perform the TUG on a hard floor, using a wooden straight back kitchen chair without his cane. The initial and follow-up tests values were as follows.

OUTCOME MEASURES

Category	Tests or Measures	Exam	4 weeks	Comments
Performance-Based Functional Measures	Timed Up and Go Test	22.5 sec	18.1 sec	Performed using kitchen chair (18") on hard floor without an assistive device on follow-up.

What is your interpretation of the results? Did the patient or client improve, decline, or stay the same? To answer this question you must first understand the minimal detectable change (MDC) value for the TUG for a frail older adult man. The MDC represents the smallest difference between the test values from initial exam to follow-up that is necessary to be confident that a true change has actually occurred. The MDC is a statistical value based on the standard error of measurement discussed previously. The MDC value for a test or measure is population and procedure specific. For example, the MDC for the TUG in an 89-year-old male who independently lives at home and is recovering from a total knee arthroplasty performed 6 weeks ago is different than the MDC in a frail 89-year-old man living at home who was recently discharged from a 6-week hospital stay. The MDC value is based on how much variability is normally expected when a test is repeated and no change has occurred. Therefore, if a difference exists between your patient or client and the patient or client population in the research study, or your procedure and the procedure performed in the research study, the interpretation of the MDC value for the test or measure should be made with caution.

Revisit the scenario above. Your patient or client is consistent with the sample population studied by Mesquita et al to assess the reliability of the TUG in those with chronic organ failure.[14] Since the specifics of the procedure utilized during the initial examination of your patient or client were not documented, you are unsure how to compare the procedure to the one utilized in the study. Furthermore, you are unsure if the procedure utilized in the follow-up assessment was consistent with those performed on the initial examination. Therefore, you are unable to judge the change in TUG score to make any informed interpretation regarding the progress of the patient or client over the last 4 weeks.

Using the same TUG values for your patient or client reported above, assume that at the initial examination your patient or client performed the TUG on hard floor from the kitchen chair (18 inches) and utilized his cane. During the re-examination you performed the TUG in the same manner but did not use the cane and found that your patient or client improved his time by 4.4 seconds. Mesquita and colleagues report the MDC for the TUG in individuals with congestive heart failure as 5.46

seconds.[14] In other words, when an individual performs the TUG multiple times the score may fluctuate by as much as 5.46 seconds without a true change in performance ability actually occurring. This suggests that your patient or client did not make any change on the TUG with the interventions implemented over the last 4 weeks. However, since your patient or client initially used an assistive device he did not use during the re-examination, you do not know if the 4.4 second improvement actually represents a statistical improvement. Remembering that the patient or client was able to ambulate without an assistive device at initial examination but self-selected to utilize his cane, it is possible that the patient or client could have taken greater than 23.5 seconds to complete the test without an assistive device at the initial examination, making the decrease to 18.1 seconds a statistically significant improvement.

Now assume that your patient or client was assessed using the same testing procedures at initial examination and re-examination, and that a 5.5 second decrease in time was recorded at the follow-up as compared to the initial examination. This result represents a statistically significant improvement in the test performance based on the MDC. However, can this 5.5 second improvement be interpreted as a meaningful improvement in the patient or client's level of function? To answer this question we would have to know the minimal clinically important difference (MCID) for the TUG. The MCID represents the smallest amount of change in the results of a test or measure that would be perceived by the patient or client as a meaningful change in the attribute being assessed (p.112).[4] As compared to the MDC, which is based on statistical procedures involving test–retest performance, the MCID is based on a comparison of results from a test or measure to a group of research participants' self-report of perceived change. The MDC and MCID may or may not be similar for a given test or measure. In general, the MCID is found to represent a greater degree of change in a test or measure score. Further discussion related to the comparison of MDC and MCID can be found elsewhere.[4] In our scenario, the MCID has not been established for the TUG in a frail older adult man with congestive heart failure. This limits our interpretation of the follow-up assessment results by decreasing the degree of confidence we can have in reporting a meaningful change in functional status based on the TUG.

DOCUMENTING TEST INTERPRETATION

Your interpretation of the results of the outcome measures you collect for your patient or client during the course of an initial examination can be included in the goals you create for your patient or client within the plan of care. In other words, your goals can reflect your patient or client's expected change in performance in response to the skilled physical therapy care you deliver. As previously noted, the MDC of a measure must be known to make a judgment as to whether a true change occurred in your patient or client on that measure. Furthermore, to determine if your patient or client's function changed as indicated by the measure, the MCID of the measure must be known. Consider the following scenario.

> You are working with a 20-year-old female who is recovering from an anterior cruciate ligament reconstruction. During your initial examination you administer the Lower Extremity Functional Scale to determine her perception of her ability to perform everyday tasks. You find that her score has improved to a 24/80. You are aware that the MDC and the MCID in women recovering from ACL reconstruction is 9 points.[15]

Given this information you might decide to incorporate the MCID into the goals that you establish as part of her plan of care as follows.

> Improve the Lower Extremity Functional Scale score by at least 9 points to indicate a clinically relevant improvement in patient's ability to perform everyday tasks.

Documenting test interpretation can also be thought of as documenting intervention effectiveness, which provides an excellent opportunity to demonstrate your clinical reasoning and decision-making skills and can be included in the daily note, a progress note, a re-examination note, or a conclusion of the episode of care summary. Documenting intervention effectiveness should include a statement addressing the statistical significance (MDC) as well as the clinical relevance (MCID) of the changes observed in the test or measure. Using the scenario above, you may choose to document in your re-examination as follows.

> The patient or client's 5.5 second improvement on the TUG represents a statistically significant improvement in performance. Although the MCID for the TUG has not been established, this change combined with the decreased use of the assistive device for in-home ambulation and increased participation in community ambulation demonstrates an overall improvement in functional mobility.

If you consider your patient or client's entire health record, and assuming you thoroughly documented test selection and performance details, then your documentation will demonstrate the validity of your test selection, the degree of reliability of your test performance, and your interpretation of the results.

Summary

The basic principles of measurement—validity, reliability, and responsiveness—are utilized by physical therapists in all settings to inform clinical decisions regarding a patient or client's status and progression of the plan of care. Current documentation practices are frequently ineffective in providing the information necessary to understand the clinical reasoning behind these decisions or to make subsequent clinical decisions based on prior documentation. This chapter provides recommendations for including the information necessary to demonstrate your knowledge and expertise as well as the requisite data needed to include evidence-based clinical decision making in your documentation (TABLE 8-3). Providing this level of detail does not have to be burdensome on the already busy clinician. Although some initial work may be required to develop documentation templates and clinic policies that facilitate implementation of the recommended documentation practices, the resultant improvements in efficiency and effectiveness of the documentation will likely make these efforts worthwhile. As with any new skill, there is an initial learning curve that requires slower more conscientious performance of the task. However, with time the skill becomes automatic and efficient. The benefits in achieving more clinically useful documentation that enhances as well as demonstrates the clinical reasoning behind your decision making may improve patient or client care and better support the value of the services you provide.

TABLE 8-3 Summary of Recommendations for Documenting the Use of Tests and Measures

1. Utilize terminology consistent with the literature.

2. Organize lists of tests and measures into categories (screening tests, diagnostic tests, prognostic tests) that reflect the context or intended purpose of the test to allow for consistent test interpretation.

3. Determine the standard procedure and alternative procedures for tests and measures performed in your clinic. Create and keep a record of these procedures as well as psychometric properties that can be easily accessed by anyone who may access your note.

4. Implement a process to ensure that tests and measures procedures are regularly reviewed and updated.

5. If a test or measure is modified from the standard procedure, be sure to document information about the modification so that sound clinical judgments and interpretations can be made. Relevant information may include patient or client position, therapist position, equipment utilized, or other environmental factors such as floor surfaces.

6. Use the clinical impression section of your re-examination or "Intervention" section of your daily note or progress note to document your interpretation of tests and measures including acknowledgement of the psychometric properties and how the interpretation affected your clinical decisions.

BOX 8-1 The Electronic Health Record: Principles of Measurement

Regardless of the electronic system used in your facility, there will likely exist a drop-down menu or list of tests and outcome measures from which you can choose for implementation with your patient or client. As mentioned above, such a system could be set up to provide links to the psychometric profile of each test and outcome measures used in your clinic as well as the standard and alternative testing procedures utilized by you and your colleagues. Similarly, the potential results of a test and outcome measures you select may be pre-populated along with an interpretation of the score you enter. It is important to recognize that while an electronic system may be able to provide you with a standard description and interpretation of a test and outcome measures, only your expertise can match the data available within the electronic system to the correct patient or client. It is this critical step that will give meaning to the other principles of measurement used in your electronic documentation system.

Discussion Questions

1. Review the tests and outcome measures that you used to collect examination data on a patient or client you recently examined.
   a. Are you aware of the reliability and the validity for each of the tests you chose to perform during your examination?
   b. What factors do you need to consider in judging the reliability or validity of these tests and outcome measures?
   c. What statistical data do you need to locate to identify the reliability and the validity of these tests and outcome measures?
   d. Are there any tests and outcome measures you utilized on which you could not find reliability and validity data?
   e. How did you document your use of these tests and outcome measures?

2. Review an initial examination or re-examination note created by one of your colleagues or clinical instructors. Based on the documentation of the tests and outcome measures reported in the note, reproduce the test and measures outcome measures on your colleague or clinical instructor.
   a. Did you perform the test the way in which it was intended?
   b. Did you have to ask your colleague or clinical instructor any questions to clarify your implementation of the test?

3. Choose a test or outcome measure that you frequently use in your clinical practice. Compile information for inclusion in a procedure manual for your clinic. Include:
   a. The description of the procedure for performing the test or outcome measure
   b. Any alternative procedures for performing the test or outcome measure
   c. The population in which reliability and validity testing for the test and or outcome measure occurred
   d. The setting in which reliability and validity testing for the test or outcome measure occurred
   e. The psychometric properties of the test for the intended population and setting

Case Study Questions

1. You are working as a home health physical therapist and you have been asked to perform a re-examination on a patient or client for your colleague who is ill. As you review the note, you see that your re-examination is to include a Timed Up and Go Test, a Five Times Sit to Stand Test, a 10-Meter Walk Test, and a 6-Minute Walk Test. What information will you look for in the documentation to assist you in collecting meaningful data that can be used to judge this patient or client's progress?

2. Consider the following information.

OUTCOME MEASURES

Category	Tests or Measures	Exam	6 weeks	Comments
Performance-Based Measures	Manual Muscle Test: lower trapezius	3/5 with substitutions noted (scapular elevation, trunk rotation)	4/5 without substitutions	Performed in prone with head in neutral

a. How will you include this information in your re-examination documentation?
b. How will you include this information in your conclusion of the episode of care documentation?

3. Consider the following information.

OUTCOME MEASURES

Category	Tests or Measures	Exam	4 weeks	Comments
Performance-Based Measures	Single Limb Stance	11 sec	18 sec	Assume position and hold without upper extremity assist; terminate test when foot touches ground or other leg, or if excessive trunk or limb motion occurs.

a. How will you include this information in your re-examination documentation?
b. How will you include this information in your conclusion of episode of care documentation?

References

1. American Physical Therapy Association (APTA) Education Division. *A Normative Model of Physical Therapist Professional Education.* Alexandria, VA: American Physical Therapy Association; 2004.

2. APTA. *Interactive Guide to Physical Therapist Practice 3.0.* Alexandria, VA: American Physical Therapy Association; 2014.

3. APTA. *Physical Therapy Documentation Reform.* House of Delegates of the American Physical Therapy Association; October 1, 2013. Available at www.APTA.org. Accessed on January 4, 2014.

4. Portney LG, Watkins MP. *Foundations of Clinical Research: Applications to Practice.* Upper Saddle River, NJ: Pearson Prentice Hall; 2009.

5. Evidence-Based Medicine Working Group. Evidence-based medicine: a new approach to teaching the practice of medicine. *J Am Med Assoc.* 1992, November 4;268(17):2420–2425.

6. Straus SE, Richardson WS, Glasziou P, Haynes RB. *Evidence-Based Medicine: How to Practice and Teach EBM,* 3rd ed. Edinburgh, UK: Elsevier Churchill Livingstone; 2005.

7. Gupta, M. A critical appraisal of evidence-based medicine: some ethical considerations. *J Eval in Clin Prac.* 2003;9(2):111–121.

8. Centers for Medicare & Medicaid Services (CMS). Physician Quality Reporting System. Baltimore. MD: CMS; August 23, 2013. Available at www.cms.gov/Medicare/Quality-Initiatives-Patient-Assessment-Instruments/PQRS/index.html?redirect=/pqri. Accessed on August 31, 2013.

9. Kokmeyer DJ, van der Wurff P, Aufdemkampe G, Fickenscher TC. The reliability of multitest regimens with sacroiliac pain provocation tests. *J Manipulative Physiol Ther.* 2002;25(1):42–48.

10. van der Wurff P, Buijs EJ, Groen GJ. A multitest regimen of pain provocation tests as an aid to reduce unnecessary minimally invasive sacroiliac joint procedures. *Arch Phys Med Rehabil.* 2006;87:10–14.

11. APTA. *Defensible Documentation General Guidelines.* Alexandria, VA: American Physical Therapy Association; last updated March 8, 2012. Available at www.apta.org/Documentation/DefensibleDocumentation/. Accessed on July 15, 2014.

12. Woolf AD. History and physical examination. *Best Pract Res Clin Rheumatol.* 2003;17(3):381–402.

13. Kim MJ, Seino S, Kim MK, et al. Validation of lower extremity performance tests for determining the mobility limitation levels in community-dwelling older women. *Aging Clin Exp Res.* 2009;21(6):437–444.

14. Mesquita R, Janssen DJ, Wouters EF, Schools JM, Pitta F, Spruit MA. Within-day test-retest reliability of the Timed Up & Go Test in patients with advanced chronic organ failure. *Arch Phys Med Rehabil.* 2013 Nov;94(11):2131–2138.

15. Alcock, G. K., Werstine, M. S., et al. Longitudinal changes in the lower extremity functional scale after anterior cruciate ligament reconstructive surgery. *Clin J Sport Med.* 2012;22(3):234–239.

CHAPTER 9

Interprofessional Communication

CHAPTER OBJECTIVES

1. Determine what communications with a patient or client or caregiver should be documented in the health record.
2. Determine how and where to document verbal or electronic communications with a patient or client or caregiver outside the context of a scheduled encounter.
3. Recognize how to document the results of a verbal or electronic consultation or inquiry with a healthcare provider on behalf of your patient or client.
4. Recognize how to document requests for documents from other healthcare providers on behalf of your patient or client such as operative reports, imaging results, or referrals.
5. Recognize the components required to create a letter of medical necessity for durable medical equipment.

KEY TERMS

Electronic communication
Letter of medical necessity

Nonverbal communication
Verbal communication

Introduction

Effective communication is a valuable adjunct to effective documentation. Because there are likely multiple consumers of your physical therapy documentation it is important to have a fundamental understanding of how to document various situations that may affect the care of your patient or client. Therefore, this chapter presents a clinical decision-making algorithm to assist you with determining which communications with a patient or client should become a part of the patient or client's health record. In addition, suggested ways of documenting verbal or electronic communications that may occur between you and your patient or client or those that occur between you and another individual on your patient or client's behalf are presented. Lastly, details regarding documenting requests to or from other healthcare providers on your patient or client's behalf, documenting refusals of service, or writing letters of medical necessity are also offered.

Communication is the cornerstone of a successful organization, whether that entity is a nonprofit group or a for-profit establishment. Without it, a business simply cannot operate. In addition to merely being present however, communication must also be detailed and timely to be effective. The medium via which communication occurs can vary as long as some mechanism exists to relay information. Equally important is a mechanism designed to receive that communicated information. In the healthcare sector, before the era of electronic health records, the contents of a health record became part of this legal document via transcription. For example, the contents of an entry were either handwritten or dictated, printed, and subsequently included in the record. The contents of a physical therapy daily visit was recorded on a prefabricated template utilizing a "SOAP" note acronym or was simply a blank page for the therapist to create the note. Likewise, when a healthcare provider spoke to a patient or client or a colleague by phone, the details of the conversation were logged and became part of the patient or client's health record. The purpose of these types of entries was to maintain a record of all communications that occurred on behalf of the patient or client so that future questions or inquiries could be managed. It is important to recognize that communications with patients or clients, caregivers, and other members of the healthcare team continue to occur despite evolutions in technology. It is not the interactions that have changed; it is the means with which they are recorded. Although technology has evolved and these processes have largely become electronic, the core goal of communication has remained the same: to facilitate the exchange of information.

Clinical Decision Making in Communication

As a healthcare provider, communication is an integral part of patient- or client-centered care. As a physical therapy professional, you have a unique responsibility to be an effective and efficient communicator simply because of the increased amount of time you spend with each patient or client compared to other members of a patient or client's healthcare team. Furthermore, you have an additional responsibility to implement a decision-making process to determine which communications between you and your patient or client make it into the legal document that is the health record. Consider the following scenario.

During her session today, your 15-year-old patient or client demonstrated and verbalized that she understood the details of the home exercise program that she is to perform over the next 3 days before coming back to your outpatient clinic for her next visit. The next day you receive a message from your front office administrator to call the patient or client as she has some questions about her exercises and would like to ask you about a pain that she has developed since her last session. You call her and have a brief conversation where you discover that she appropriately performed her exercises and is experiencing delayed onset muscle soreness. You educate

her about this phenomenon and provide some detail about how she should dose her home exercises over the next 2 days.

Is it necessary to document the contents of this phone call? Take a moment to reflect on your answer. Consider an alternative situation where you discern, based on the contents of the phone conversation, that your patient or client injured herself when *inappropriately* performing the home exercise program you prescribed. Is this situation different from the previous scenario? Do you think that both scenarios warrant inclusion into the patient or client's health record?

Regardless of how communication occurs between you and your patient or client, it is your responsibility to capture in the health record any information that could potentially impact the physical therapy plan of care created with your patient or client. You could consider the plan of care to be a sort of contract, and therefore *any* communication that occurs that could affect the implementation and outcome of that contract should be recorded. Examples of this type of content include inquiries from the patient or client, caregiver, or healthcare provider about any aspect of the plan of care. Perhaps your patient or client's parent or sports coach inquires about the activities your 15-year-old patient or client should be doing with the sports team at school. Perhaps your patient or client's referring physician, nurse, or case manager calls to ask about the content of a re-examination you recently conducted. **FIGURE 9-1** depicts an algorithm you can utilize to assist your decision making regarding communications you may have on behalf of your patient or client.

APPROPRIATE COMMUNICATION

Because of your patient or client's right to privacy, the *appropriateness* of the communication is a proper initial factor to consider when determining the need to document communication in the health record. Consider that it is pertinent to first know if you are permitted to communicate with certain individuals on your patient or client's behalf before determining the need to capture the communication in the patient or client's health record. First ask yourself, "Is this communication appropriate?" To answer "yes" to this question, you must first identify with whom you have permission to communicate on your patient or client's behalf. If you

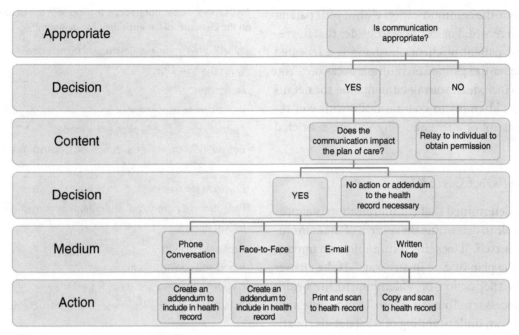

FIGURE 9-1 Communication Algorithm.

are engaged in communication with the patient or client in a clinical setting than you likely have his or her consent to do so. However, if you are approached by any other individual regarding the care of your patient or client, you must determine if your patient or client has consented to your communicating with that individual on their behalf prior to engaging in the conversation. This is an important part of your patient or client's right to privacy under the Health Insurance Portability and Accountability Act of 1996. Generally, your patient or client will have signed a form consenting to receive intervention from the healthcare providers employed at your facility. There will likely be a statement on this consent that includes the exchange of the patient or client's health information with providers outside your facility on their behalf. Your patient or client will also sign a disclosure indicating those individuals with whom you can communicate regarding their care. It is your responsibility to know who these individuals are, not only as a professional courtesy, but also because failure to do so is a violation of the law. Consider the following scenario.

You are a physical therapist or physical therapist assistant in a busy outpatient clinic. You go to the waiting room to greet your patient or client and to walk into the clinic with her hoping to analyze her gait

without her realizing it. As you walk behind your patient or client into the clinic gym, your patient or client's husband taps you on the shoulder and indicates that you should call his cell phone later that day. He states briefly that he has left his number with your front office administrator and that he wants to relay some concerns he has about his wife.

As the algorithm in Figure 9-1 suggests, you should first determine if it is appropriate for you to contact your patient or client's husband and begin communicating with him on her behalf. To do this you would have to refer to your patient or client's intake paperwork to determine if her husband is included on her disclosure as someone with whom you can communicate regarding her care. If you find that he is not listed, then you are not permitted to communicate with him on her behalf. In this case, you would indicate to your patient or client's husband that he would need to obtain permission from his wife before you could communicate with him regarding her health care. Because there was no information exchanged that could impact the plan of care or your patient or client's right to privacy, there is no need to include this communication within the patient or client's health record. Alternatively, if you feel concern that your communication with an individual regarding your patient or client may have the potential to impact the plan of care at some point, then it is relevant to include the communication within your patient or client's health record. For example, consider that the request from your patient or client's husband is a repeated request that you have explained on multiple occasions. You might decide to include in your documentation the details of the husband's attempts to communicate with you regarding your patient or client and why you are restricted from doing so.

COMMUNICATION CONTENT

Once you have determined that communication is appropriate, it is suitable to determine the *content* of the communication. Ask yourself, "Does this communication impact, alter, or affect the plan of care in any way?" If the answer is "no," then further action or addendum to the health record is not necessary. To answer "yes" to this question you must possess an understanding of what details constitute meaningful communication that potentially impacts your patient or client's plan of care. It is straightforward to identify as communication any activity that identifies the care or service you provide during an encounter with a patient or client. These items, which include details of the elements of patient or client management as defined in the American Physical Therapy Association (APTA) *Guide to Physical Therapist Practice*, should clearly be included in the patient or client's health record (TABLE 9-1).[1] These details include the contents of the initial examination, evaluation and plan of care, as well as any outcome measures collected and interventions prescribed including the home exercise program. Daily notes, progress notes, re-examination notes, and conclusion of episode of care summaries are also clearly relevant content for the health record. Additional information such as medication lists, physician referrals, payer information, and content from any prior healthcare provider should also be included. It is not as straightforward, however, to identify as communication those activities that are appropriate to include in the health record that occur *outside* the context of a scheduled encounter with that patient or client (TABLE 9-2). Consider the following scenario.

You are working in a skilled nursing facility where you are working with an older adult who is recovering from spine surgery. When you walk by his room you see that he is leaning over his bed to smooth out the blankets. You see that he is not wearing his thoracolumbosacral orthosis (TLSO). You enter the

TABLE 9-1 Communications to Include in the Health Record Based on the Elements of Patient/Client Management*

Initial examination, evaluation, and plan of care
Outcome measures
Daily notes
Progress or reassessment notes
Conclusion of episode of care summaries
Exercise flow sheets; intervention logs; postsurgical protocols
Home exercise programs
Physician referrals
Patient/client history and demographic information, medication lists
Informed consent
Payer information
Billing and coding information
Case management activities

* As defined by the American Physical Therapy Association.

TABLE 9-2 Communications to Include in a Health Record that May Not Be Part of a patient or client Encounter

Phone calls with the patient or client, caregiver, and/or other healthcare professionals
E-mail communications with the patient or client, caregiver, and/or other healthcare professionals
Face-to-face conversations with a patient or client, caregiver, and/or other healthcare professionals
Observations made of a patient or client that could impact the plan of care
Requests to healthcare providers for: ○ Operative reports   ○ Imaging results   ○ Referrals
Cancellations
Refusals of service
Conflicts with other appointments
Letters of support of letters of medical necessity

room and assist him with making the bed as well as donning the TLSO. You speak with the nursing team regarding your interaction with the patient or client.

Do you think that you should document this encounter in this patient or client's health record? If so, how did you decide? What information will you include in the record? Because the communication with the nursing team has the potential to impact the patient or client's plan of care, the encounter with the patient or client should be documented in the health record including the conversation that occurred with the nursing staff such as is indicated in the narrative below.

> Addendum to Daily Note for Mr. X on *insert date here:* At approximately 3pm, Mr. X was seen leaning over his bed. He was not wearing his TLSO. I entered his room, helped him don the TLSO, and made his bed for him. He stated that he was not having any pain and was hot, which is why he took off the TLSO. He stated that he had taken it off about 1 hour after his lunch was over at 1:00pm. He indicated that he often takes the TLSO off in the afternoon after lunch when he is resting in his room. I educated the patient or client on the importance of wearing his TLSO at all times including during sleep except when showering. I reiterated that he will need to wait for assistance from his nurse or occupational therapist for showering and bathing activities. I also educated Mr. X on how to change the thermostat in his room. Mr. X indicated that he understood the need for the continued use of the TLSO until he follows up with his surgeon in 2 weeks. I spoke with Mr. X's nurse immediately after speaking to Mr. X to relay the details above. The nurse indicated that she will check in on Mr. X more often and also reinforce the importance of wearing the TLSO to him as well as to her nursing staff.

This addendum relays the facts of what you witnessed and is devoid of any opinion. In addition, the actions you took on the patient or client's behalf including assisting him with the task he was attempting, educating him regarding his attempt to engage in this task without wearing his TLSO, and alerting his nurse are included. In addition to including your interaction in your patient or client's health record, it is important that you follow up in person with his care team, especially his nurse, to assure that the nurse is aware of an event involving a patient or client for whom she is responsible. Taking the time to create such an addendum in your documentation could further indicate, for example, details that assist other healthcare providers or the patient or client's family members to understand if the patient or client's recovery is not progressing as expected. Therefore, leaving this communication out of the health record has the potential to negatively impact the patient or client's plan of care.

Now consider that you are working in a busy outpatient clinic. You run out to your car to get your sweater and you see your patient or client who has had recent back surgery leaning into the trunk of his car to get his TLSO. It is your understanding that the patient or client is to wear this brace for at least 6 weeks. As you start your session, you see that the patient or client is wearing the TLSO. He indicates to you during your conversation that his surgeon told him that he does not have to wear the TLSO to drive.

Do you think that you should document this communication in this patient or client's health record? If so, how did you decide? Because this patient or client's behavior has the potential to impact his plan of care, it is relevant to include your observation and conversation in the health record. Equally important is your decision to follow up with the surgeon to verify any instructions regarding the TLSO and to subsequently include this conversation in the health record as well. Your daily note might look like the note below.

> Mr. Y reports a 7/10 pain across his central low back that started while he was getting dressed this morning. He states that he does not recall any specific action or position that increased his pain. He notes that he felt minimal pain (1/10) after his physical therapy session 2 days ago, which continued until this morning.
>
> Provided education to Mr. Y regarding the importance of wearing TLSO at all times except when showering including when driving and performing other activities. Mr. Y was observed retrieving his TLSO from the trunk of his car after exiting the driver's side of his car without wearing it. When questioned about the wear schedule for the TLSO, Mr. Y relayed that his surgeon told him he did not have to wear the TLSO while driving. Subsequently, Mr. Y was advised to wear the TLSO while driving or to make alternative arrangements for transportation until an alternative TLSO wear schedule could be confirmed with his surgeon. Positioning for dressing tasks was also reviewed and revised per flow sheet. Bending and stooping mechanics while wearing the TLSO were also included per flow sheet.
>
> Mr. Y demonstrated the ability to don his TLSO independently as well as perform bending and stooping to retrieve at least a 5-pound object from the floor without increased pain and without postural compensations while wearing his TLSO. He also indicated that he will attempt to wear his TLSO today while driving home but reports that this will be difficult because he

does not feel that he can safely drive while wearing it. He also states that he will speak with his wife about driving him to his medical appointments if he is to continue to wear the TLSO to drive.

Will place a call to Mr. Y's surgeon today to clarify TLSO wear schedule. Continue to address poor motor control at lumbar extensors to increase standing tolerance for grooming tasks and meal preparation.

A further addendum to this patient or client's health record can be included to reflect your communication with the patient or client's surgeon.

Addendum to Daily Note for Mr. Y on *insert date here*:

Spoke with surgeon's nurse, *insert name here*, via phone this afternoon who relayed that Mr. Y is to wear his TLSO at all times except when showering or bathing for the next 5 weeks until his follow-up appointment with the surgeon on *insert date here* at *insert time here* pm. The nurse indicated that he would contact Mr. Y today to reiterate this wear schedule. I also spoke with Mr. Y via phone after speaking with *insert name here* to reiterate the TLSO wear schedule. Mr. Y indicated that he understood and thanked me for calling.

As noted above, it can be challenging to identify the information your patient or client shares or exhibits in communications and interactions that occur outside the context of a scheduled encounter that should be included in the health record. Equally challenging is determining the content of communication exchanged with your patient or client that may not need to be included in the health record. This type of information can occur within the context of a scheduled encounter with a patient or client or outside the context of a scheduled encounter. Consider the following scenario.

During the physical therapy session, your postsurgical patient or client from the outpatient scenario above further discusses with you details about his friend who had a similar back surgery and who subsequently was prescribed a TLSO to wear for 6 weeks after the surgery. Your patient or client indicates that his friend only wore the brace for 3 weeks and fully recovered and returned to his job without wearing the TLSO for the prescribed 6 weeks.

Do you think that this detail should be included in this patient or client's health record? One could argue that your patient or client may make decisions about his own care based on the information he shared with you about his friend and with this rationale you might decide to include this detail in the health record. However, the content that is likely more appropriate for your patient or client's record is the education you provide about your patient or client's particular situation and wearing his TLSO as indicated.

Now consider that you encounter this same patient or client as you are waiting in line at the post office. He indicates that he was exhausted after his last physical therapy session. You chat about the weather, the traffic, and his work schedule where he indicates that his hours at work have increased again this week.

Do you think that you should document this communication in this patient or client's health record? If so, how did you decide? You may decide that based on your plan of care, your patient or client's mention of increased work hours is relevant to your plan of care. However, you may decide simply to make a point to ask him about his increased work hours and how it is affecting him and his current condition at his next session with you rather than document the conversation you had with him at the post office.

COMMUNICATION MEDIUM

Once you have determined that the content of your communication is relevant to include in the patient or client's health record, it is important to recognize that the mode of communication or the medium through which communication occurs (Figure 9-1) can also influence how the communication is recorded. Forms of communication that may affect the plan of care you have established with your patient or client include verbal, nonverbal, and written forms of communication. **Verbal communication** via a phone conversation or a face-to-face conversation can occur outside the context of the patient or client's actual visit but have an impact on the plan of care. In this case, the content of the verbal communication should be included in the patient or client's health record. **Nonverbal communication** can be expressed with gestures and other facial or body movements and may become important to you when the nonverbal message relayed is different than the verbal communications you may have had with your patient or client. Consider the following scenario.

You are working with an 85-year-old patient or client in a skilled nursing facility who is recovering from a stroke he suffered during cardiac surgery. He is surrounded by his loved ones and appears to have a large supportive family network. He appears motivated and positive when his family is present; however, you notice that his demeanor and energy level deteriorate when he is not with his family.

Do you think that this nonverbal behavior impacts your plan of care with your patient or client? Will you document the presence of this behavior? Why or why not? Because this nonverbal behavior has the potential to impact the plan of care you have established with this patient or client, you may decide that it is relevant to include it in your documentation, which may look like the following in your patient or client's daily note.

> Mr. Z indicates that he practiced walking outside with his rollator that his family brought in today during his occupational therapy session.
>
> See flow sheet for gait reassessment including TUG and 10MWT with and without the rollator. Vital signs show normal response at rest and with activity per flow sheet. Mr. Z appears lethargic and uninterested when using rollator for gait. Gait scores were significantly slower with use of the rollator than without per flow sheet; however patient or client demonstrated safety while maneuvering the rollator around turns and obstacles and over changes in floor surfaces.
>
> Reassess gait during tomorrow morning's session to determine impact of fatigue on gait with rollator vs. no device. Monitor observed lethargy and low energy level.

Alternatively, Mr. Z's nonverbal behavior may trigger you to have a verbal conversation with the patient or client to determine the change in behavior that you observed, the results of which are indeed relevant to include in the health record. An alternative addition to Mr. Z's health record might appear as follows.

> Addendum to Daily Note for Mr. Z on *insert date here*:
>
> Mr. Z was observed today to be motivated and positive regarding his progress with physical therapy in the presence of his family this morning; however when his family left for the day, Mr. Z appeared unmotivated, lethargic, and uninterested in participating in any further

activities. When asked about his change in demeanor, he relayed that his family does not want him to come home unless he uses the rollator that they brought in for him today. I discussed with Mr. Z that we would further evaluate his gait and balance and based on his progress would determine recommendations to share with his family regarding safety with ambulation and balance upon returning home. Mr. Z was agreeable to this plan and stated that his family was due to visit again in 2 days.

Written communication is most likely to occur in the form of an e-mail (a form of **electronic communication**), but can also come to you from the patient or client in a handwritten format. Assume that your 15-year-old patient or client from the scenario above sends you an e-mail communication rather than a phone call regarding her concern with her home exercise program and the pain she developed as a result. If you decide to reply to your patient or client via e-mail, should that reply be included along with the original e-mail from your patient or client as a permanent part of the health record?

Assume that you did not include in the health record your e-mail reply regarding your patient or client's inquiry. At her next appointment, your patient or client continues to complain of pain after doing the home exercises you prescribed. You ask her to perform the program so that you can ensure that she is utilizing proper form as well as to identify if she has made the appropriate adjustments that you relayed to her in your e-mail response. As you observe her form, you see that she has not incorporated the information you shared via your e-mail communication. Because she has incorrectly done this activity she has developed a persistent pain that is more than delayed onset muscle soreness. Leaving the e-mail communication out of the patient or client's health record omits an important part of the educational intervention that you delivered to your patient or client even though the educational intervention occurred outside the context of a scheduled encounter. In other words, you have not included an important part of the plan of care into the health record.

Revisit the scenario above, where your patient or client's husband asks you to call him to discuss his wife, your patient or client. Professionally, it would be appropriate to document the conversation as it is taking place. If you are not able to do this directly into the health record, it would be appropriate to take notes during the conversation so that you can accurately create an addendum to the patient or client's health record as soon as you are able to ensure the accuracy of the information you include in the record. A similar approach to recording handwritten or verbal communication can occur during communication with a healthcare provider on your patient or client's behalf. Consider the following scenario.

You have been working in the home of a patient or client who has Parkinson's disease. She is experiencing a decline in her executive functioning that is affecting her ability to prepare meals and organize her medications. She is going to visit her neurologist the following day. You decide with her permission to write down a few important points that should be brought up to the neurologist. She agrees to take this note to her physician for review during the visit. Later that day, the neurologist calls you to further discuss the patient or client's medical management as well as the care this patient or client is receiving in physical therapy.

Ideally, as indicated above, the documentation of the phone call with the physician should occur in real time in the patient or client's health record. However, circumstances may affirm that this is not feasible. Therefore, you should take notes so that you can either scan these notes as a permanent part of the health record or so that you can create an addendum to the health record based on the notes you took during the actual phone conversation. The addendum to your patient or client's health record may appear as below.

Received a phone call from Dr. A, Mrs. B's neurologist this afternoon. She indicated that she saw Mrs. B for an office visit and thanked me for helping the patient or client with her list of concerns. The neurologist indicated that the patient or client will start on an alternative dosing schedule for her anti-Parkinson's medications tonight which should address the patient or client's complaint of fatigue and poor mobility upon waking in the morning. I will follow up with the neurologist per her request in 2 weeks to relay Mrs. B's mobility abilities in the morning hours to determine the effectiveness of new medication dose.

Additionally, a copy or recreated list of the details you asked the patient or client to share with the neurologist at her visit should also be included in the health record.

Reflect for a moment on the value of including this information in the health record. Why would this detail be valuable to you and the neurologist or other members of the patient or client's healthcare team?

Regardless of the setting in which you practice, you will likely encounter a situation where you would like to initiate communication with another healthcare provider on behalf of your patient or client for information such as operative reports, imaging results, and referrals. Consider the following scenario.

You are working with a patient or client after a rotator cuff repair. She suffered a major tear when she fell in her bathroom. She is progressing well and you are now interested in continuing her plan of care so that you can perform a fall risk assessment and subsequent fall prevention interventions based on her history. You call her physician's office to request a referral for a fall risk assessment and intervention. You leave a message with a nurse regarding this request.

Do you think it is important that you document this phone conversation in the patient or client's health record? Why or why not? Because obtaining this referral helps to determine how your plan of care will develop over time and how the patient or client's health insurance is utilized, it is important to include that you initiated communication to obtain this referral in the patient or client's health record. Alternatively, you may decide that it is beneficial to request information such as referrals or requests for supporting documents on behalf of your patient or client via written communication instead of a verbal or electronic request. Consider the following written communication to request a referral for additional physical therapy services on behalf of the patient or client in the above scenario.

Date:

Dear Dr. _____,

I am the physical therapist who has been working with your patient or client, *insert patient or client's name here*, for a right rotator cuff repair after she suffered a tear due to a fall in her bathroom on *insert date here*. I have treated Mrs. A three times per week for 3 weeks. She is progressing towards her goals as outlined in her initial examination (attached). Her pain and function have improved to the point that we are able to address her fall risk and initiate fall prevention intervention. Please sign and return the attached referral for fall assessment and intervention. Thank you.

Sincerely,

Insert your name and credentials here

A letter such as this may be necessary in the event that you did not include a desired assessment or intervention in your initial plan of care. This request could, alternatively, be imbedded in a re-examination note that you created during a reassessment of your patient or client. In this case, you would report on your patient or client's progress to date as well as report on newly collected outcome measures that identify your patient or client as being at risk for falls and create an appropriate plan of care to reflect this new information. Your electronic documentation system may allow you to create a status update or a report addendum to an initial examination or re-examination note in which objective data can be incorporated into a report that can then be faxed, e-mailed, or printed and given directly to the patient or client for delivery to the intended recipient.

Another communication that would warrant inclusion into your patient or client's health record is a cancellation or refusal of physical therapy services. Consider that you are working in an outpatient clinic and are expecting a patient or client for whom you are performing a re-examination today to determine his ability to actively move his ankle and ambulate since he no longer is required to wear a walking boot. Below is the addendum that you include in this patient or client's health record.

> Mr. A cancelled his appointment today via message he left with front office due to his report of feeling nauseous. I called the patient or client to verify his next appointment tomorrow, *insert date here* at *insert time here*. I also indicated that today was to be the visit where I would have assessed his ability to move his ankle and ambulate without his walking boot and advised him to continue wearing the boot until our re-examination tomorrow.

It is likely that there is a location in a paper-based health record or a mechanism in an electronic record for recording cancellations and no-shows. It is also likely that this communication is entered into the patient or client's health record by the individual who received the message.

However, due to the details that were to happen at the cancelled appointment, it is pertinent to ensure the patient or client's safety by following up with the patient or client and recording this additional communication in the patient or client's record. In addition, it is important to accurately document somewhere in the patient or client's health record that he or she cancelled or did not come to the scheduled appointment since policies regarding the termination of physical therapy services are based on this information.

If you practice in a setting such as an inpatient rehabilitation facility or a skilled nursing facility it is possible that you will experience a situation where your patient or client either refuses your services or has a scheduling conflict with another appointment. Consider that you enter your patient or client's room for his 8:30am physical therapy session. He indicates that he is exhausted because he did not sleep well the night before. Despite your efforts, your patient or client is not willing to participate in your session. You indicate to your patient or client that you will try back again right after his lunch at 1:00pm for a 30-minute session. Your documentation of your patient or client's refusal may look as follows.

> Mr. A refused his morning and afternoon physical therapy sessions due to report of being exhausted and not being able to sleep last night. I initiated a conversation with his nurse regarding Mr. A's report and she indicated that if his vital signs are stable this evening that she will indicate to her staff to allow restorative sleep and not wake him between the hours of midnight and 6am.

Including this detail in the patient or client's health record will assist you as well as other members of the patient or client's healthcare team to understand and address any barriers that may exist to the patient or client meeting his recovery potential.

Creating Letters of Support or Medical Necessity

As a physical therapist, you may be asked to write a letter of support or medical necessity on a patient or client's behalf. This communication may be requested to support your patient or client's return to work, school, or sports activity; to recommend the suspension or termination of certain job, school, or work-related activities; or to relay the need for disability license plates or paratransit services. Written communication may also be necessary to substantiate the need for durable medical equipment such as an ankle foot orthosis, a bedside commode, or a wheelchair. Requests for such written communication may come from a variety of sources such as another healthcare professional, an insurance provider, a durable medical equipment vendor, the patient or client's employer or school, or directly from the patient or client. Because the document you create will likely be used to make important decisions on your patient or client's behalf, it is important that all of the relevant information needed to make an informed decision be included in your communication. In addition, your letter should be written in such a way that it is appropriate for multiple audiences. Those making decisions on your patient or client's behalf may or may not be physical therapists or even healthcare providers; therefore, you should include enough detail about your patient or client's physical abilities that allows you to succinctly generate your clinical opinion and relay your recommendations. Consider the following communication on behalf of your patient or client to support that she is unable to perform her current work duties.

Date:

United States Department of Labor

Office of Workers' Compensation Programs

P.O. Box 1234

Washington , DC 20210

To Whom It May Concern:

I am a physical therapist writing in response to a request from Ms. B to write a letter on her behalf regarding her physical status. I treated Ms. B at *insert your clinic name here* for a total of seven visits from *insert date here* to *insert date here* for neck pain. Her physical therapy examination (attached) is consistent with a repetitive strain injury at her cervical spine with concurrent headaches that appear to be cervicogenic (coming from the cervical spine) in nature. Ms. B describes her job duties to include heavy lifting, repeated reaching and sorting, and repeated use of her arms overhead in a mailroom. She reports that she currently works 8-hour shifts 4–5 days per week and that she has been taking personal leave to attend physical therapy sessions.

Ms. B makes intermittent and limited progress with physical therapy intervention. Any gains achieved are negated after 2–3 days of performing her current work duties.

At this time I recommend that Ms. B avoid lifting parcels and boxes > 10 pounds and to avoid any overhead lifting or sorting. She would likely benefit from a postural change such as sitting every 30–45 minutes and the use of a step stool so that she can be eye level with the areas she is required to reach. These modifications will likely assist her so that she can continue to be productive on her shift.

Please contact me at with any further questions.

Sincerely,

Your name and credentials here

The above letter opens with brief and important detail regarding the purpose of the letter followed by your interpretation of the problem as well as your recommendations. It is also pertinent to invite the recipient to contact you should any further questions develop.

Additional guidelines for the content that is relevant to include in a **letter of medical necessity** is relayed in **TABLE 9-3**. Your success in your ability to communicate via a letter of medical necessity will lie in your ability to briefly translate your clinical findings such that a

TABLE 9-3 Content of a Letter of Medical Necessity

Brief statement of the purpose of the communication
Brief narrative of relevant history and current condition   ○ Health condition   ○ Activity limitations and participation restrictions   ○ Contextual factors that affect function
Results of relevant objective tests and outcome measures performed
Interpretation of relevant objective tests and outcome measures performed
Summary of findings that interfere with function and that necessitate need for assistance   ○ Statement of why certain activity limitations and participation restrictions are listed   ○ Statement as to why alternative equipment or services are inferior   ○ Statement as to why the recommended equipment or service will assist with current limitations and restrictions
Recommendations based on presented data and clinical judgment
Contact information for further inquiries

nonclinical professional can recognize and concur with your recommendations. Furthermore, a succinct and informative opening sentence will improve the likelihood that the remainder of the letter will be read. Consider the following letter of medical necessity for a power wheelchair.

Date:

To Whom It May Concern:

Insert name here is a 52-year-old man who was referred to *insert your name or clinic name here* for a wheelchair assessment performed on *insert date here*. Mr. C was diagnosed with MSA 2 years ago. He is limited in all ADLs. He relies on his wife for assistance with bed mobility and transfers. He is extremely bradykinetic and rigid throughout his body. He experiences resting tremor in both UEs and LEs that is more prominent and physically limiting when fatigued. He experiences pain in his neck, back, hips, legs, and feet. Mr. C is able to ambulate short distances with a cane. He experiences freezing episodes and requires assistance to stop his festinating gait pattern and loss of balance. It takes Mr. C several minutes to ambulate as little as 50 feet. Mr. C has a history of frequent falls. As a result Mr. C is interested in obtaining a power wheelchair to assist him in performing ADLs with less pain, and increased safety and independence. Please see the objective data from Mr. C's physical assessment below.

Observation/Posture: Forward head, protracted c-spine, rounded shoulders, increased t-spine kyphosis; decreased lumbar lordosis.

Pain: Constant 8/10 pain throughout neck, back, hips, legs, and feet B.

Sitting Balance: Limited by pain and poor postural strength.

Standing Balance: Min to mod A needed to stand from sitting depending on the height of the sitting surface.

Transfers/Bed Mobility: Mod to max A due to muscular rigidity and pain.

Gait: With straight cane for very short distances (910 feet) with mod to min A X 1, requires sitting rests due to fatigue; toe-heel pattern noted.

UE AROM/PROM: Limited AROM of B shoulder flexion, abduction, and extension; all limited by pain.

UE Strength: UE strength is grossly 3+/5 to 4−/5 B; limited by pain.

LE AROM/PROM: AROM of B LEs limited by pain. B passive hip extension = 5 degrees; B knee extension = −10 degrees indicating knee flexion contractures. Ankle DF = 10 degrees R; 5 degrees L.

LE Strength	Right	Left
Hip flexion	3+/5	3+/5
Hip extension	4−/5	4−/5
Hip abduction	3+/5	4−/5
Hip int rotation	4/5	4/5
Hip ext rotation	3+/5	4−/5
Knee flexion	4−/5	4−/5
Knee extension	3+/5	3+/5
Ankle dorsiflexion	4/5	4/5
Ankle plantarflexion		Unable to raise up on toes

Tone: Increased in B UEs, LEs, and trunk.

Coordination/Fine Motor Control: Undershooting targets observed.

Based on the findings outlined above, I recommend a power wheelchair to meet Mr. C's needs.

Sincerely,

Insert your name and contact information here

Is the detail provided here valuable enough to warrant that this patient or client receive a power wheelchair? Why or why not? Is there any additional information you would you use to determine if this patient or client would benefit from a power wheelchair? What components as indicated in Table 9-3 are missing from this letter?

Table 9-3 indicates that a brief statement of the purpose of the letter should be included. The above letter indicates that a wheelchair assessment was performed at the encounter. However, a separate opening sentence that briefly connects the reader to you as the communicator is warranted. By adding this sentence, the patient or client's healthcare provider or insurance carrier can immediately identify that the letter requires their attention. Mr. C's history and current condition in the narrative that follows are not provided in enough detail for the reader to understand the activity limitations, participation restrictions, and contextual factors present that affect Mr. C's function. The letter does refer the reader to the objective data from Mr. C's physical assessment; however, an interpretation of these findings is absent. This critical information will help the reader draw the link between the stated activity limitations and participation restrictions and the impairments in body functions and structures identified during the physical examination. In addition, many sentence fragments and abbreviations are used throughout the physical examination findings, which further limit the ability to synthesize the presented data. A narrative summary of the findings that interfere with Mr. C's function and that necessitate need for assistance is also absent from this letter of medical necessity. Detail regarding why equipment or services alternative to that which are recommended is also needed. If your audience is the entity who is paying for the needed equipment or service, an explanation as to why a lower-cost option is not appropriate for the patient or client will be sought. It is important to re-summarize why the recommended equipment or service will assist with the patient or client's current limitations and restrictions at the end of the letter so that the reader is not required to scour the letter for details of your assessment to find information relevant to the decision at hand. It is also important to invite the reader to contact you should any questions about your recommendations remain. This sentence will help relay that your letter was not a computer-generated form letter, but a communication specific to the needs of your mutual patient or client. Now consider the more detailed scenario below.

Date:

To Whom It May Concern:

I am a physical therapist writing today to support a request from your client, *insert name here*, for *insert reason for communication here*.

Insert name here is a 52-year-old man who was referred to *insert your name or clinic name here* for a wheelchair assessment performed on *insert date here*. Mr. C was diagnosed with multiple system atrophy, a Parkinson's disease-like progressive movement disorder 2 years ago. The complications of this disorder have limited Mr. C's ability to perform activities of daily living such as dressing, grooming, bathing, toileting, and ambulating. He relies on his wife for assistance with bed mobility and transfers as he is unable to independently perform these activities due to the symptoms of this disorder. He is severely bradykinetic during any physical movement and therefore the activities he performs

are severely slowed. This slowed movement is inefficient and contributes to Mr. C's constant complaint of fatigue. Bradykinesia not only affects skeletal muscle but also smooth muscle. Mr. C, therefore, lacks a cough reflex and has slowed digestive motility. He is extremely rigid throughout his body, especially his neck and trunk, which contributes to his swallowing difficulties. He experiences resting tremor in both upper extremities and both lower extremities that is more prominent and physically limiting after his musculoskeletal system has been stressed as in during any movement or when he is fatigued. He experiences constant and deep aching pain in his neck, back, hips, legs, and feet due to muscular rigidity and neuropathy. Mr. C is only able to ambulate short distances, up to 50 feet, with a straight cane. However, he experiences freezing every two to three steps and requires the assistance of another person or object such as walls or furniture to stop his festinating gait pattern. It therefore takes 3–4 minutes to ambulate 50 feet. As mentioned, his tremor, rigidity, and bradykinesia increase as his effort level increases. Mr. A has a history of frequent falls and reports falling four times in the last week. All of these falls occurred during ambulation to the commode or when trying to ambulate in his home. As a result of these limitations and restrictions, Mr. C is interested in obtaining a power wheelchair to assist him in performing activities of daily living with increased safety and independence. Please see the objective data from Mr. C's physical assessment below.

Observation/Posture: Mr. C has a forward and protracted cervical spine, rounded shoulders, and an increased thoracic kyphosis. When sitting in a backed chair, Mr. C's posterior shoulders and upper thoracic spine do not contact the chair given his severe forward leaning posture. He lacks a significant lumbar lordosis and therefore sits in a slumped sacral sitting position. This posture forces Mr. C to extend his thoracic and lumbar spine in order to direct his gaze at someone sitting in front of him. Additionally, this posture suppresses Mr. C's cough reflex, swallowing mechanism, and ability to project his voice to be heard. This posture is not adequate for propelling a manual wheelchair as he loses his balance forward when attempting to contact the wheels for propulsion. He also lacks the flexibility to use his arms to advance the chair. See upper extremity range of motion findings below.

Bradykinesia and rigidity prevent him from propelling the chair with his legs and feet.

Pain: Mr. C complains of constant pain throughout his neck, back, hips, legs, and feet bilaterally. He is unable to move freely due to muscular rigidity and cramping. He also experiences burning neuropathic pain in both feet. He is able to find minimal relief of his back pain sitting in a reclined position. A power wheelchair is the only mobility device that has the adjustability in the seating system to tilt or recline allowing Mr. C the ability to locate a position that will minimize his pain and allow him the opportunity to complete daily activities such as grooming, dressing, and eating.

Sitting Balance: Mr. C's sitting balance is limited by pain and poor postural strength. He requires both upper extremities on the seat to impart support in sitting. His forward posture as previously mentioned is such that he slumps forward and looks down. He is unable to independently adjust his position to provide pressure relief due to bradykinesia and rigidity. He is able to sit without back support for less than 5 minutes before requiring the assistance of another person to move to a reclined position.

Standing Balance: Mr. C requires minimum to moderate assistance to stand from sitting depending on the height of the sitting surface due to muscular rigidity, pain, bradykinsesia, and difficulty planning volitional movements. A functional balance assessment was not possible due to the above mentioned impairments.

Transfers/Bed Mobility: Mr. C requires moderate to maximum assistance with bed mobility and transfer tasks due to muscular rigidity, pain, bradykinsesia, and difficulty planning volitional movements.

Gait: At the evaluation, Mr. C ambulated with a straight cane in his right hand 25 feet before needing a sitting rest due to the fatigue of developing a festinating gait pattern and freezing every two to three steps. He utilized a toe-heel pattern often catching his toe on the floor during the swing phase of gait. He consistently required the assistance of another person to stop his momentum to prevent a fall. He is unable to use a standard or a rolling walker as it increases his tendency to freeze by becoming an obstacle in his path. He is unable to coordinate the movement patterns necessary to advance one foot in front of the other while also advancing the walker.

UE AROM/PROM: Mr. C has limited active range of motion (ROM) of bilateral shoulder flexion, abduction, and extension to approximately 140 degrees, 150 degrees, and 40 degrees, respectively. All ROM measures are limited by pain. As previously noted, he has a severely forward posture such that the posterior shoulders and upper back do not contact the back of the seat in which he is sitting. These limitations would prevent Mr. C from propelling an optimally configured manual wheelchair.

UE Strength: Upper extremity strength is grossly 3+/5 to 4–/5 bilaterally. All planes are limited by pain.

LE AROM/PROM: Active ROM of bilateral lower extremities is limited by pain. Passive hip extension is limited to approximately 5 degrees bilaterally. Bilateral knee extension is limited to –10 degrees indicating knee flexion contractures. Ankle dorsiflexion is 10 degrees on the right and 5 degrees on the left.

LE Strength: Lower extremity strength is grossly 3+/5 to 4–/5 bilaterally. All planes at the knee and hip are limited by pain.

Tone: There is increased resistance to passive movement of Mr. C's bilateral upper and lower extremities and trunk, especially, hip flexion, internal rotation, external rotation, knee flexion, and hip adduction. Trunk rigidity is apparent when Mr. C attempts to initiate a movement such as leaning forward to get out of a chair or when initiating rolling which compromises his balance and therefore his ability to complete daily activities.

Coordination/Fine Motor Control: Mr. C has upper extremity motor control deficits, as he tends to undershoot targets and misjudge distances. He is unable to coordinate the fine motor skills involved in brushing his teeth, and fastening buttons and zippers for dressing. He also requires assistance to eat as he has difficulty using utensils to cut food and bring food to his mouth. Mr. C also lacks lower extremity motor control apparent when attempting to place his foot near a target in sitting or standing. The deficits in motor coordination cited above would interfere with Mr. C's ability to propel and maneuver a manual wheelchair. He does however possess the physical and mental ability (Mini-Mental State Exam = 27) to operate a power wheelchair with a joystick device on his dominant side in the home, as trunk and extremity movement would be minimized with the operation of this type of device. A power scooter is inappropriate for reasons previously mentioned such as Mr. C's need for a seating system that can provide a tilt or recline. A scooter is also insufficient for assisting Mr. C with pressure relief or postural repositioning as it does not possess the supportive system needed to accommodate Mr. C's postural rigidity and tone.

Based on the findings outlined above, I recommend a power wheelchair with a joystick, a seating system that allows for a tilted and reclined sitting position, and elevating leg rests. These features will allow Mr. C the ability to independently maneuver around his home so that he can gain control over activities of daily living such as grooming and dressing. As previously noted, abnormal tone, poor postural structure, limited range of motion, muscular weakness, and pain prevent Mr. C from independently maneuvering a manual wheelchair around his home. Parameters such as speed, acceleration, and joystick sensitivity can be programmed electronically to allow Mr. C the opportunity to freely move through the rooms of his home including his bedroom, bathroom, and kitchen. Additionally, the electronics for a tilt and recline system at the joystick will afford Mr. C the opportunity to independently manage his sitting posture for pressure relief and for basic needs such as swallowing and eating.

Thank you for your assistance in meeting Mr. C's needs. Please contact me at *insert information here*, if I can be of any further assistance.

Sincerely,
Insert your name and credentials here

Clearly, this letter is more detailed than the first. The opening statement briefly directs the reader to the purpose of the communication. The narrative format of the letter relays Mr. C's health condition as well as the factors that currently limit his ability to function. The narrative format of the physical assessment also relays important detail and connects Mr. C's limitations and participation restrictions with his impairments in body functions and structures. An interpretation of how these impairments will affect Mr. C is also included. Explanations supporting the recommended equipment and supporting why lower cost equipment would not benefit Mr. C is provided. A summary paragraph concludes the letter re-emphasizing the most relevant reasons why the recommendation is being made.

Summary

The ability to create and translate verbal and written communication clearly and succinctly will supplement your proficiency as a physical therapy professional. As

---

BOX 9-1 Electronic Health Record: Interprofessional Communications

Some electronic systems may have a mechanism for you to create an addendum to the patient or client's health record should the communication you wish to include occur outside the context of a scheduled encounter. You may have an opportunity within your system to copy and paste the details of communication such as an e-mail into this section. Alternatively, you could print the e-mail communication and scan it into the patient or client's record much like an external document such as a fax communication from a referring physician's office or a paper-based outcome measure that you collected at the initial examination. If communication comes to you in the form of a handwritten note, you could similarly scan this document to your electronic system for inclusion into the patient or client's health record.

There may be an opportunity within an electronic documentation system to create a report or template so that an outline of the desired information for a letter of medical necessity for a certain piece of equipment is provided to you as the examining therapist. This template could be used as a guide to follow during an examination to ensure that all relevant data is considered and collected so that the content of the letter of medical necessity is optimal. Even if you have the opportunity to collaborate with a professional whose primary function is to obtain the desired durable medical equipment, it is important to possess an understanding of the content of a letter of medical necessity in the event you are asked to create one.

technology evolves and electronic documentation systems are implemented, the need to consistently develop the framework for your communications may dissolve. However, you are still responsible as a physical therapy professional to recognize and understand how to effectively and efficiently document the content of professional communication. This includes:

○ Distinguishing which communications with patients or clients and caregivers should be documented within a health record and which communications should not.
○ Determining where in the health record communications should be recorded should they occur outside the context of a scheduled encounter with a patient or client.

○ Recognizing how to document communications with other professionals on behalf of your patient or client.
○ Creating the framework and content of letters of support and medical necessity on behalf of your patient or client.

The templates for creating the communications included in your documentation such as letters of medical necessity may be prefabricated. However, as a physical therapist you should be informed and aware of how to create these documents as if the protocol or template did not exist. In the event that an electronic system does not exist or fails, your patient or client may still call on you to communicate on his or her behalf. You will then be required to do so effectively and efficiently.

Discussion Questions

1. Choose an orthopedically focused examination you performed recently in the clinical setting in which you practice.
   a. Write a mock letter of medical necessity for a brace or splint.
   b. Exchange letters with one of your peers or colleagues. Assume that you are the party responsible for determining if this patient or client receives the brace or splint. Based on the letter you read, would you accept or deny the request? Provide specific support from the letter to support your decision.
2. Choose a neurologically focused examination you performed recently in the clinical setting in which you practice.
   a. Write a mock letter of medical necessity for a wheelchair.
   b. Exchange letters with one of your peers or colleges. Assume that you are the party responsible for determining if this patient or client receives the wheelchair. Based on the letter you read, would you accept or deny the request? Provide specific support from the letter to support your decision.
3. You evaluate a 30-year-old man 2 weeks after he experienced a whiplash injury in a car accident. He

states that he has had an x-ray and an MRI but he does not know the results of these tests. Write a letter on your patient's behalf requesting this information.
4. Your 16-year-old baseball player is recovering from a labral repair on his pitching arm and is eager to participate in strength and conditioning practices. His coach contacts you and wants to know what activities are safe to perform in these practices. Create an addendum to your re-examination note to your patient or client's coach relaying your recommendations.
5. Your patient or client is a 42-year-old contractor who fell off a ladder while at work and injured his back. He has been participating in physical therapy with you three times per week for 12 weeks. He indicates that he needs a letter from you recommending a functional capacity examination before his employer will allow him to return to work. Create this letter on behalf of your patient or client.
6. You are working in an inpatient rehabilitation facility. You learn from your occupational therapy partner that your patient or client left in the middle of the OT session to have an EKG performed. Your patient or client has still not returned by the end of your day and as a result you missed 60 minutes of physical therapy intervention with him. How will you document this situation in your patient or client's health record?

Case Study Questions

1. You are treating your patient or client in a busy inpatient rehabilitation hospital when the patient or client's son approaches you and asks why he was not notified about his mother's admission to the

emergency room the day before for a hypertensive episode. He further relays to you that his mother's sister, his aunt, was notified. He indicates that his aunt is not on his mother's disclosure and consent as someone your company is authorized to discuss your patient or client's health information. You apologize for this oversight and assure your patient or client's son that you will relay this problem to the healthcare team to determine how this mistake was made. Based on this scenario, create the documentation you would include in the patient or client's health record of the conversation you had with her son.

2. You are working in a busy outpatient clinic and are awaiting the arrival of one of your patients or clients. She is late and you are concerned since she is never late. Just then, you see an ambulance outside of your facility in the parking lot and realize that your patient or client's caregiver is standing there as well. You go outside and learn from your patient or client and her caregiver that she fell in the parking lot. You see that she is scraped and cut on her head above her right eye, on her right shoulder, and on her right knee. She states that she is very painful at her shoulder, but is otherwise just embarrassed. She states that she will call you later with an update on her status.

   a. Should the communication you had with your patient or client and the caregiver be included in the patient or client's health record?

   b. If you decide to include this communication in the health record, what will you write?

   c. If you decide not to include this communication in the health record, indicate your reasoning for your decision.

3. You are shopping at the grocery store one afternoon and you run into one of your current patients or clients who you are treating in your outpatient clinic for shoulder pain. You notice that she is using her shoulder with many of the postural compensations that you spent her previous physical therapy session working to address. She mentions to you that she is still having pain and that she is not sure that physical therapy is helping her. You mention your observations about how you see her using her shoulder and offer some suggestions on how she might change her positioning to facilitate the use of her arm in a less painful way. She indicates an understanding of and an appreciation for what you have shown her and states that she will see you tomorrow at her next appointment.

   a. Should the communication you had with your patient or client and the caregiver be included in the patient or client's health record?

   b. If you decide to include this communication in the health record, what will you write?

   c. If you decide not to include this communication in the health record, indicate your reasoning for your decision.

   d. Your patient or client arrives for her appointment the day after you spoke with her about her body

mechanics and postural positioning of her shoulder at the grocery store. She states that she is in more pain than she was when she saw you in the store yesterday. She indicates that it was the advice that she followed from your suggestions that increased her pain. After reassessing her movement and further educating her, she now understands what activities to avoid and how to position herself. How will you document this information in your daily note?

4. You are working in an acute hospital setting with a gentleman who suffered a hip fracture after a fall that was surgically fixated 4 days ago. The patient or client's surgeon stops you in the hall and indicates that he has removed any weight-bearing precautions that were initially in place. How should you incorporate this communication with the surgeon into the health record?

5. You are attending a case conference on behalf of a patient or client with whom you are working in his home. The case manager asks you about the content of a re-examination you performed 2 days ago. She indicates that you as the physical therapist are the only discipline that performed a re-examination to continue his care. The case manager reports that nursing and occupational therapy have concluded the episode of care for the patient or client. She questions if you still think that this patient or client requires home health physical therapy intervention and seems to be implying that she would like you to conclude the physical therapy episode of care for the patient or client. You present your findings again and substantially support why you are continuing physical therapy services with this patient or client.

   a. Should you document the conversation with the case manager in the patient or client's health record?

   b. If you decide to include this communication in the health record, what will you write?

   c. If you decide not to include this communication in the health record, indicate your reasoning for your decision.

6. You receive a phone call from a local football coach who is inquiring about the status of your patient or client who is also one of his star players. You determine from the patient or client's informed consent that you are not permitted to disclose health information to the coach about your patient or client.

   a. Should you document this conversation in the patient or client's health record?

   b. If you decide to include this communication in the health record, what will you write?

   c. If you decide not to include this communication in the health record, indicate your reasoning for your decision.

7. Consider the following letter of medical necessity.

   Date:

   To Whom It May Concern:

   Insert name here is a 77-year-old female who was referred to *insert your name or clinic name here* for a power wheelchair assessment performed on *insert date here*. Ms. Z's medical history includes macular degeneration, osteoporosis, and osteoarthritis. She had a right total knee replacement 5 years ago and currently experiences limitations as a result of left knee osteoarthritis. Approximately 1 year ago, Ms. Z experienced a fall resulting in a left hip fracture. Since this time she has used a standard manual wheelchair. Ms. Z experiences pain, weak trunk musculature, a thoracic kyphosis, and poor shoulder extension ROM that severely limit her ability to propel the manual wheelchair. Please see below for the objective findings from Ms. Z's *physical* assessment.

   Observation/Posture: Forward, protracted cervical spine, rounded shoulders, increased thoracic kyphosis. Lateral R trunk lean, elevated L iliac crest in sitting. Standing limited to 2 minutes. Tends to have loss of balance to R when standing regardless of UE support.

   Pain: Constant throughout upper and lower back, L hip, knee.

   Sitting Balance: Limited by poor postural strength.

   Standing Balance: Ms. Z requires SBA to CGA during standing without UE support. Unable to stand safely for greater than 8 seconds with upper extremity support, or her cane, without also reaching out for assistance with her other hand. BBS = 25/56.

   Transfers/Bed Mobility: Mod I for transfers, bed mobility.

   Gait: Ambulates with a straight cane in R hand and her son at her L side. He provided Ms. Z with mod to max A for approximately 75 feet before she required a wheelchair due to the fatigue and pain. Ms. Z also relied on her son for direction during ambulation, as she is unable to see the details of a change in flooring such as tile to carpet or a doorway threshold due to macular degeneration.

   UE AROM/PROM: UE AROM WFL except shoulder extension, which is limited B to approximately 45 degrees by her thoracic kyphosis.

   UE Strength: Grossly 4/5 bilaterally.

   LE AROM/PROM: L knee AROM limited by pain. R knee AROM WFL. L knee extension lacks 20 degrees. Passive hip extension is limited to approximately −10 degrees B.

LE Strength	Right	Left
Hip flexion	4/5	3+/5
Hip extension	4−/5	4−/5
Hip abduction	3−/5	3−/5
Hip adduction	2+/5	2/5
Hip internal rotation	3/5	3/5
Hip external rotation	4−/5	4−/5
Knee flexion	4−/5	4−/5
Knee extension	4/5	4−/5
Ankle dorsiflexion	4/5	4/5
Ankle plantarflexion		Unable to raise up on toes

   Based on the findings outlined above, I recommend a standard power wheelchair to meet Ms. Z's needs.

   Sincerely,

   Insert your name and credentials here

   Is the detail provided here valuable enough to warrant that this patient or client receive a power wheelchair? Why or why not?

   How would you change the letter so that the detail provided is meaningful to an audience who may not be a physical therapist or even a healthcare provider?

References

1. American Physical Therapy Association (APTA). *Guide to Physical Therapist Practice*, 1st ed. Arlington, VA: American Physical Therapy Association; 2014.

CHAPTER 10

Electronic Health Records: The Medium for Documentation

Jacqueline Osborne PT, DPT, GCS, CEEAA
and Marilyn Moffett PT, DPT, GCS, CEEAA, PhD(c)

CHAPTER OBJECTIVES

1. Identify how electronic health records are used in the healthcare sector.
2. Recognize relevant features unique to paper-based documentation systems.
3. Recognize the challenges of using paper-based documentation and electronic documentation systems.
4. Recognize the benefits of using electric health records.
5. Recognize the disadvantages of using electronic health records.

KEY TERMS

Electronic health record
Health Information Technology for Economic and Clinical Health (HITECH) Act

Paper-based documentation

Introduction

Electronic documentation is becoming an integrated component of nearly every healthcare provider's clinical practice. This chapter will identify how electronic health records are being used in the healthcare sector and how information in an electronic system can be utilized by physical therapists and physical therapist assistants. Common elements unique to paper-based documentation systems as well as those features that are important considerations for both paper-based and electronic systems are also presented. Lastly, common advantages and disadvantages to using electronic documentation systems are introduced.

Healthcare Reform and the Shift to Electronic Documentation

The **Health Information Technology for Economic and Clinical Health (HITECH) Act** was signed into law on February 17, 2009 and is designed to promote the adoption and meaningful use of health information technology. One goal of the HITECH Act is to strengthen enforcement of the Health Insurance Portability and Accountability Act (HIPAA) rules and regulations including the use of private health information within the context of electronic documentation systems. Specifically, the HITECH Act delineates a revised penalty scheme for violations of the security and protection of health information.[1] Additional programs were also created under the HITECH Act to provide assistance and technical support to healthcare providers, to enable coordination of healthcare information among states, to connect the public health community to needed resources in case of emergencies, and to ensure that that providers are properly trained and equipped to be meaningful users of **electronic health records**.[2] These programs include grant money and funding:

○ For communities to build and strengthen information technology infrastructure

○ To assist states in establishing health information exchange capabilities among healthcare providers and hospitals

○ To establish regional technical support centers for providers using electronic health records (EHRs)

○ To support research to develop the security of health information technology and the secondary use of EHR data

○ To develop a workforce of highly skilled health information technology experts who can assist providers with EHR implementation and use

○ To increase a consumer's ability to access his or her own health information with the goal of empowering individuals to actively participate in their own health care[2]

As a healthcare provider in the physical therapy profession, it is paramount for you to recognize the new responsibilities that accompany the exposure and vulnerability of the health information you use in your daily clinical practice. In other words, the exposure of protected health information in electronic-based systems is far greater than the exposure generated by paper-based systems. Therefore, you will be responsible for adopting certain habits and behaviors when using electronic systems in your clinical practice that maximize privacy to your patient or client.

As of 2015, eligible healthcare providers who have not transferred from paper-based documentation methods to certified electronic health record technology face reimbursement reductions from the Centers for Medicare & Medicaid Services (CMS) that progressively increase every year that an EHR is not in place.[3] Furthermore, if an eligible healthcare provider has also demonstrated meaningful use of that EHR system, than he or she will receive incentive payments for every year that EHRs are implemented.[4] While physical therapists and physical therapist assistants were not considered "eligible" providers under the CMS EHR Incentive Program as of 2014, those healthcare providers with whom you collaborate for the interdisciplinary care of your patients or clients are considered eligible providers. In response to this mandate, many physical therapy providers have adopted or are adopting EHRs to keep up with this technological evolution. Therefore, you will have to demonstrate your competence in using an electronic system, not only for retrieving health information to incorporate into the comprehensive care of your patient or client, but also for creating it.[5]

Using Information in an Electronic Documentation System

As a physical therapist or physical therapist assistant it is important to realize how EHRs can impact you in your practice as a *passive recipient* of information from an EHR, an *active investigator* of the information housed within an EHR, and an *active contributor* to the physical therapy documentation within an EHR. Being a passive recipient of information from an EHR involves your ability to accurately search and seek information for an individual patient or client. This requires baseline computer navigation skills as well as the ability to recognize the structural organization of an EHR so that you might know where in an electronic database to look or how to define search terms that will return the information you are looking for. Therefore, you must be aware of how the data entered into an electronic record is represented when you read your patient or client's note in its entirety. Being an active investigator of the information housed within an EHR involves an ability to collate and organize multiple data points from many different patients or clients to generate reports to perform cost analyses, identify practice patterns, or determine scheduling details such as cancellation rates or frequency and duration of care patterns. This skill also requires an understanding of the framework used to produce the end products of an EHR. Being an active contributor to the actual content of an EHR requires a clear understanding of the anatomy of your documentation. This understanding is fundamental to all documentation whether the medium is paper-based or electronic. Thus, the framework that constitutes *creating* successful documentation (TABLE 10-1) is applicable to paper-based documentation or to documenting in an electronic system. The documentation you create depends on your ability to transfer your clinical reasoning processes from your thoughts to your documentation, on your ability to use a feedforward process to identify the content relevant to your documentation, your ability to include the details in your note that can be used to

TABLE 10-1   Key Elements for Creating Successful Documentation

Transfer clinical reasoning processes from thoughts to health record.
Use a feedforward framework.
Include details required to make well-informed decisions.
Provide support for why physical therapy services are needed.

TABLE 10-2   Definitions of ICF Components

Component	Definition
Health Condition	Disease, disorder, or injury analogous to the medical diagnosis
Body Functions	Physiological functions of body systems (including psychological functions)
Body Structures	Anatomical parts of the body such as organs, limbs, and their components
Impairments	Problems in body functions or structure such as a significant deviation or loss
Activity	Execution of a task or action by an individual
Participation	Involvement in a life situation
Activity Limitations	Difficulties an individual may have in executing activities
Participation Restrictions	Problems an individual may experience in involvement in life situations
Contextual Factors **Environmental factors** **Personal factors**	The physical, social, and attitudinal environment in which people live and conduct their lives

Reproduced from World Health Organization. International Classification of Functioning Disability and Health: ICF. Geneva, Switzerland: World Health Organization; 2001.)

make well-informed decisions, and the evidence that supports why your physical therapy services are necessary for your patient or client. Your knowledge of the content of the initial examination, the daily note, the intervention flow sheet, the home exercise program, progress notes or re-examination notes, and the conclusion of the episode of care summary, as well as your ability to thread *The International Classification of Functioning, Disability, and Health* (ICF) model terminology (**TABLE 10-2**) throughout these components to organize the plan of care for your patient or client, will also assist in your ability to excel as a successful documenter. In other words, your ability to create successful documentation does not depend on the medium that houses this data.

Elements of a Paper-Based Documentation System

While much of the healthcare sector is moving towards or has already implemented electronic documentation systems, many providers still use **paper-based**

TABLE 10-3   Documentation Issues in Paper-Based Systems

Storage
Access
Legibility
Error correction
Data organization

documentation formats. Therefore, it is important to have an understanding of the elements that present unique issues when utilizing a paper-based documentation format for physical therapy documentation such as storage, access, legibility, error correction, and data organization (**TABLE 10-3**).

STORAGE

A paper-based health record has tangible requirements such as paper, a mechanism to hold its parts together, and a location for storage. Healthcare providers are required to keep paper-based health records for a certain period of years after the conclusion of the patient or client's episode of care. For example, the CMS requires that Medicare beneficiaries' records be kept for up to 6 years after the termination of services.[6] However, there are record retention requirements that are mandated at the state level and include differences depending on the type of medical information retained, the setting in which the information was gathered, and the party responsible for reimbursement.[7] Furthermore, there are costs associated with ensuring that additional space is available to house these materials as well as costs associated with the eventual disposal of paper-based health records.

ACCESS

Access to paper-based documentation can impose limitations in many ways. Challenges in multidisciplinary settings occur when more than one user wants to access a health record simultaneously. For example, you may want to obtain your patient or client's health record so that you have access to information you created at the initial examination in order to structure your re-examination. However, if another provider has the paper-based record for another purpose, not only have you lost valuable time searching for the record, but now you are forced to create temporary documentation that you must transcribe to the actual record at a later time. Furthermore, access to information may be delayed if a member of the patient or client's healthcare team seeks information from a colleague whose data has not been written or dictated and subsequently filed into the record. Access to paper-based information can also be significantly delayed because a patient or client's paper-based information is likely stored in multiple locations such as with a referring physician's office, a hospital records department, a radiologist's office, or a prior physical therapy provider. Sharing and exchanging paper-based information then requires faxing, mailing, or using a courier service to move information between locations thus delaying access to pertinent information.

LEGIBILITY

Handwriting legibility in paper-based documentation can also be problematic. Poor handwriting can lead to improper interpretation of recorded information and subsequent errors based on the need of the user to interpret or assume the data's meaning to the best of his or her ability. Furthermore, time spent attempting to decipher poor handwriting is time taken away from the comprehensive care of your patient or client. Signatures can also be illegible, making it difficult to determine which healthcare provider authored the entry into the documentation system. Illegible signatures can disrupt a collaborative communication process with your patient or client's healthcare team, as well as interfere with practice standards if it is unclear which level of practitioner signed a note or who might be the therapist of record.

ERROR CORRECTION

Error correction in a paper-based health record requires a specific procedure. Black permanent ink is the expected standard manner in which information should be written in a paper-based record. Black ink should also be used to correct any errors made when handwriting documentation. The incorrect word or phrase would be indicated with a single line through it and then dated and initialed by the note's author adjacent to the error. It is important to ensure that no information is removed from or concealed in the record, and therefore no other correction mechanism such as erasing or using correction fluid is permitted.

DATA ORGANIZATION

Data organization is also an issue to consider when using paper-based documentation. The way in which you might organize information in a paper-based record may

be different than the way in which another healthcare provider from an alternative discipline might organize the information he or she records in a paper-based record. This "disorganization" can lead to wasted time looking for relevant information or can lead to assumptions that the information is not available. Therefore, it can be valuable to have policies and procedures in place regarding the standard and accepted arrangement of the paper-based record that is appropriate for the setting in which you practice. Again, the non-value-added time spent looking for relevant information is valuable time taken away from your patient or client.

Issues Common to Paper-Based and Electronic Documentation Systems

In addition to the unique issues present when using paper-based documentation systems, there are also issues that exist among paper-based and electronic documentation systems that are important to consider as a physical therapist or physical therapist assistant (TABLE 10-4).

INTERFACE FOR CLINICAL DECISION MAKING

The algorithms used in computer software that generate the content of physical therapy documentation are very different than the algorithms that might exist in your head for creating a paper-based note. When you generate a paper-based written document, you present it in an order that makes logical sense to you. On the contrary, an electronic system utilizes fragmented data entry code from many different locations within the software's structure that does not exist tangibly in real time as an ordered collection of information and events.[5] There are also many

TABLE 10-4 Documentation Considerations in Paper-Based and Electronic Systems

Interface for clinical decision making
Content of documentation notes
"Documenting by exception" strategy
Use of abbreviations
Documenting time spent in patient or client care
Privacy and security of patient or client data
Documenting at the point-of-service
Data entry

features in an EHR such as drop-down menus, check boxes, and prefabricated sentence structures that may interfere with your clinical decision-making paradigm. An EHR template tends to include areas within the documentation that allow for much more information than you might actually need to capture with your particular patient or client. Therefore, while the features of an EHR were actually intended to be timesavers, they may add time and effort to your ability to create successful documentation. Thus, the inability to apply the fundamental framework indicated above to your documentation may inhibit your ability to retrieve information and create successful documentation within an electronic health record.[5]

CONTENT OF DOCUMENTATION NOTES

Documentation generated in an EHR tends to be lengthier than handwritten notes in a paper-based system.[8] As indicated above, this can be because the amount of information available from pre-populated templates and drop-down menus in an EHR creates a lengthier end product. Conversely, writing paper-based notes may be self-limiting due to the availability of space in a paper-based template or due to the inability to consider any additional thought processes that might be triggered by a pre-populated electronic template. It can also be challenging to proofread your electronically created note in real time due to the fact that the final narrative format of the note emerges via a conglomeration of pre-populated sentence structures, drop-down menus, and free-text areas. Therefore, it is imperative as a user of an EHR that you are aware of the final formatting of a note you create so that you are able to apply a specific framework and organized structure to ensure that you are creating a succinct but complete piece of documentation.

DOCUMENTING BY EXCEPTION

To control the amount of writing in a paper-based note, a documentation strategy known as "documenting by exception" has been utilized. Similarly, the organizational structure within an electronic system facilitates the use of a "documenting by exception" strategy. Documenting in this way refers to applying an examination and intervention protocol that includes predetermined assessment tools, goals, outcomes, and frequency and duration of the episode of care for a patient or client. Thus, the only unique documentation that would occur in either a paper-based system or an EHR when using this strategy is any status

or event not indicated by the protocol.[9] Consider that your patient or client is a 52-year-old female with activity limitations and participation restrictions consistent with adhesive capsulitis of the right shoulder. A "documenting by exception" protocol would indicate range of motion loss at the glenohumeral joint in a certain expected pattern, joint mobility loss in certain expected planes, a predetermined list of expected limitations and restrictions, prefabricated goals, and predetermined timing of the duration and frequency of the episode of care that likely does not accurately reflect the actual impairments in body functions and structures, activity limitations and participation restrictions, contextual factors, or goals unique to your patient or client. Documenting in this way is not recommended since it is not a patient- or client-centered approach that considers the unique needs of a patient or client. Additionally, use of a generic protocol does not relay the medical necessity of why your skilled services are warranted for your unique patient or client.

USE OF ABBREVIATIONS

Another strategy employed to decrease the amount of writing in a paper-based note is the use of abbreviations. The organizational structure of an EHR also facilitates the use of abbreviations. While the use of abbreviations can lead to errors in interpretation[10] and is not generally supported by the American Physical Therapy Association (APTA),[9] there may be an appropriate way to use them in an electronic system without compromising quality of care or patient or client safety. For example, an organization might publish an accepted list of abbreviations available to any provider in that healthcare system via a policies and procedures document. The meanings of these approved abbreviations could then be pre-populated and selected from a drop-down menu any time you decide to use the abbreviation. Thus, the full meaning of the abbreviation would be revealed in the final product of your documentation eliminating the need for an interpretation of the abbreviation by the note's user.

DOCUMENTING TIME WITH THE PATIENT OR CLIENT

Determining the timing of your interventions is also an important consideration in your documentation regardless of the system you use but that requires a different process in a paper-based system than an EHR. Electronic systems include the capability to capture *any* activity that occurs within the EHR such calculating the timing of access and cataloguing exact keystrokes within a patient or client's record. It is important to be aware when using an EHR that the system would be able to track your entry into or exit out of a note, but not the actual time that you spent delivering care to your patient or client. Therefore, a specific method for determining actual treatment time may need to be built into the system you use if this is an element of data you are aiming to collect in your clinical practice. A method for tracking actual treatment time may also be necessary in a paper-based documentation system; however, there is not an additional mechanism in a paper-based system for tracking who accesses the record to retrieve data from it or to add data to it.

PRIVACY AND SECURITY OF PATIENT OR CLIENT DATA

Access to a paper-based health record can theoretically be obtained by anyone who has the physical capability to open and read its contents. Your responsibility regarding the privacy and security of a paper-based note includes ensuring that the physical record is in a secure and safe location even when it is in your possession. Additionally, you are responsible for ensuring that all identifying information on copies made of any part of a paper-based record is obscured. As an EHR user, you will also have the responsibility to maintain the privacy of the health records you access. For example, if your facility uses devices such as laptop computers or tablets for documentation, then it will be important that you secure access to that device before walking away from it. It will be equally important that you do not allow any other EHR user to access health information via your personal access information since the only way an electronic system can identify the user of its contents is through login information. Furthermore, it is possible that you might share hardware with other providers. If you walk away from a computer terminal or device but forget to logout, you may either become locked out of the system or leave your EHR access available to any other individual who uses that device.

DOCUMENTING AT THE POINT-OF-SERVICE

As you become proficient at navigating and creating data within the electronic system you use, it will be important to also become proficient at creating documentation for your patient or client in real time, at the point-of-service.

It may be important for you to plan on "catching up" with your documentation at certain points during your work day so that you are not inundated at the end of the day with documentation that you are creating based on your memory of the details of each of your patient or client's sessions. This is an appropriate practice regardless of the type of documentation system you utilize.

DATA ENTRY

Information entered into your patient or client's physical therapy record can occur at multiple points in time by different members of the patient or client's immediate physical therapy team. This includes office support personnel who may be entering your patient or client's note to record a phone call cancellation or a conversation regarding insurance coverage. Similarly, nonprofessional personnel such as a therapy aide may be involved in documenting collected vital signs or the provision of certain modalities such as hot packs or cold packs. Furthermore, your physical therapist assistant partner may be entering your patient or client's note to record the results of the patient or client's reported history or the results of performance on collected outcome measures. Because electronic systems are set up to allow only one user to access a patient or client's record at any given time, it is extremely important to communicate with your team to determine who should have access to a note, the timing of that access, what information he or she is responsible for recording, and what circumstances are not appropriate for anyone other than a physical therapist or physical therapist assistant to record. Additionally, if you as a physical therapist share a schedule with a physical therapist assistant during the day, then you will need to agree which person is responsible for the completion of each patient or client's documentation. This situation is different from the scenario where you and your physical therapist assistant colleague are familiar with the same patients or clients but carry a separate case load for the day.

Advantages and Benefits to Using EHRs

Advancements in communications and information exchange technology has infiltrated the healthcare sector facilitating advancements unprecedented in the history of

TABLE 10-5 Advantages of Electronic Documentation Systems

Availability of clinical decision support
Ability to perform data analysis

Immediate access to information
  ○ Facilitates communication.
  ○ Improves documentation efficiency.

medicine. EHRs are among the technologies expected to assist providers in delivering higher quality care to their patients or clients.[11] EHRs are also expected to support increased access to health records and health information by providers.[12] However, as with any innovation, barriers to implementation and use exist. Alternatively, important benefits to using EHRs have also been recognized. **TABLE 10-5** reviews the advantages and benefits to using an electronic documentation system.

AVAILABILITY OF CLINICAL DECISION SUPPORT

Electronic documentation systems can be equipped with clinical decision support (CDS) tools such as the use of computerized reminders. This technology has been used in preventative medicine and prophylactic care in hospitalized patients or clients at risk for deep vein thrombosis (DVT). For example, computerized alerts resulted in an increase in the use of anticoagulation therapy leading to a reduced risk of DVT or pulmonary embolism 90 days after a patient or client was discharged from the hospital setting.[13] In physical therapy, computerized alerts may be used to remind you when your patient or client is scheduled for a follow-up visit with another healthcare provider, to serve as a reminder to create re-examination documentation for your patient or client, or to alert other members of your patient or client's healthcare team of the presence of precautions or contraindications for your patient or client.

The inherent organizational structure of an EHR can also be an asset to you in your documentation affording you the potential to improve your efficiency with your documentation. If you lack a framework around which to build your documentation, then the features of an EHR such as drop-down menus and pre-populated fields can halt your clinical reasoning process. However, these features could guide your decisions and help to improve your documentation time, accuracy, and efficiency as long as you preserve your professional obligation to create meaningful and usable information. In other words, you should use a drop-down alphabetized menu of tests and measures to quickly select those relevant to your patient or client based on your sound clinical reasoning process rather than scroll through a list of tests and measures searching for those that seem like a good idea to collect for your patient or client.

DATA ANALYSIS ABILITY

An additional benefit of EHRs includes the ability to analyze collected data over time. For example, data can be gathered and reports generated regarding clinicians practice patterns to help identify inefficiencies in practice, to determine patient or client satisfaction rates, and to inform clinicians of coding and billing practices. Furthermore, research can be conducted within organizations as well as across patient or client communities and populations to identify public health needs.[14]

IMMEDIATE ACCESS TO INFORMATION

EHR utilization also allows for immediate access to your patient or client's health information that may include important history, medication or imaging information, as well as documentation from prior services your patient or client may have received. Furthermore, your patient or client, other healthcare providers, and third-party payers can become aware of the data you collect for your patient or client immediately upon your entering it into an electronic system for more efficient, quality care and for faster reimbursement for the services you delivered.

Disadvantages and Barriers to Using EHRs

In addition to the benefits of utilizing electronic documentation systems, barriers to the implementation and use of EHRs have also been identified (**TABLE 10-6**).

TABLE 10-6 Disadvantages of Electronic Documentation Systems

Ongoing costs
Intermittent disruptions in workflow
Learning curve for users
Error correction
Inherent composition of the system

ONGOING COSTS

Aside from the large costs associated with the initial implementation of EHRs, there are large ongoing hardware and software maintenance costs as well as ongoing training costs associated with continuing successful use of an electronic system. To offset start-up costs, you may be required to share a laptop or tablet with your colleagues rather than have a device of your own.

INTERMITTENT DISRUPTIONS IN WORKFLOW

Unscheduled disruptions in workflow are another disadvantage of using electronic documentation systems. For example, technology requires maintenance as well as power to operate. You must be prepared and able to continue care for your patient or client in the event of a technical problem with your electronic documentation system. Therefore, it is important to be aware of your clinical affiliation site or your employer's policies regarding how documentation should be recorded when the electronic documentation system is down. This includes identifying preferred practices utilizing paper-based forms or templates and a process for recording information. For example, it would be valuable to fill out a paper-based template designed for a specific type of patient or client encounter that could be scanned into the electronic system at a later date. Alternatively, disruptions in workflow can also occur due to user error stemming from new employees and practitioners using a new system resulting in temporary losses in productivity.[11]

LEARNING CURVE FOR USERS

Demonstrating proficiency at using EHRs both for retrieving information and creating documentation is a skill that must be learned and practiced over time. Your ability to successfully and consistently use an EHR is dependent upon many dynamic components. These components include the inherent structure of an EHR, the steps required to gain access to an electronic system, the need for technological support, your inherent computer navigation and typing skills, and your ability to adapt and translate your clinical reasoning processes to an electronic format. Therefore, these fundamental characteristics of an EHR create a learning curve for users.

ERROR CORRECTION

Another disadvantage of using an EHR is the lengthy process required to correct an error within electronic documentation. There are a certain series of steps that exist in an EHR for making an entry into the documentation a permanent part of the record. For example, after creating your note you may have to save it just like any other piece of electronic data that you create. However, saving the data may only allow you to see the documentation again rather than being available to other users of the note. There are likely additional steps such as declaring your entry as an official visit or proceeding with the billing component of the process that ultimately makes your entry into the system a permanent record. Thus, if you identify an error in your documentation after you have completed these steps, there is an alternative set of processes that you must follow to alter the contents of a note you previously created. In some systems, an option to reopen a note that has already been completed will not be available. Therefore, it is imperative to understand prior to using the electronic system the process for correcting any documentation errors. Transmittal 442 from the CMS, effective January 8, 2013, indicates that any correction or addendum to a paper-based or electronic health record must clearly and permanently identify any correction or addition to the documentation as well as clearly indicate the date and author of the altered documentation. Therefore, documentation as it was originally created must be preserved.[16]

INHERENT COMPOSITION

As indicated above, features inherent to an EHR such as drop-down menus, prefabricated sentence structures, and pre-populated data fields can be considered an asset to such a system. However, these characteristics were designed with the goals of increasing efficiency, saving time, and improving the quality of your documentation. Therefore, if these features are applied to every single component of your documentation, then a fragmented note that does not possess the key elements necessary for successful documentation will be created. In other words, your documentation will be so efficient that quality will be compromised because the note lacks content. It is extremely important that you are able to employ these features inherent to an EHR appropriately throughout your documentation by supplementing areas where you choose these features with narrative content to provide the clinical rationale for your selections and to ensure that you have created meaningful and comprehensive documentation.

Summary

Electronic health records are an inevitable part of physical therapy practice and therefore your ability to successfully communicate within EHRs will ensure that you are able to completely participate in the comprehensive care of your patient or client. Ongoing training in the proficient use of an electronic system for documentation is necessary as continuous efforts are made to improve EHRs and as understanding of such complex systems evolve to meet the needs of different clinicians with different specialties in different healthcare settings.[15] It will be important for you to utilize the technical support offered by your clinical affiliation site, your employer, or the EHR's vendor, as well as to maintain an open communication with your colleagues about the challenges you encounter in using your system. It is also important to recognize the ease with which you could become overwhelmed and inundated with healthcare information especially when utilizing a documentation system that may be integrated into a larger healthcare system. For example, there may be multiple locations of information such as vital signs and the results of imaging studies. There may be different levels of care within your organization where the individual received care across the continuum such as in an intensive care unit, acute care, inpatient rehabilitation, and home health care. Thus, it will be paramount that you communicate with your team to identify how to determine multiple locations of different health information to optimize efficient use. Lastly, it may be valuable as you continue to use electronic health systems to revisit resources such as this text, to exchange and critique samples of documentation with your colleagues, and to engage in self-reflection regarding your documentation on a regular basis to develop your efficiency with the documentation system you use.

Discussion Questions

1. What are the challenges with using electronic health records? How will you overcome these challenges?
2. What are the advantages and disadvantages to using electronic health records?
3. What is meant by using a "documentation by exception" strategy? Why is this strategy not supported by the American Physical Therapy Association?
4. What does it mean to document at the point-of-service? What are the challenges you may potentially face or have actually experienced when trying to implement this real-time documentation strategy?
5. Challenge yourself to create some or all of the components of your documentation without the use of a paper-based or electronic template (such as what you might have to do if your electronic system was not functional). What were the barriers to doing this? Were there areas that you rely on more than others to create certain components of your documentation?

References

1. The United States Department of Health and Human Services. HITECH Act Enforcement Interim Final Rule. *Federal Register*. 2009;74(209):56123–56131. Available at www.hhs.gov/ocr/privacy/hipaa/administrative/enforcementrule/enfifr.pdf. Accessed on October 17, 2014.
2. The United States Department of Health and Human Services. HITECH Programs and Advisory Committees. HealthIT.gov. Available at http://www.healthit.gov/policy-researchers-implementers/hitech-programs-advisory-committees. Accessed on October 17, 2014.
3. Centers for Medicare & Medicaid Services. *An Introduction to the Medicare EHR Incentive Program for Medical Professionals*. Available at www.cms.gov/Regulations-and-Guidance/Legislation/EHRIncentivePrograms/downloads/Beginners_Guide.pdf. Accessed on July 19, 2014.
4. Centers for Medicare & Medicaid Services. Medicare Electronic Health Record Incentive Payments for Eligible Professionals, May 2013. Available at www.cms.gov/Regulations-and-Guidance/Legislation/EHRIncentivePrograms/Downloads/MLN_MedicareEHRProgram_TipSheet_EP.pdf. Accessed on July 19, 2014.
5. Han H, Lopp L. Writing and reading in the electronic health record: an entirely new world. *Med Educ Online*. 2013;18:18634. Available at http://dx.doi.org/10.3402/meo.v18i0.18634. Accessed on July 20, 2014.
6. Centers for Medicare & Medicaid Services, *MLN Matters*: SE1022. Available at www.cms.gov/Outreach-and-Education/Medicare-Learning-Network-MLN/MLNMattersArticles/downloads/SE1022.pdf. Accessed on July 20, 2014.
7. University of Minnesota, School of Public Health, Health Policy and Management. *State Regulations Pertaining to Clinical Records*. Available at www.hpm.umn.edu/nhregsplus/NH%20Regs%20by%20Topic/NH%20Regs%20

Topic%20Pdfs/Clinical%20Records/category-administration-clinical%20records-final.pdf. Accessed on July 20, 2014.

8. Payne TH, Hirschmann JV, Helbig S. The elements of electronic note style. *J AHIMA*. 2003; 74: 68–70.

9. American Physical Therapy Association. *Defensible Documentation. Frequently Asked Questions.* Arlington, VA: American Physical Therapy Association; 2011.

10. Sinha S, McDermott F, Srinivas G, Houghton PW. Use of abbreviations by healthcare professionals: what is the way forward? *Postgrad Med J.* 2011;87(1029):450–452.

11. Menachemi N and Collum TH. Benefits and drawbacks of electronic health record systems. *Risk Management and Healthcare Policy.* 2011;4:47–55.

12. American Physical Therapy Association. *PT in Motion.* April 2013; 27. Available at www.multivu.com/mnr/50965-level-3-independent-cio-survey-confidence-=lacking-in-network-security.

13. Kucher N, Koo S, Quiroz R, et al. Electronic alerts to prevent venous thromboembolism among hospitalized patients. *N Engl J Med.* 2005;352(10):969–977.

14. Kukafka R, Ancker JS, Chan C, et al. Redesigning electronic health record systems to support public health. *J Biomed Inform.* 2007;40(4):398–409.

15. Blavin F, Ramos C, Shah A, Devers K. *Lessons Learned from the Literature on Electronic Health Record Implementation.* Office of the National Coordinator of Health Information Technology of the U.S. Department of Health and Human Services; 2013. Available at www.healthit.gov/sites/default/files/hit_lessons_learned_lit_review_final_08-01-2013.pdf. Accessed on July 20, 2014.

16. Centers for Medicare and Medicaid Services Pub 100-08 Medicare Program Integrity, 2012. Available at http://www.cms.gov/Regulations-and-Guidance/Guidance/Transmittals/downloads/R442PI.pdf. Accessed March 28, 2015.

CHAPTER 11

The Impact of Healthcare Reform on Physical Therapy Documentation

CHAPTER OBJECTIVES

1. Recognize the elements necessary to supplement the components of your physical therapy documentation to ensure reimbursement for the physical therapy services you provide.
2. Define International Classification of Diseases (ICD) codes and Current Procedural Terminology (CPT) codes and recognize how these codes are used by the physical therapy profession.
3. Define functional limitation reporting (FLR) and recognize how G-codes are used by the physical therapy profession.
4. Recognize efforts by the Centers for Medicare & Medicaid Services to develop quality reporting initiatives such as the Physician Quality Reporting System (PQRS).
5. Recognize that billing procedures are setting specific and that rules and regulations that mandate billing procedures are updated annually.
6. Discuss the therapy cap and the exceptions process.
7. Define direct access and recognize how it impacts physical therapy practice.

KEY TERMS

Accountable care organizations
Current Procedural Terminology codes
Direct access
Functional limitation reporting
G-codes

International Classification of Diseases
Physician Quality Reporting System
Reimbursement
Therapy cap

Introduction

This chapter relays the current status of healthcare reform and how this reform affects physical therapy documentation. First, accountable care organizations are defined. Second, recognizing reimbursement patterns as a learning tool within clinical practice to advance documentation skills is relayed. Third, the use of coding schemes in physical therapy practice such as the International Classification of Diseases (ICD) codes, Current Procedural Terminology (CPT) codes, and Functional Limitation Reporting (FLR) codes are introduced. Next, recently implemented quality initiatives in various practice settings are reviewed. Billing practices in outpatient settings and consolidated billing are also described. Finally, the therapy cap, the KX modifier, and direct access are defined and related to documentation in physical therapy practice.

Accountable Care Organizations

Healthcare reform does not signify a compilation of new ideas, but rather includes revisions of old ideas that have been a part of healthcare reform for decades. Healthcare reform of the 21st century calls for the widespread, cost-effective delivery of quality healthcare services that require physical therapists and physical therapist assistants to be integral contributors to the approaches that define this reform. The Affordable Care Act, signed into law in 2010, was developed to initiate comprehensive healthcare reform over a period of years to implement new consumer protections, improve quality, lower costs, and increase access to affordable healthcare. **Accountable care organizations** (ACOs), networks of healthcare providers who are financially incentivized to provide high-value quality care to Medicare beneficiaries,[1] is one such example of this reform. Specifically, ACOs are charged with slowing their patient or client's healthcare spending by emphasizing quality and prevention.[1] The goal of an ACO is to function as the mediator who integrates healthcare between all of the settings a beneficiary might encounter when attempting to manage his or her own healthcare. In other words, ACOs are a form of managed care. Some examples of services provided by ACOs that are intended to improve quality of care while reducing overall healthcare costs include:

○ Providing weekend and evening shift physical therapy services in various settings[2]
○ Utilizing physical therapy services in emergency departments[3]
○ Promoting interdisciplinary care[4,5]
○ Performing early mobility in intensive care units[6,7]

Sound documentation practices in all settings will help to relay the value of the services physical therapists and physical therapist assistants provide and how these services are paramount to the success of increasing access to quality healthcare.

Additional reform approaches such as bundled payment and pay-for-performance reimbursement models are approaches that also affect physical therapist practice and documentation. It is important to recognize that the details of some of these methods are transient and are likely to change quickly. Therefore, it is pertinent to have a cursory understanding of some of the methods that define current healthcare reform rather than to have an in-depth understanding of how key provisions in the law might be implemented or how each might affect physical therapists and physical therapist assistants in a variety of practice settings. Therefore, the remainder of this chapter provides an overview of selected healthcare reform issues, how each might impact physical therapists and physical therapist assistants, and when available, how additional information regarding these issues can be obtained.

Reimbursement

You likely became a physical therapist or physical therapist assistant because you want to help people maximize their health potential. Furthermore, you likely feel a sense of satisfaction for assisting your patient or client in setting goals, reaching milestones, and navigating unprecedented territory as physical potential is realized and abilities are achieved. Hopefully, you feel a similar sense of validation for getting paid for the services you provide. This aspect of job satisfaction may be imperceptible to you however because the entity providing your salary and benefits and the entity providing **reimbursement** for the services you deliver are different. If you have the opportunity to learn of your own reimbursement patterns in your clinical practice, as one does in private practice, it may be natural for you to feel that services not reimbursed were for reasons or circumstances beyond your control. For example, you may receive notice that you were not paid for services you rendered because a referring physician did not sign your plan of care in a timely manner, as is a requirement for some third-party payers, or a date of service was incorrectly entered into an electronic health record (EHR) by an administrator. However, in the midst of healthcare reform in the 21st century, you as a physical therapist or physical therapist assistant are held accountable for the value of the services you provide, which includes operational details outside the context of the actual patient or client encounter. Alternatively, other reasons for claim denials may be directly related to the content of the information you provided in the patient or client's health record such as scant details relaying support for the frequency and duration of care indicated or providing interventions for impairments in body functions and structures, activity limitations, or participation restrictions that you did not assess. Therefore, knowing the reasons for reimbursement denials can help you to improve your documentation skills so that you can infuse greater value and quality into your documentation. Thus, the portal into determining this value is directly linked to your documentation. Well-written information that justifies the necessity of the services you deliver to your patient or client includes the outcomes achieved during an episode of care. In other words, tests and measures and outcome tools that relay your patient or client's functional abilities will communicate the quality and value of your services to the payer source. The payer may include the patient or client, known as "self-pay"; your employer, known as "pro-bono" service; you, in the case of private practice; or most commonly, a third-party payer such as a private insurance, Medicare, Medicaid, or Tricare. Regardless of the source and mechanism for how the value of your services is determined, your documentation should be successfully written to relay that quality healthcare services were needed and delivered. Ultimately, the payer either reimburses a flat rate regardless of the services you provide or the payer analyzes your documentation for the evidence that supports that the services they are funding are truly valuable to your patient or client.

Most third-party private insurance programs use federal rules and regulations as the "gold standard" for determining quality documentation. While the Centers for Medicare & Medicaid Services (CMS) provide specific requirements for documenting the delivery of physical therapy services in each care setting, the fundamental basis of this "gold standard" includes guidelines for documenting care (TABLE 11-1). It is also important to recognize that most states have documentation requirements delineated in their practice acts that override guidelines recommended by the CMS. Ultimately, underscoring these state or federal guidelines are the key elements for creating successful documentation (TABLE 11-2) such as ensuring that your documentation reflects your clinical reasoning, using a feedforward framework in your documentation so that no one section of your note is left unsubstantiated, including details required for a user to make well-informed decisions, and clearly indicating why physical therapy services are needed for the amount of time recommended. Ensuring that these components are present in your documentation will help to relay that your physical therapy services were skilled and necessary regardless of the changing legislation in the healthcare environment.

TABLE 11-1   Medicare Guidelines for "Reasonable and Medically Necessary" Documentation of Therapy Services

Physical therapy services rendered must be:
Safe and effective.
Not experimental or investigational.
Appropriate in duration and frequency.
In accordance with the standards of practice for the patient or client's condition.
Provided in the appropriate setting to match the patient or client's medical needs and health condition(s).
Ordered and delivered by qualified personnel.
Appropriate to meet but not exceed the patient or client's medical needs.
At least as beneficial as an existing and available medically appropriate alternative.

Data from CMS. *Medicare Program Integrity Manual*, Chapter 13, 13.5.1- Reasonable and Necessary Provisions in LCDs (Rev. 473, Issued: 06-21-13, Effective: 01-15-13, Implementation: 01-15-13). Baltimore: Centers for Medicare & Medicaid Services. Available at www.cms.gov/manuals/downloads/pim83c13.pdf.

TABLE 11-2   Key Elements for Creating Successful Documentation

Transfer clinical reasoning processes from thoughts to health record.
Use a feedforward framework.
Include details required to make well-informed decisions.
Provide support for why physical therapy services are needed.

Coding

Ensuring that you are reimbursed for the physical therapy services you provide requires a team approach including coding specialists and a systematic coding structure including the **International Classification of Diseases** (ICD), Current Procedural Terminology (CPT) codes, and functional codes required by the CMS. In addition, the *International Classification of Functioning, Disability, and Health* (ICF) model includes a coding structure that has not yet been adopted nationally for coding health-related information. By way of review, the ICF model is a conceptual framework developed by the World Health Organization (WHO) in 2001 to classify an individual's functioning and ability, and is therefore referred to as an "enablement" model. In other words, the ICF model provides a mechanism to describe how an individual functions in life given a certain set of abilities rather than describing a pathology and how it affects that individual or results in disabilities. This model can therefore be used to organize information gathered from your patient or client and then to further synthesize it into a cohesive physical therapy plan of care.

INTERNATIONAL CLASSIFICATION OF DISEASES

The International Classification of Diseases (ICD) is a diagnostic coding schema created by the World Health Organization to organize and code health information used for epidemiology, national mortality and morbidity statistics, resource allocation, research, primary care, prevention, healthcare management, and reimbursement.[8] The ICD, first developed in 1855, was revised several times to eventually become the International List of Diseases and Causes of Death by 1886.[9] By 1948, the sixth revision of the International List of Diseases and Causes of Death, revised over the first half of the 20th century, was redefined by the WHO and became ICD-6. This revision contained two volumes including a tabular list of diagnostic categories, the form of the medical certificate cause of death, the rules for classification, and an alphabetical index of diagnostic terms coded to the appropriate categories.[10] According to the World Health Organization Family of International Classifications (WHO-FIC) Network, the main objectives of the ongoing ICD update and revision process are to:

- Reflect advances in medicine and all health sciences including compatibility with electronic health records.
- Support clinical decisions while eliminating redundancy.
- Be readily integrated into routine clinical practice in any healthcare setting.
- Assist in public health policy, resource allocation, and monitoring outcomes by recording population statistics.[11]

Currently, the physical therapy profession uses code sets known as the International Classification of Diseases, Clinical Modification (ICD-CM) and Procedure Coding System (ICD-PCS). As of October 1, 2015, the federal government plans to replace the ninth version of the classification system (ICD-9) used to report diagnoses and procedures with ICD-10 codes. In addition, the release of the eleventh revision is planned for 2017. A specific goal of the ICD-11 revision is to combine disorders and diseases (ICD) with ability and functioning (ICF) to ensure that functioning is reflected in the new definitions of diseases and disorders.[12] Just as the ICF model provides a common language for successful and meaningful physical therapy documentation that can be used by multiple entities for decision making, the ICD serves as a common language for reporting and monitoring diseases and health conditions internationally for data analysis and evidence-based decision making.[13]

In any given setting, ICD codes are used by coding professionals to create a complete and accurate patient or client record. In other words, clear and open communication must occur between you and the coding and billing team to ensure that the documentation in the patient or client's health record matches the code that categorizes the reason the patient or client is seeking physical therapy services. Online resources and search engines are available to assist your team in determining which codes to apply to your patient or client. In addition, resources are available to convert ICD-9-CM codes to ICD-10-CM codes. For example, abnormality of gait is coded 781.2 according to the ICD-9 classification and as R26.9 according to ICD-10 (for ICD-10 codes see www.icd10data.com).

CURRENT PROCEDURAL TERMINOLOGY CODES

In addition to ICD codes, Current Procedural Terminology (CPT) codes are required in order to receive payment from the payer source for skilled services provided. These codes, originally created by the American Medical Association (AMA) in 1966, are used by healthcare professionals to report medical procedures and services under public and private payer sources.[14] In 1977 the fourth CPT edition was published and in 1983 this version was adopted as part of the CMS Healthcare Common Procedure Coding System (HCPCS).[14] There are two primary levels of the HCPCS. In physical therapy, Level I HCPCS codes are five-digit codes that contain CPT codes. These are commonly referred to as the "97000 series" and labeled as "Physical Medicine and Rehabilitation" codes. There are other codes that exist outside of the 97000 series, however, that can be used by physical therapists and physical therapist assistants. Level II HCPCS codes include codes for services that do not have a corresponding Level I HCPCS/CPT code such as durable medical equipment, medical supplies, prosthetics, and orthotics. These are four-digit numerical codes that are preceded by a letter.

CPT codes are intended to be used to determine what skilled services were provided during an encounter, not what products or equipment were used in the delivery of the skilled service. However, certain services such as providing an ultrasound (97035) and issuing a hot or cold pack (97010) during a physical therapy encounter still have CPT codes associated with them. It is important to recognize that simply because a service has a CPT code associated with it does not mean that it is a reimbursable code according to a payer source. Therefore, you must be aware of the CPT codes that are reimbursable by your patient or client's payer source so that you can inform your patient or client of the potential for an out-of-pocket cost despite the fact that he or she has insurance, or discuss with your employer your decision to deliver a service that is not covered. Ethically, you must deliver the skilled services that you professionally determined to be clinically necessary and valuable for the physical therapy care of your patient or client, not the services that have reimbursable codes per your patient or client's payer source.

At times, some commonly used CPT codes and Level II HCPCS codes are billed together either erroneously or fraudulently. A CPT modifier known as modifier 59 was created by the CMS to define a "distinct procedural service" and to prevent providers from unbundling a service so that it could be billed twice. In other words, modifier 59 was to be attached to a CPT code to represent services that are typically bundled, but due to a special circumstance, are billed separate and distinct from each other, such as when a service is performed on two different regions of the body on the same day.[15] According to the CMS, however, as of January 2015, modifier 59 will be replaced by four new codes, called –X modifiers (TABLE 11-3) intended to clarify the distinct and separate

TABLE 11-3   X-Modifiers

Code	Definition
XE	Separate Encounter: A service that is distinct because it occurred during a separate encounter; used to describe separate encounters on the same date of service
XS	Separate Structure: A service that is distinct because it was performed on a separate organ/structure
XP	Separate Practitioner: A service that is distinct because it was performed by a different practitioner
XU	Unusual Non-overlapping Service: Use of a service that is distinct because it does not overlap usual components of the main service

Data from Centers for Medicare & Medicaid Services (CMS). MLN Matters. Number: MM8863. August 2014; MM8863.

reasons that two codes generally considered to be bundled are billed separately.[15]

Consistent with other healthcare payment reform initiatives, in 2013 the American Physical Therapy Association (APTA) proposed to transition from the currently utilized payment system where services are reimbursed based on the procedures delivered over a certain period of time to a per session payment system termed the Physical Therapy Classification and Payment System (PTCPS).[16] Under this system, CPT codes would be redefined and a new coding structure based on a patient or client's severity level would be implemented. The APTA continues efforts to reform the current payment system for outpatient physical therapy services to align with the goals of achieving greater reporting accuracy, promote quality care, and reduce coding and billing fraud and abuse.[16]

FUNCTIONAL LIMITATION REPORTING

In addition to ICD codes and CPT codes, the CMS requires the use of nonpayable **functional limitation reporting** (FLR) represented by **G-codes** that allow for the collection of information regarding a Medicare beneficiary's health condition and level of functioning. Currently, these codes are required for outpatient physical therapy services rendered. The CMS intends to use this information in the future to reform payment for outpatient physical therapy services. Therefore, it is important for physical therapists and physical therapist assistants to have a working knowledge of this system. FLR is intended to be a marker for capturing information about a patient or client's activity limitations and participation restrictions. As of July 1, 2013, G-codes must be collected for any physical therapy, occupational therapy, or speech language pathology service billed under Medicare Part B including acute care hospitals, critical access hospitals, skilled nursing facilities, comprehensive outpatient rehabilitation facilities, rehabilitation agencies, home health agencies, and private outpatient practices at the initial examination visit, every re-examination visit or tenth visit thereafter, and at the conclusion of the episode of care. There are three levels to the functional limitation codes reported: the G-code descriptor, based on ICF terminology; a severity modifier; and a therapy modifier. The G-code descriptors applicable to physical therapy services include Mobility: Walking and Moving Around, Changing and Maintaining Body Position, Carrying and Handling Objects, Self-Care,

Other Physical Therapy/Occupational Therapy Primary Functional Limitation, and Other Physical Therapy/Occupational Therapy Subsequent Functional Limitation (**TABLE 11-4**).[17] Currently, the CMS requires that G-code reporting occur for only the primary functional limitation measured even if your patient or client presents to you with more than one functional limitation that fits into the categories in **TABLE 11-4**. The Centers for Medicare & Medicaid Services has also defined specific criteria for selecting the "Other" codes which include:

○ A patient or client's functional limitation is not defined by one of the four specific categories.

○ A patient or client's episode of care is not intended to treat a functional limitation such as is the case in prevention and wellness.

○ A functional assessment tool is used that does not clearly represent a functional limitation defined by one of the four specific categories.[18]

TABLE 11-4 Functional Limitation G-Code Descriptors for Physical Therapy Services

Functional Limitation Descriptor*	G-Code
Mobility: walking and moving around	Current status: G8978 Projected status: G8979 Actual status: G8980
Changing and maintaining body position	Current status: G8981 Projected status: G8982 Actual status: G8983
Moving and handling objects	Current status: G8984 Projected status: G8985 Actual status: G8986
Self-care	Current status: G8987 Projected status: G8988 Actual status: G8989
Other PT/OT primary functional limitation	Current status: G8990 Projected status: G8991 Actual status: G8992
Other PT/OT subsequent functional limitation	Current status: G8993 Projected status: G8994 Actual status: G8995

*There are seven additional functional limitation descriptors with codes that may be used by physical therapists if any of these specific categories represent the primary limitation of the patient or client: swallowing, motor speech, spoken language comprehension, spoken language expressive attention, memory, and voice. (APTA. Arlington, VA: American Physical Therapy Association. Available at www.apta.org/Payment/Medicare/CodingBilling/FunctionalLimitation/FAQs/General/. Accessed on August 11, 2014.)

Modified from *G-Codes for Claims-Based Functional Reporting for Calendar Year 2013, PT in Motion, Endurance Tested, The Personal and Professional Benefits of Extreme Athleticism*, March 2013, with permission of the American Physical Therapy Association. © 2013 American Physical Therapy Association.

Many facilities use specific functional outcome tools to satisfy the definition of a specific G-code descriptor and to represent a patient or client's primary functional limitation. For example, a Timed Up and Go, a 10-Meter Walk Test, or the Dynamic Gait Index are performance-based outcome tools that could be used to relay the "Mobility: Walking and Moving Around" descriptor. Similarly, self-report outcome tools such as the Neck Disability Index, the Oswestry Low Back Disability Questionnaire, or performance-based outcome tools such as the Functional Independence Measure could be used to relay the "Self-Care" descriptor. Other facilities incorporate the patient or client's subjective complaints, examination findings, and the physical therapist's clinical impression to meet the functional limitation reporting requirement. It is important to recognize, however, that if you create documentation based on a sound clinical decision-making rationale from your history to your evaluation, you will meet this requirement by default.

If through the course of your intervention, your patient or client's primary functional limitation on which you have reported G-codes resolves then you should either conclude the episode of care with that patient or client or you should report on the functional limitation that remains that has now become the primary focus of your intervention. The "Other PT/OT Subsequent Functional Limitation" descriptor should only be used when the "Other PT/OT Primary Functional Limitation" descriptor was reported to be resolved in the same episode of care.[18] Guidance regarding which of the G-code categories describes your patient or client's functional limitations is delineated in a document created by APTA called *Clarification of the ICF Categories* (**APPENDIX 11-A**). An additional document created by the CMS called *Quick Reference Chart: Short and Long Descriptors for Therapy Functional Reporting G-codes* is also available (**APPENDIX 11-B**).

As shown in Table 11-4, "Current status" indicates your patient or client's current level of ability or functional limitation within the descriptor on which you are reporting. For example, if after your examination you determined that your patient or client's primary functional limitation can be categorized by the mobility descriptor, then you would include the nonpayable G-code G8978 in your billing. "Projected status" and "Actual status" refer to the level of ability you will aim for your patient or client to achieve as the episode of care progresses and by the conclusion of the episode of care, respectively. Therefore,

TABLE 11-5 G-Code Functional Limitation Severity Modifiers

Modifier	% Functional Limitation Restriction
CH	0%
CI	1 to 19%
CJ	20 to 39%
CK	40 to 59%
CL	60 to 79%
CM	80 to 99%
CN	100%

Modified from Smith HL, New funtional limitation reporting requirements. *PT in Motion.* 2013;5(2): 42-45, with permission of the American Physical Therapy Association. © 2013 American Physical Therapy Association.

the projected status mobility G-code is G8979 and the actual status determined at the conclusion of the episode of care mobility G-code is G8980.

The second level of the code includes a severity modifier (**TABLE 11-5**),[17] which is intended to reflect the percentage of the functional limitation of your patient or client. Your choice of the severity modifier for your patient or client should be based on sound clinical rationale that is not only shown in the objective data you have collected, but is also reflected in your documentation of appropriately selected and interpreted tests and measures and outcome tools. For example, consider that your patient or client achieves the following scores on the balance and mobility measures you administered at the initial examination:

○ Timed Up and Go = 17.4 seconds
○ 10-Meter Walk Test = 0.89 m/s
○ Berg Balance Test = 37/56

Based on your clinical interpretation and judgment of these scores along with other data you collect at your initial examination, you might categorize your patient or client as having a functional limitation restriction in mobility of 45%. Then assume that after your evaluation, you determine that your patient or client can likely achieve an improvement to 30% by the re-examination in 4 weeks (or at the tenth visit). Therefore, the G-codes that would accompany this patient or client's billing claim for the initial examination would be as follows: G8978CK and G8979CJ. Currently, the CMS is only looking for the

completion of the correct G-code reporting for each patient or client and is not making any judgments regarding reimbursement based on how the G-code is supported at this time. However, as indicated above, your ability to translate your interactions with your patient or client into sound documentation will ensure that you are paid for the services you render when FLR evolves to include reimbursement based on the quality of the information you report to support your patient or client's functional limitations.

The third level of the code includes a therapy modifier. This modifier signals which therapy discipline is submitting the code. For example, "GP" identifies physical therapy, "GO" identifies occupational therapy, and "GN" identifies speech language pathology. It is important to note that the therapy modifier is used on all billing claims, not just in FLR, to distinguish which therapy discipline provided the service billed.

Generally, two G-codes are billed at required intervals for a Medicare beneficiary. The G-code billed depends on the type of visit within the episode of care you have created for that patient or client (**TABLE 11-6**). For example, if you are a physical therapist conducting an initial examination, the G-codes you record include the current status and the projected status or goal status codes as in the scenario above. Two G-codes should also be recorded at every re-examination visit or at every tenth visit: the current status at the re-examination visit and the projected or goal status. During this time, the severity modifier level of the G-code can be altered based on your patient or client's progress. At the conclusion of the episode of care visit, two G-codes should also be billed: the G-code indicating your patient or client's projected or goal status and the patient or client's status at the conclusion of the episode of care. Consider the following scenario.

You have determined the frequency and duration of your patient or client's episode of care to be two

TABLE 11-6 Frequency of Functional Limitation Reporting

Type of Visit	G-Codes Recorded
Initial examination visit	Current status, projected or goal status
Re-examination visit	Current status, projected or goal status
Tenth visit	Current status, projected or goal status
Conclusion of the episode of care visit	Projected or goal status, conclusion of episode of care status

times per week for 4 weeks. At the initial examination, you determined that your patient or client was 65% limited in his self-care and you projected an improvement in self-care to 15%. At the eighth visit, you performed a re-examination and found his self-care limitation to now be at 20%. You continued the episode of care for an additional two times per week for 2 weeks. At the twelfth visit you decided to conclude the episode of care because he was able to independently manage his remaining self-care deficits, which you estimate to be 10% limited.

The G-codes reported for this patient or client's episode of care are as follows:

○ Initial Examination: G8987CL GP; G8988CI GP
○ 8th visit: G8987CJ GP; G8988CI GP
○ 12th visit: G8988CI GP, G8989CI GP

In the scenario above, once a re-examination has been performed the reporting period starts over. In other words, G-codes would not have to be reported again on the tenth visit because a re-examination was done on the eighth visit. This schedule would be in alignment with Medicare's requirement that re-examinations are to be done at least every tenth visit. Therefore, the next time G-codes would be required is at the 18th visit, which is 10 visits since the last re-examination visit. Alternatively, if the patient or client's episode of care is ending at the twelfth visit, which is the original plan for the conclusion of the episode of care, a projected or goal status code and a conclusion of the episode of care G-code would be reported along with the appropriate documentation.

You may determine at the initial examination that your patient or client is not appropriate for physical therapy services and you conclude the episode of care on the same day. In this case, you would report three G-codes: the current status code, the projected status or goal status code, and the conclusion of the episode of care code. In the case where no functional limitation could be identified, the severity modifier for each code would be the same. Consider the following scenario.

Assume that your 75-year-old patient or client comes to you with complaints of low back pain. After your examination the only significant finding is tenderness with percussion over the right kidney. After explaining your findings, you recommend that the patient or client speak to his primary care provider and you

agree to communicate with this provider on his behalf to relay your concerns regarding the lack of physical and mechanical findings and the potential kidney dysfunction that is referring pain to the low back.

The G-codes reported for this patient or client's one-day episode of care are as follows:

○ Current Status: G8990CH GP
○ Projected/Goal Status: G8991CH GP
○ Conclusion of the Episode of Care Status: G8992CH GP

The G-codes for the functional limitation descriptor "Other PT/OT Primary Functional Limitation" is used in the example above because the patient or client's functional limitation is not defined by one of the four specific categories.

In the event that your patient or client does not return for the last scheduled physical therapy session, you would document your conclusion of the episode of care summary as usual but without billing CPT or nonpayable G-codes since no services were actually rendered. Examples of how to apply G-codes to alternative clinical scenarios are available to members of the APTA at www.apta.org/payment/medicare/codingbilling/functionalLimitation.

Some organizations may elect to record G-codes at every visit rather than every tenth visit to decrease the potential that G-codes are mistakenly omitted from the billing claim at the tenth visit, at a visit when a re-examination is performed, or at the conclusion of the episode of care visit. If this is the policy for your employer, then a physical therapist assistant is also responsible for correctly reporting G-codes. It is important to note however that physical therapist assistants are unable to determine the actual G-codes. This determination is the sole responsibility of the physical therapist because assigning the G-code requires an evaluation of the patient or client's status and progress. Thus, a physical therapist assistant would be responsible for ensuring that a G-code, previously determined by the physical therapist, is carried over to the patient or client's billing claim for that session as well as communicating with the physical therapist the timing of the tenth visit, re-examination visit, or conclusion of the episode of care visit.

Quality Initiatives

It is important to recognize that new programs will be implemented as understanding of healthcare utilization, delivery, and payment evolve. Additionally, several existing programs will be modified and alternative rules and regulations will be mandated as healthcare reform evolves. For example, the **Physician Quality Reporting System** (PQRS), a pay-for-reporting (P4R) program created by the CMS in the early 2000s, incentivized eligible healthcare providers including physical therapists to ensure the delivery of quality services by reporting on the use of quality measures. As of 2015, this program will have evolved to a pay-for-performance (P4P) program that will penalize eligible healthcare providers including physical therapists for not reporting the actual use of quality measures in the documentation of outpatient services furnished under Medicare Part B. Thus, the same settings that are required to report functional limitations via non-payable G-codes are also required to submit quality measures through the PQRS. Unlike G-codes, however, the PQRS program is linked to CPT codes. Acceptable PQRS quality measures for 2014 include:

○ Documented communication with the physician managing the ongoing care of an older adult after a fracture that the patient or client was or should be assessed for osteoporosis

○ Documentation of current medications in a health record

○ Documentation of a pain assessment using standardized tools on each visit and documentation of a follow-up plan if pain is present

○ Documentation of a physical exam at an initial visit for back pain using standardized tools

○ Documentation of a falls risk assessment for those with a history of falls

○ Documentation of a change in functional status for those with knee, hip, lower leg, ankle, foot, lumbar spine, shoulder, elbow, wrist, hand, thoracic spine, ribs, head, or neck deficits

○ Documentation of caregiver support and education on dementia management and documentation of referral to additional supportive services

○ Documentation of screening for hypertension and documentation of a recommended follow-up plan

○ Documentation of functional status for those with total knee and hip replacements[19]

According to the CMS, participation in the PQRS program will "improve the care of patients served through the evidence-based measures that are based upon clinical guidelines." Therefore, if you implement successful documentation strategies as previously described including substantiating your findings with reliable, valid, and measurable outcome tools, you will always be in compliance with this federal program.

In addition to the PQRS in outpatient settings, the CMS has developed or is developing similar quality reporting programs for inpatient rehabilitation, skilled nursing facilities, home health, and hospital settings (**TABLE 11-7**).[20] For example, acute care settings are required to participate in the inpatient quality reporting (IQR) program and the value-based purchasing (VBP) program as well as reporting hospital readmission rates. The IQR program requires reporting on the care of and mortality of those admitted with myocardial infarction, heart failure, pneumonia, or stroke; patient or client satisfaction, safety, hospital-associated infections, hospital-acquired conditions, immunization measures, emergency department throughput, and cost efficiency.[21] The value-based purchasing program rewards hospital systems with higher performance on clinical process and patient or client experience measures with higher payments than those paid to lower performing hospitals. Skilled nursing facilities are required to use the Minimum Data Set (MDS 3.0) to report and document quality measure use. Home health agencies are required to use the Outcome Assessment and Information Set (OASIS-C) to report on emergency department use without hospitalization, and to administer the Home Healthcare Consumer Assessment of Healthcare Providers and Systems (HHCAHPS). The HHCAHPS is a survey designed to measure the experiences of Medicare beneficiaries who receive home health services.

In October 2014, The Improving Medicare Post-Acute Care Transformation (IMPACT) Act was passed. This legislation requires post-acute care providers including home health agencies, skilled nursing facilities, inpatient rehabilitation facilities, and long-term care hospitals to begin reporting standardized patient assessment data at admission and discharge and to collect information on quality measures including functional status, cognitive function, skin integrity, medication reconciliation, incidence of major falls, patient preference when transitioning to and from care settings, resource use, and hospital readmission rates.[22] According to the US Senate Finance Committee and the House Ways and Means Committee, the IMPACT Act will enable the CMS to compare quality across

TABLE 11-7 Centers for Medicare & Medicaid Services Quality Programs

Setting	Programs	Mandatory Reporting	Payment Incentive/Penalty
Outpatient	PQRS	Yes	Yes; P4P Incentive 0.5% until 2014 Penalty 1.5% in 2015
Acute care hospitals	IQR, Readmissions VBP	Yes	Yes; P4R and P4P in 2013
Skilled nursing facilities	MDS 3.0	Yes	No
Home healthcare	OASIS, HH CAHPS	Yes	Yes; P4R penalty 2%
Inpatient rehabilitation facilities			
Long-term care hospitals		Beginning in 2014	
Hospice care			

PQRS = Physician Quality Reporting System

P4P = Pay-for-Performance

P4R = Pay-for-Reporting

IQR = Inpatient Quality Reporting

VBP = Value-Based Purchasing

MDS= Minimum Data Set

OASIS = Outcome Assessment and Information Set

HHCAHPS = Home Healthcare Consumer Assessment of Healthcare Providers and Systems

Modified from Centers for Medicare and Medicaid Services. *Quality Summary Table, Medicare Quality Measures in Every Setting*, with permission of the American Physical Therapy Association. Available at http://www.apta.org/Payment/Medicare/PayforPerformance. © 2015 American Physical Therapy Association.

different post-acute settings, to improve hospital and post-acute care discharge planning, and to use this information to reform reimbursement to post-acute care settings.[23]

Billing

OUTPATIENT REHABILITATION PROVIDERS

Reimbursement for outpatient physical therapy services is currently rendered via a fee-for-service, procedural-based payment system and is used in settings that deliver outpatient physical therapy services (**TABLE 11-8**). **Current Procedural Terminology codes** provide the vehicle for relaying to third-party payers how you spend your time with your patient or client and therefore how you bill a provider for the physical therapy services you deliver. CPT codes include untimed codes and timed codes each with specific definitions and time increments for how the code should be applied. These specifics can be found along with CPT codes in a resource provided by the APTA or the AMA. Included in the code definitions are details regarding requirements such as one-on-one patient or client contact or patient or client supervision.

For example, Initial Examination has an untimed code billed as 97001 and Therapeutic Exercise has a timed code billed as 97110. When billing an untimed code, only one unit of service can be billed for that code regardless of the amount of time you spent delivering that service. In other words, an initial examination that took you 60 minutes

TABLE 11-8 Outpatient Rehabilitation Settings

Setting	Comment
Hospitals	Inpatients and outpatients who are not covered under Medicare Part A
Skilled nursing facilities (SNF)	○ Residents not covered in a Part A stay ○ Nonresidents who receive outpatient services from the SNF
Home health agencies (HHA)	Individuals who are not homebound and therefore not under a home health plan of care
Comprehensive outpatient rehabilitation facilities (CORFs)	Previously termed "rehabilitation agencies" or "outpatient physical therapy facilities" by CMS
Private practice	

Data from CMS. *Medicare Claims Processing Manual*, Chapter 5 – Part B Outpatient Rehabilitation and CORF/OPT Services. Baltimore: Centers for Medicare & Medicaid Services; revised February 6, 2014.

to complete, not including documentation time after the encounter, and an initial examination that took you 20 minutes to complete, not including documentation time after the encounter, are each billed as one unit of service and reimbursed at the same rate. Alternatively, most timed CPT codes are billed in 15-minute increments and require direct one-on-one contact with the patient or client. For example, if you are working with two patients or clients simultaneously you would have to keep track of the amount of time spent one-on-one with each patient or client so that you could appropriately bill for the services you provided. For rehabilitation services billed under Medicare Part B, the "Eight-Minute Rule" or "Rule of Eight" guideline for billing timed CPT codes is utilized (**TABLE 11-9**).[22] For example, if you spent 22 minutes delivering therapeutic exercise to your patient or client, you would bill one unit of 97110. However, if you spent 23 minutes delivering therapeutic exercise, you would bill two units of 97110. Consider the following scenario.

You are a physical therapist conducting an initial examination for a resident who is a Medicare Part B beneficiary in a skilled nursing facility. You have 60 minutes to spend with the patient or client. You complete your examination in 22 minutes. You spend 20 of the remaining 38 minutes gait training the resident both in the room, the bathroom, and out in the hallway. You spend the remaining 18 minutes educating the patient or client on an exercise program and instructing the patient or client how this program can be performed in the room. You also create and administer a written copy of this program to leave with the patient or client.

TABLE 11-9 Medicare "8-Minute Rule" Guideline for Billing Timed CPT Codes for Physical Therapy Services Furnished Under Medicare Part B

# of Units	Minimum # of Intervention Minutes Provided
1	8 minutes to < 23 minutes
2	23 minutes to < 38 minutes
3	38 minutes to < 53 minutes
4	53 minutes to < 68 minutes
5	68 minutes to < 83 minutes
6	83 minutes to < 98 minutes
7	98 minutes to < 113 minutes
8	113 minutes to < 128 minutes

Reprinted from CMS. *Medicare Claims Processing Manual*, Chapter 5, page 38. Baltimore: Centers for Medicare & Medicaid Services; 2014.

The CPT codes that would be applied to this patient or client's billing claim include the following:

○ 97001 × 1 – Initial Examination (untimed code) = 22 minutes
○ 97116 × 2 – Gait training (timed code)
○ 97535 × 1 – Self-care instruction (timed code)

In the example above, since the total time spent in timed-based interventions is 38 minutes, then according to the Eight-Minute Rule it is appropriate to bill three units for the interventions delivered. When billing more than one timed CPT code on a calendar day, the total number of units that you can bill is limited by the total treatment time. According to the CMS, it is appropriate in this situation to assign more timed units to the service that took the most time.[23] Therefore, in the example above you would bill two units for gait training and one unit for self-care.

Capturing accurate billing codes requires you to be cognizant of the amount of time you spend delivering each service to your patient or client. Alternatively, you may have decided to spend 45 minutes performing an initial examination. You may have then decided to spend the remaining 15 minutes between gait training (5 minutes) and self-care (10 minutes) minutes in which case you would only bill one unit for the initial examination and one unit of self-care. It is paramount to recognize that the decisions you make regarding your billing practices must be ethically driven. It is equally important to remember that the "Eight-Minute Rule" has evolved from a foundation of billing in 15-minute increments as initially defined by the AMA with the introduction of CPT codes.

While many payer sources model their policies after Medicare guidelines, it is pertinent to always be aware of the contract you or your employer and the payer have negotiated regarding the initial time required to bill one unit of service as well as the additional time required to bill an additional unit of service. For example, a private payer contract may utilize a billing guideline that allows you to bill in 5-minute increments, meaning that an additional unit of service may be billed after 5 minutes of services have been delivered. Alternatively, a payer may not utilize a minute requirement but instead pay a flat rate for any procedure or service provided within the entire treatment session. Thus, the services delivered within a 30-minutes session would be reimbursed at the same rate as the services delivered in a 60-minutes session. When a billing guideline is not stipulated in a payer contract, the

CPT guideline of billing in 15-minute increments must be followed. Thus, it is very important to keep track of your time that you spend with your patient or client so that you can appropriately bill for the services you provide. It is also important to be mindful that certain physical therapy services that are within the scope of your physical therapy practice may not be recognized as covered services by certain payer sources and therefore are not reimbursable. You must be aware of these services, which differ by state and payer source, so that you can proactively initiate a discussion with your patient or client regarding the relative need for the non-covered service and the need to pay for this service out-of-pocket. One consequence of not being aware of your patient or client's insurance requirements would be that you and your employer do not receive payment for this service you rendered because you billed for a non-covered service. Being aware of billing requirements as it applies to an individual patient or client also includes being aware of the rules and regulations as it pertains to group therapy, providing physical therapy services to more than one individual at the same time, and as it pertains to co-treatments, providing care to one patient or client with another member of your patient or client's healthcare team such as the occupational therapist or certified occupational therapist assistant. It is equally important to be aware of your state's rules and regulations regarding billing when you work in a team with a physical therapist assistant, physical therapy aide, or physical therapy student. Medicare also provides guidelines when you as a physical therapist bill for services that are delivered by these other providers under your supervision. For example, only the services of a physical therapist or physical therapist assistant can be billed under Medicare Part B. A physical therapy student or physical therapist assistant student can participate in the delivery of physical therapy services to the Medicare Part B beneficiary but only when:

○ The session and service delivery is directed by the physical therapist or physical therapist assistant.
○ The physical therapist or physical therapist assistant is in the room for the entire session.
○ The physical therapist or physical therapist assistant is not engaged in treating another patient or client or in doing alternative tasks at the same time.[24]

It is important to recognize that where state regulations are more restrictive than Medicare rules and regulations, it is the state regulations that must be followed.

CONSOLIDATED BILLING

Medicare certified home healthcare agencies and skilled nursing facilities who serve Medicare Part A beneficiaries utilize consolidated billing. For example, rather than tracking the minutes spent providing each skilled procedure such as therapeutic exercise or manual therapy, you would document the total time spent with your patient or client by documenting the beginning time and ending time of your provision of skilled care. Therefore, the services billed in settings providing care under Medicare Part A (TABLE 11-10) would include medical expenses with a few exceptions such as a physician's professional services, plus room and board.[25] School-based settings who serve Medicaid beneficiaries or who receive school funding utilize a flat per-session rate and therefore minutes of skilled services are not recorded for billing purposes. Physical therapy services provided through early intervention programs or in private schools, however, can utilize private or federal funding sources in which case the billing guidelines utilized by that payer would be followed. It is also important to recognize that if your patient or client pays out of pocket for the services you deliver that you charge a fair rate for the service. In other words, many providers institute a policy that charges a self-pay rate that is comparable to a rate charged by a third-party payer in the same geographic region.

THE THERAPY CAP AND THE "KX" MODIFIER

The Balanced Budget Act passed in 1997 included an annual cap on outpatient physical therapy services delivered to Medicare beneficiaries. In other words, as a result of this legislation, there is a predetermined cap that, when reached, terminates payment for outpatient physical, occupational, and speech therapy services to a Medicare beneficiary on an annual basis. Thus, when the new year rolls over, the cap reloads to the annual amount. On a

TABLE 11-10   Settings Providing Medicare Part A

Setting	Comment
Hospitals	
Skilled nursing facilities (SNF)	Residents not covered in a Part B stay
Home health agencies (HHA)	Individuals who are homebound and therefore under a home health plan of care
Hospice care	

nearly annual basis, physical therapy advocates have fought to repeal the cap or to stall the implementation of the cap for the next year by imposing moratoriums so that services will not be hindered or interrupted by the provisions of the cap. The presence of a cap for outpatient services not only limits Medicare beneficiaries' access to critical services, but also inhibits ongoing preventative care. In 2014, the annual amount for physical and speech therapy services combined was capped at $1920 with an additional $1920 for occupational therapy services. If you assume a cost per visit of $100, then approximately 19 visits per calendar year would be covered for the Medicare beneficiary who requires either physical therapy or speech therapy services. This translates to a plan of care frequency and duration of approximately two times per weeks for 9 weeks or three times per week for 6 weeks for both physical and speech therapy services. An additional 19 visits would be available to this beneficiary for occupational therapy services. There are situations in which a Medicare beneficiary may continue to receive services after the cap has been exhausted however. This is known as an automatic exceptions process in which a "KX" modifier is attached to the billing codes to signify that the Medicare beneficiary requires medically necessary care that exceeds the cap. It is important to be mindful that "use of the 'KX' modifier is considered to be the therapist's attestation that services provided above the cap are medically necessary and that there is documentation in the record to justify the necessity of services delivered."[26] Documentation for any patient or client, not just those in whom a **therapy cap** will be exceeded, should link and identify the relationships that exist among the patient or client's health condition, impairments in body functions and structures, activity limitations, participation restrictions, and contextual factors. Subsequently, these details gathered from the history, systems review, tests and measures, and outcome tools, should be related to the therapy goals and utilized to determine prognosis and to direct the development of the intervention plan. In other words, your documentation should clearly state what factors and circumstances impact your patient or client's recovery or progress within the plan of care you created on their behalf. Ensuring that this fundamental content exists in each of your patient or client's health records will help to ensure payment for the services you deliver as well as ensuring uninterrupted quality care for your patient or client. The CMS cautions clinicians to recognize that

routine use of the "KX" modifier is not an appropriate use of the modifier and that it should only be used when a patient or client requires care that exceeds the cap.

It is also important to recognize that the "KX" modifier cannot be added to claims retrospectively. The modifier must be added to a billing claim prior to rendering the physical therapy services that exceed the therapy cap.[22]

A second level to the exceptions process requires a health record review of therapy services that exceed an annual amount of $3700 for physical and speech therapy services combined and a separate $3700 for occupational therapy services. The manual medical review process requires that you as the physical therapy provider submit your documentation for review when requested by the CMS to make a final determination as to why the services you rendered were justified as medically necessary. This process applies to claims submitted with and without the "KX" modifier. Consider the following scenario.

Your 79-year-old patient or client suffers from a systemic muscle disease called inclusion body myositis. She was diagnosed 8 years ago and since then has experienced marked muscle atrophy in her extremities that has affected her grip strength, triceps strength, and plantar flexor strength bilaterally leading to functional decline and recurrent injurious falls. Eight months ago, she experienced a fall onto her left side that resulted in a scapular fracture. She was immobilized at the glenohumeral joint with a removable shoulder immobilizer for 6 weeks and subsequently required 8 weeks of outpatient physical therapy (two times per week) to regain her upper extremity mobility and improve her ability with activity limitations and participation restrictions. Three months later she experienced a fall onto her left knee that resulted in a tibial plateau fracture. She was immobilized at the tibiofemoral joint for 6 weeks with a removable long leg brace and was required to be toe touch weight bearing with a wheeled walker. Due to lack of upper extremity and grip strength to maneuver an assistive device she spent most of this time using a manual wheelchair as her primary means of mobility. Subsequently, she required 8 weeks of physical therapy (3 × per week for 3 weeks and 2 × per week for 5 weeks) to regain knee range of motion and lost function with her basic activities of daily living. You realize towards the end of the second episode of care that you want to implement a fall prevention plan of care with the goal of decreasing this patient or client's fall risk. After a thorough fall-risk assessment, you determine that a minimum of 12 additional weeks (2 × per week for 4 weeks and 1 × per week for 8 weeks) of skilled physical therapy intervention is required based on the literature and based on her current ability level for implementing an exercise program to decrease fall risk.

Because over the course of 8 months within the same year this patient or client received outpatient physical therapy services for a total of 51 visits over the course of 28 weeks, she will have exceeded the therapy cap. It would be appropriate therefore in this scenario to append the "KX" modifier to any billing submitted for the fall-risk reduction plan of care since this patient or client will have had 35 visits over the course of the first two plans of care. She will likely have also exceeded the $3700 threshold that triggers a manual medical review. As long as your documentation reflects medical necessity, however, the services you provided, although over and above average utilization, would be deemed appropriate and would be funded by Medicare.

If you question if the services you want to provide to your patient or client are medically necessary, then it is appropriate to initiate communication with your patient or client regarding alternative payment options such as paying a self-pay rate, paying an out-of-pocket cost from the provider for a non-covered service, or issuing a mandatory Advanced Beneficiary Notice (ABN) (**FIGURE 11-1**). This form indicates that the Medicare beneficiary will agree to pay out of pocket or via a secondary insurance provider for physical therapy services received in the event that Medicare does not cover the services provided. The CMS requires that the ABN be issued prior to providing services that exceed the cap. In the scenario above, it would not be necessary for you to obtain a signed ABN from this patient or client if you are able to show with sound documentation that the services to be rendered are indeed medically necessary services in order for the patient or client to regain her abilities with her basic activities of daily living (ADLs) and to prevent a subsequent injury due to a fall. Therefore, use of the "KX" modifier and the ABN requires you to have an understanding of when the services you would like to deliver to your patient or client are not expected to be covered by Medicare because they are deemed to be unnecessary. Consider that your patient or

client in the scenario above is earlier in her disease process and would like to start on a preventative exercise and mobility program. In this situation, you may not be able to identify activity limitations and participation restrictions that would warrant a 12-week plan of care even though you are aware that the literature supports this duration of exercise to reduce fall risk. Therefore, you would consider obtaining an ABN. Clearly, your ability to successfully document will serve to not only benefit you as you are reimbursed for the services you deliver, but will also benefit your patient or client who will continue to have covered access to the services they need.

Direct Access

Direct access allows a physical therapist to be the practitioner of choice as one's entry point into the healthcare system. This process is regulated by each state. Therefore, the actual meaning of "direct access" varies widely from state to state. For example, some states allow a patient or client to visit a physical therapist without first visiting their physician to obtain a referral. However, that state may then require a physician's signature if the beneficiary is still receiving physical therapy services after 21 consecutive days of physical therapy service. In 2005, federal legislation ruled that physical therapy services were available to Medicare beneficiaries without a physician's referral. However, even though the law eliminated the need for a physician visit or referral prior to seeking the services of a physical therapist, the law also stipulated that the beneficiary must be under the care of a physician. This requirement is met by obtaining a physician's signature on the plan of care. As indicated above, each state has different requirements regarding how that physician's signature is obtained and therefore has differing definitions of direct access. Several limitations imposed by state legislatures ultimately mean that open and unrestricted access to the physical therapy profession is not as straightforward as it might seem. For example, a physician may require a visit with the patient or client prior to signing a physical therapy plan of care or it may take several days to obtain a physician's signature interrupting or even completely halting the provision of physical therapy services. Furthermore, other third-party payers may not reimburse for services provided by a physical therapist without a physician's referral, or payers that require preauthorization

A. Notifier:

B. Patient Name: C. Identification Number:

Advance Beneficiary Notice of Noncoverage (ABN)

NOTE: If Medicare doesn't pay for **D.** _____ below, you may have to pay.

Medicare does not pay for everything, even some care that you or your healthcare provider have good reason to think you need. We expect Medicare may not pay for the **D.** _____ below.

D.	**E. Reason Medicare May Not Pay:**	**F. Estimated Cost**

WHAT YOU NEED TO DO NOW:

- ○ Read this notice, so you can make an informed decision about your care.
- ○ Ask us any questions that you may have after you finish reading.
- ○ Choose an option below about whether to receive the **D.** _____ listed above.

NOTE: If you choose Option 1 or 2, we may help you to use any other insurance that you might have, but Medicare cannot require us to do this.

G. OPTIONS: **Check only one box. We cannot choose a box for you.**
☐ **OPTION 1.** I want the **D.** _____ listed above. You may ask to be paid now, but I also want Medicare billed for an official decision on payment, which is sent to me on a Medicare Summary Notice (MSN). I understand that if Medicare doesn't pay, I am responsible for payment, but **I can appeal to Medicare** by following the directions on the MSN. If Medicare does pay, you will refund any payments I made to you, less co-pays or deductibles.
☐ **OPTION 2.** I want the **D.** _____ listed above, but do not bill Medicare. You may ask to be paid now as I am responsible for payment. **I cannot appeal if Medicare is not billed**.
☐ **OPTION 3.** I don't want the **D.** _____ listed above. I understand with this choice I am **not** responsible for payment, and **I cannot appeal to see if Medicare would pay.**

H. Additional Information:

This notice gives our opinion, not an official Medicare decision. If you have other questions on this notice or Medicare billing, call **1-800-MEDICARE** (1-800-633-4227/**TTY:** 1-877-486-2048).

Signing below means that you have received and understand this notice. You also receive a copy.

I. Signature:	**J. Date:**

Form CMS-R-131 (03/11)   Form Approved OMB No. 0938-0566

FIGURE 11-1 Advanced Beneficiary Notice.
Reprinted from from the U.S. Department of Health and Human Services, Centers for Medicare & Medicaid Services.

BOX 11-1 The Electronic Health Record: Billing

The format and location of the billing template for the documentation system you utilize will determine when you can actually enter the billing codes for any given patient or client encounter. Therefore, it may be beneficial for you to jot down on a piece of paper the specific time frames you spent with your patient or client on each task so that you can accurately allocate the units of service to the appropriate codes at the end of the encounter. It is possible that your patient or client's billing information may be built into your intervention flow sheet, which is likely linked to your note for that encounter. Thus, if the EHR you use has a feature that carries forward the last session's note, it is important for you to notice if the billing information from last session also carried forward. In this case, it will be necessary for you to develop a system for deleting the units of service that corresponded to the prior session so that they are not inadvertently applied to the current session. It is also important as you utilize an EHR's "copy forward" feature that you do not carry forward the exact content of the last session's note and utilize it as the documentation for the current session. You must show why each session is medically necessary for the continued care of your patient or client. A note written exactly as the prior note will not relay this message. Additionally, if you are not the author of the prior note, copying forward the contents and passing it off as your own is a form of plagiarism. Rather, tailor the note to the current session and make it unique to your patient or client's current encounter.

Your patient or client's payer information may be housed in a location within the EHR that is not intuitive or easily accessible from the platform you use to create your documentation. Therefore, it will be important for you to identify the location of information such as covered and non-covered services, date of service and visit limitations, and therapy cap details so that you can quickly access and refer to this information.

Electronic health systems utilize different templates to generate reports based on the type of encounter you have with your patient or client. For example, a form letter is likely generated after you populate an initial examination template that is sent to your patient or client's referral source to relay the information of the encounter as well as to obtain a signature on the plan of care. A similar letter is likely generated after you collect and record information at a patient or client's conclusion of the episode of care visit. Likewise, if you work with a patient or client who comes to you directly without a referral or without having a prior physician's visit, it will be valuable for you to know if a template exists that generates a direct access letter relaying that your patient or client has come to you directly.

---

prior to obtaining covered services may not recognize direct access to the physical therapy profession. Therefore, it is important to continue to be aware that your documentation includes all the necessary elements to ensure that you are imparting maximum benefit to your patient or client and to ensure your reimbursement for the services you provide as the healthcare system continues to reform and evolve.

Summary

As a physical therapist or a physical therapist assistant you have a responsibility to provide quality care for your patient or client. In today's changing healthcare environment, this means that you should have a working knowledge of federal and state regulations that potentially impact your ability to provide this quality care. At the core of such legislative reform is your attention to the detail of your documentation. Consider viewing your documentation from the perspective of your patient or client's payer. Based on what you have created in your documentation, would you pay for the services you delivered? Can you discern from the detail you have included in your documentation the value or the quality of the services you delivered? Are your services truly necessary and justified? Ultimately, your successful documentation can serve to authorize you as a practitioner of choice who delivers consistent, quality, medically necessary care. Strong documentation should therefore solidify your success as a physical therapist or physical therapist assistant within a reforming healthcare system.

Discussion Questions

1. Inquire to your employer or to your clinical instructor regarding the processes in place to:
   a. Receive feedback on documentation.
   b. Learn of reimbursement patterns for services delivered.
2. What steps are involved in identifying the appropriate ICD-9 or ICD-10 codes that are applied to your patient or client's health record? Who are the staff members involved in this process?
3. Review the insurance information for one of your patient or clients. Are you able to quickly identify information about covered and non-covered services, visit, or therapy cap limitations? If not, what steps were involved in determining this information and what changes might you suggest for this process?
4. What is the purpose of functional limitation reporting and the use of G-codes in an outpatient physical therapy environment?
5. As a physical therapist, what information would you use to determine your patient or client's severity status when creating a G-code?
6. What is the difference between consolidated billing and a procedural-based payment system?
7. Explain what is meant by the therapy cap exceptions process.
8. Discuss with your employer or with your clinical instructor the use of the "KX" modifier in that particular clinic. What was the patient or client scenario that indicated the use of the "KX" modifier? Share this scenario with your peers or your colleagues in an effort to increase understanding of this billing code.
9. When is it appropriate to issue an Advanced Beneficiary Notice to a Medicare beneficiary?
10. Discuss with your employer or with your clinical instructor the use of an Advanced Beneficiary Notice in that particular clinic. What was the patient or client scenario that indicated the use of the ABN? Share this scenario with your peers or colleagues in an effort to increase understanding of this federal mandate.

Case Study Questions

1. You have determined the frequency and duration of your patient or client's episode of care to be three times per week for 6 weeks. At the initial examination, you determined that your patient or client was 85% limited in mobility, specifically ambulation and transfers. You project an improvement in mobility to 60%. At the tenth visit, you performed a re-examination and found his mobility limitation to now be at 50%.
   a. Will you continue the episode of care with this patient or client? Why or why not?
   b. What G-codes will you report at the initial examination?
   c. What G-codes will you report at the tenth visit?
2. Assume that your 85-year-old patient or client comes to you after being referred by his physician for balance training and gait training with an appropriate assistive device. He indicates to you during your attempt at an initial examination that the only reason he is in your clinic is because his wife made him come. He states that he is not interested in participating and will not use a walker or a cane like the doctor suggested. He allows you to perform an examination to identify his needs, however as you explain your findings regarding his mobility restrictions which you estimate to be about 50%, he decides that he does not want to participate in physical therapy and leaves the clinic. What G-codes will you report related to this encounter?
3. Assume in the scenario above that your patient or client agrees to participate in physical therapy as you have recommended for three times per week for 8 weeks. Assume also that you have projected an improvement for this patient or client from 50% to 25%. However, he never returns to your clinic after the initial examination. What G-codes will you report in this situation?
4. You are a physical therapist or physical therapist assistant working with a 90-year-old patient or client in an outpatient clinic. Of your 45-minute treatment session, you spend 20 minutes on strengthening exercises. The remaining time is spent working on transfer training into and out of the passenger side of her car. Determine the units of service you will bill for this patient or client using Medicare's "Eight-Minute Rule."

References

1. Sherwin J. Contemporary Topics in Healthcare: Accountable Care Organizations. *PT in Motion*. February 2012;4(1):28–32.
2. Peiris CL, Taylor NF, Shields N. *Arch Phys Med Rehabil*. September 2011;92(9):1490–1500.
3. Fleming-McDonnell D, Czuppon S, Deusinger SS, Deusinger RH. Physical therapy in the emergency department: development of a novel practice venue. *Phys Ther*. 2010;90:420–426.

4. Smith BA, Fields CJ, Fernandez N. Physical therapists make accurate and appropriate discharge recommendation for patients who are acutely ill. *Phys Ther.* 2010;90:693–703.

5. Jette AM. Toward a common language for function, disability, and health. *Phys Ther.* 2006;86:726–734.

6. Clark DE, Lowman JD, Griffin RL, et al. Effectiveness of an early mobilization protocol in a trauma and burns intensive care unit: a retrospective cohort study. *Phys Ther.* 2013;93:186–196.

7. Hopkins RO, Miller RR III, Rodriguez L, et al. Physical therapy on the wards after early physical activity and mobility in the intensive care unit. *Phys Ther.* 2012;92:1518–1523.

8. World Health Organization (WHO). *ICD Information Sheet.* Geneva: World Health Organization. Available at www.who.int/classifications/icd/factsheet/en/. Accessed on July 30, 2014.

9. Moriyama IM, Loy RM, Robb-Smith AHT. *History of the Statistical Classification of Diseases and Causes of Death.* Rosenberg HM, Hoyert DL, eds. Hyattsville, MD: National Center for Health Statistics; 2011.

10. WHO. *Manual of the International Statistical Classification of Diseases, Injuries, and Causes of Death*, 6th revision. Geneva: World Health Organization; 1949.

11. WHO. Family of International Classifications (FIC) Network. *Production of ICD-11: The Overall Revision Process.* Geneva: World Health Organization; March 2007. Available at www.apta.org/uploadedFiles/APTAorg/About_Us/Vision_and_Strategic_Plan/Research_Conference/Article ProductionofICD11.pdf#search=%22ICF Coding%22. Accessed on August 2, 2014.

12. WHO. ICD-11 ICD-ICF ICAMP Meeting, January 2010. Available at youtu.be/Sx7RkiVU8Dg. Accessed on August 2, 2014.

13. WHO. *ICD-11: Frequently Asked Questions.* Geneva: World Health Organization. Available at www.who.int/classifications/icd/revision/icd11faq/en/. Accessed on July 30, 2014.

14. American Medical Association. *CPT Process: How a Code Becomes a Code.* Chicago: American Medical Association; 2014. Available at www.ama-assn.org/ama/pub/physician-resources/solutions-managing-your-practice/coding-billing-insurance/cpt/cpt-process-faq/code-becomes-cpt.page. Accessed on August 2, 2014.

15. Centers for Medicare & Medicaid Services (CMS). *MLN Matters. Specific Modifiers for Distinct Procedural Services, 1-3.* August 2014; MM8863.

16. American Physical Therapy Association (APTA). *Physical Therapy Classification and Payment System (PTCPS) Overview.* Arlington, VA: American Physical Therapy Association; 2013. Available at www.apta.org/PTCPS/Overview/. Accessed on August 10, 2014.

17. Smith HL. Compliance matters: new functional limitation reporting requirements. *PT in Motion.* March 2013;5(2):42–45.

18. APTA. *FAQ: Functional Limitation Reporting General Information.* Arlington, VA: American Physical Therapy Association. Available at www.apta.org/Payment/Medicare/CodingBilling/FunctionalLimitation/FAQs/General/ Accessed on August 11, 2014.

19. CMS. *Physician Quality Reporting System (PQRS) Measures List*, Version 8.1. Baltimore: Centers for Medicare & Medicaid Services; 2014.

20. APTA. *Physician Quality Reporting System: General Information.* Arlington, VA: American Physical Therapy Association; 2014. Available at www.apta.org/PQRS/. Accessed on August 18, 2014.

21. APTA. *Acute Care Hospital: Quality Reporting Program Details.* Arlington, VA: American Physical Therapy Association; 2014. Available at www.apta.org/Payment/Medicare/PayforPerformance/. Accessed on August 18, 2014.

22. Centers for Medicare and Medicaid Services. IMPACT Act of 2014 & Cross Setting Measures. Available at www.cms.gov/Medicare/Quality-Initiatives-Patient-Assessment-Instruments/Post-Acute-Care-Quality-Initiatives/IMPACT-Act-of-2014-and-Cross-Setting-Measures.html Accessed 4/23/2015.

23. The United States Senate Committee on Finance. Bipartisan, bicameral bill strengthens Medicare's Post-acute Care. Available at www.finance.senate.gov/newsroom/ranking/release/?id=cec94759-c44a-4c7d-9d88-cf38ab4b7dfc Accessed April 23, 2015.

24. CMS. *Medicare Claims Processing Manual* (Chapter 5). Baltimore: Centers for Medicare & Medicaid Services; revised February 6, 2014. Available at https://www.cms.gov/Regulations-and-Guidance/Guidance/Manuals/downloads/clm104c05.pdf. Accessed on August 10, 2014.

25. APTA. Chart: *Supervision of Students Under Medicare.* Arlington, VA: American Physical Therapy Association; 2013. Available at www.apta.org/Payment/Medicare/Supervision/. Accessed on August 31, 2014.

26. CMS. *SNF Consolidated Billing.* Baltimore, MD: Centers for Medicare & Medicaid Services; 2013. Available at www.cms.gov/Medicare/Billing/SNFConsolidatedBilling/. Accessed on August 31, 2014.

27. APTA. *Ensuring Appropriate Payment by Using Modifiers* (podcast transcript). *PT in Motion*; August 6, 2012. Available at www.apta.org/PTinMotion/NewsNow/?blogid=10737418615&id=10737427706.

Functional Limitation Reporting Categories and the International Classification of Functioning, Disability and Health (ICF)

The functional limitations categories selected by CMS are from the International Classification of Functioning, Disability and Health (ICF). The ICF is a classification of health and health-related domains. The ICF model acknowledges that every human being can experience some level of "disability" and views functioning and disability as an interaction between health, the environment, personal and social factors. For more information on the ICF, please see the APTA ICF web site. The way that CMS is using the term "functional limitation" is within the context of the areas of the ICF relating to "activity limitations" and "participation restrictions."

The definitions of the terms described below come from the *International Classification of Functioning, Disability and Health, World Health Organization, 2001, Geneva*. You may also find all of the descriptions of the components classified in the ICF using the ICF Browser.

1. **Mobility**: Moving by changing body position or location or by transferring from one place to another, by carrying, moving or manipulating objects, by walking, running or climbing, and by using various forms of transportation.
   a. Walking: Moving along a surface on foot, step by step, so that one foot is always on the ground, such as when strolling, sauntering, walking forwards, backwards, or sideways. Inclusions: walking short or long distances; walking on different surfaces; walking around obstacles
   b. Moving Around: Moving the whole body from one place to another by means other than walking, such as climbing over a rock or running down a street, skipping, scampering, jumping, somersaulting or running around obstacles. Inclusions: crawling, climbing, running, jogging, jumping, and swimming
   c. Moving around in different locations: Walking and moving around in various places and situations, such as walking between rooms in a house, within a building, or down the street of a town. Inclusions: moving around within the home, crawling or climbing within the home; walking or moving within buildings other than the home, and outside the home and other buildings
   d. Moving around using equipment: Moving the whole body from place to place, on any surface or space, by using specific devices designed to facilitate moving or create other ways of moving around, such as with skates, skis, or scuba equipment, or moving down the street in a wheelchair or a walker.
   e. Moving around using transportation: Using transportation to move around as a passenger, such as being driven in a car or on a bus, rickshaw, jitney, animal-powered vehicle, or private or public taxi, bus, train, tram, subway, boat or aircraft. Inclusions: using human-powered transportation; using private motorized or public transportation

2. **Changing basic body position**: Getting into and out of a body position and moving from one location to another, such as getting up out of a chair to lie down on a bed, and getting into and out of positions of kneeling or squatting. Inclusion: changing body position from lying down, from squatting or kneeling, from sitting or standing, bending and shifting the body's center of gravity

   a. Maintaining a body position: Staying in the same body position as required, such as remaining seated or remaining standing for work or school. Inclusions: maintaining a lying, squatting, kneeling, sitting and standing position

   b. Transferring oneself: Moving from one surface to another, such as sliding along a bench or moving from a bed to a chair, without changing body position. Inclusion: transferring oneself while sitting or lying

3. **Lifting and carrying objects**: Raising up an object or taking something from one place to another, such as when lifting a cup or carrying a child from one room to another. Inclusions: lifting, carrying in the hands or arms, or on shoulders, hip, back or head; putting down

   a. Moving objects with lower extremities: Performing coordinated actions aimed at moving an object by using the legs and feet, such as kicking a ball or pushing pedals on a bicycle. Inclusions: pushing with lower extremities; kicking

   b. Fine hand use: Performing the coordinated actions of handling objects, picking up, manipulating and releasing them using one's hand, fingers and thumb, such as required to lift coins off a table or turn a dial or knob. Inclusions: picking up, grasping, manipulating and releasing.

   c. Hand and arm use: Performing the coordinated actions required to move objects or to manipulate them by using hands and arms, such as when turning door handles or throwing or catching an object Inclusions: pulling or pushing objects; reaching; turning or twisting the hands or arms; throwing; catching.

4. **Self Care**: caring for oneself, washing and drying oneself, caring for one's body and body parts, dressing, eating and drinking, and looking after one's health.

   a. Washing oneself: Washing and drying one's whole body, or body parts, using water and appropriate cleaning and drying materials or methods, such as bathing, showering, washing hands and feet, face and hair, and drying with a towel. Inclusions: washing body parts, the whole body; and drying oneself.

   b. Caring for body parts: Looking after those parts of the body, such as skin, face, teeth, scalp, nails and genitals, that require more than washing and drying. Inclusions: caring for skin, teeth, hair, finger and toe nails.

   c. Toileting: Planning and carrying out the elimination of human waste (menstruation, urination and defecation), and cleaning oneself afterwards. Inclusions: regulating urination, defecation and menstrual care.

d. Dressing: Carrying out the coordinated actions and tasks of putting on and taking off clothes and footwear in sequence and in keeping with climatic and social conditions, such as by putting on, adjusting and removing shirts, skirts, blouses, pants, undergarments, saris, kimono, tights, hats, gloves, coats, shoes, boots, sandals and slippers. Inclusions: putting on or taking off clothes and footwear and choosing appropriate clothing.

e. Looking after one's health: Ensuring physical comfort, health and physical and mental well-being, such as by maintaining a balanced diet, and an appropriate level of physical activity, keeping warm or cool, avoiding harms to health, following safe sex practices, including using condoms, getting immunizations and regular physical examinations. Inclusions: ensuring one's physical comfort; managing diet and fitness; maintaining one's health.

Appendix 11-B

Quick Reference Chart: Short & Long Descriptors for Therapy Functional Reporting G-codes

Please note: The information in this publication applies only to the Medicare Fee-For-Service Program (also known as Original Medicare).

The Middle Class Tax Relief and Jobs Creation Act (MCTRJCA) of 2012 amended the Social Security Act to require a claims-based data collection system for outpatient therapy services, including physical therapy (PT), occupational therapy (OT), and speech-language pathology (SLP) services.

The system collects data on beneficiary function during the course of therapy services to better understand beneficiary conditions, outcomes, and expenditures. Beneficiary function information is reported using 42 nonpayable functional G-codes and seven severity/complexity modifiers on claims for PT, OT, and SLP services.

G-CODES FOR FUNCTIONAL REPORTING

There are 42 functional G-codes, 14 sets of three codes each. Six of the G-code sets generally describe PT and OT functional limitations, and eight sets of G-codes generally describe SLP functional limitations.

Mobility G-code Set	Long Descriptor	Short Descriptor
G8978	Mobility: walking & moving around functional limitation, current status, at therapy episode outset and at reporting intervals	Mobility current status
G8979	Mobility: walking & moving around functional limitation, projected goal status, at therapy episode outset, at reporting intervals, and at discharge or to end reporting	Mobility goal status
G8980	Mobility: walking & moving around functional limitation, discharge status, at discharge from therapy or to end reporting	Mobility D/C status

Changing & Maintaining Body Position G-code Set	Long Descriptor	Short Descriptor
G8981	Changing & maintaining body position functional limitation, current status, at therapy episode outset and at reporting intervals	Body pos current status
G8982	Changing & maintaining body position functional limitation, projected goal status, at therapy episode outset, at reporting intervals, and at discharge or to end reporting	Body pos goal status
G8983	Changing & maintaining body position functional limitation, discharge status, at discharge from therapy or to end reporting	Body pos D/C status

Carrying, Moving & Handling Objects G-code Set	Long Descriptor	Short Descriptor
G8984	Carrying, moving & handling objects functional limitation, current status, at therapy episode outset and at reporting intervals	Carry current status
G8985	Carrying, moving & handling objects functional limitation, projected goal status, at therapy episode outset, at reporting intervals, and at discharge or to end reporting	Carry goal status
G8986	Carrying, moving & handling objects functional limitation, discharge status, at discharge from therapy or to end reporting	Carry D/C status

Self Care G-code Set	Long Descriptor	Short Descriptor
G8987	Self care functional limitation, current status, at therapy episode outset and at reporting intervals	Self care current status
G8988	Self care functional limitation, projected goal status, at therapy episode outset, at reporting intervals, and at discharge or to end reporting	Self care goal status
G8989	Self care functional limitation, discharge status, at discharge from therapy or to end reporting	Self care D/C status

ICN 908924 August 2013

Other PT/OT Primary G-code Set

Code	Short Descriptor	Long Descriptor
G8990	Other PT/OT current status	Other physical or occupational therapy primary functional limitation, current status, at therapy episode outset and at reporting intervals
G8991	Other PT/OT goal status	Other physical or occupational therapy primary functional limitation, projected goal status, at therapy episode outset, at reporting intervals, and at discharge or to end reporting
G8992	Other PT/OT D/C status	Other physical or occupational therapy primary functional limitation, discharge status, at discharge from therapy or to end reporting

Other PT/OT Subsequent G-code Set

Code	Short Descriptor	Long Descriptor
G8993	Sub PT/OT current status	Other physical or occupational therapy subsequent functional limitation, current status, at therapy episode outset and at reporting intervals
G8994	Sub PT/OT goal status	Other physical or occupational therapy subsequent functional limitation, projected goal status, at therapy episode outset, at reporting intervals, and at discharge or to end reporting
G8995	Sub PT/OT D/C status	Other physical or occupational therapy subsequent functional limitation, discharge status, at discharge from therapy or to end reporting

Swallowing G-code Set

Code	Short Descriptor	Long Descriptor
G8996	Swallow current status	Swallowing functional limitation, current status at therapy episode outset and at reporting intervals
G8997	Swallow goal status	Swallowing functional limitation, projected goal status, at therapy episode outset, at reporting intervals, and at discharge or to end reporting
G8998	Swallow D/C status	Swallowing functional limitation, discharge status, at discharge from therapy or to end reporting

Motor Speech G-code Set (Note: This code set is not sequentially numbered.)

Code	Short Descriptor	Long Descriptor
G8999	Motor speech current status	Motor speech functional limitation, current status at therapy episode outset and at reporting intervals
G9186	Motor speech goal status	Motor speech functional limitation, projected goal status at therapy episode outset, at reporting intervals, and at discharge or to end reporting
G9158	Motor speech D/C status	Motor speech functional limitation, discharge status at discharge from therapy or to end reporting

Spoken Language Comprehension G-code Set

Code	Short Descriptor	Long Descriptor
G9159	Lang comp current status	Spoken language comprehension functional limitation, current status at therapy episode outset and at reporting intervals
G9160	Lang comp goal status	Spoken language comprehension functional limitation, projected goal status at therapy episode outset, at reporting intervals, and at discharge or to end reporting
G9161	Lang comp D/C status	Spoken language comprehension functional limitation, discharge status at discharge from therapy or to end reporting

Spoken Language Expressive G-code Set

Code	Short Descriptor	Long Descriptor
G9162	Lang express current status	Spoken language expression functional limitation, current status at therapy episode outset and at reporting intervals
G9163	Lang express goal status	Spoken language expression functional limitation, projected goal status at therapy episode outset, at reporting intervals, and at discharge or to end reporting
G9164	Lang express D/C status	Spoken language expression functional limitation, discharge status at discharge from therapy or to end reporting

Attention G-code Set	Long Descriptor	Short Descriptor
G9165	Attention functional limitation, current status at therapy episode outset and at reporting intervals	Atten current status
G9166	Attention functional limitation, projected goal status at therapy episode outset, at reporting intervals, and at discharge or to end reporting	Atten goal status
G9167	Attention functional limitation, discharge status at discharge from therapy or to end reporting	Atten D/C status

Memory G-code Set	Long Descriptor	Short Descriptor
G9168	Memory functional limitation, current status at therapy episode outset and at reporting intervals	Memory current status
G9169	Memory functional limitation, projected goal status at therapy episode outset, at reporting intervals, and at discharge or to end reporting	Memory goal status
G9170	Memory functional limitation, discharge status at discharge from therapy or to end reporting	Memory D/C status

Voice G-code Set	Long Descriptor	Short Descriptor
G9171	Voice functional limitation, current status at therapy episode outset and at reporting intervals	Voice current status
G9172	Voice functional limitation, projected goal status at therapy episode outset, at reporting intervals, and at discharge or to end reporting	Voice goal status
G9173	Voice functional limitation, discharge status at discharge from therapy or to end reporting	Voice D/C status

Other Speech Language Pathology G-code Set	Long Descriptor	Short Descriptor
G9174	Other speech language pathology functional limitation, current status at therapy episode outset and at reporting intervals	Speech lang current status
G9175	Other speech language pathology functional limitation, projected goal status at therapy episode outset, at reporting intervals, and at discharge or to end reporting	Speech lang goal status
G9176	Other speech language pathology functional limitation, discharge status at discharge from therapy or to end reporting	Speech lang D/C status

SEVERITY/COMPLEXITY MODIFIERS

For each nonpayable functional G-code, one of the modifiers listed below must be used to report the severity/complexity for that functional limitation. The severity modifiers reflect the beneficiary's percentage of functional impairment as determined by the clinician furnishing the therapy services.

Modifier	Impairment Limitation Restriction
CH	0 percent impaired, limited or restricted
CI	At least 1 percent but less than 20 percent impaired, limited or restricted
CJ	At least 20 percent but less than 40 percent impaired, limited or restricted
CK	At least 40 percent but less than 60 percent impaired, limited or restricted
CL	At least 60 percent but less than 80 percent impaired, limited or restricted
CM	At least 80 percent but less than 100 percent impaired, limited or restricted
CN	100 percent impaired, limited or restricted

This Quick Reference Chart was current at the time it was published or uploaded onto the web. Medicare policy changes frequently so links to the source documents have been provided within the document for your reference.

This Quick Reference Chart was prepared as a service to the public and is not intended to grant rights or impose obligations. It may contain references or links to statutes, regulations, or other policy materials. The information provided is only intended to be a general summary. It is not intended to take the place of either the written law or regulations. We encourage readers to review the specific statutes, regulations, and other interpretive materials for a full and accurate statement of their contents.

Your feedback is important to us and we use your suggestions to help us improve our educational products, services and activities and to develop products, services and activities that better meet your educational needs. To evaluate Medicare Learning Network® (MLN) products, services and activities you have participated in, received, or downloaded, please go to http://go.cms.gov/MLNProducts and click on the link called 'MLN Opinion Page' in the left-hand menu and follow the instructions.

Please send your suggestions related to MLN product topics or formats to MLN@cms.hhs.gov.

The Medicare Learning Network® (MLN), a registered trademark of the Centers for Medicare & Medicaid Services (CMS) is the brand name for official information health care professionals can trust. For additional information, visit the MLN's web page at http://go.cms.gov/MLNGeninfo on the CMS website.

CHAPTER 12

Legal Considerations in Physical Therapy Documentation

Sheila K. Nicolson, Esquire, PT, DPT, JD, MBA, MA

CHAPTER OBJECTIVES

1. Recognize the legal expectations from documentation in the patient or client's health record.
2. Recognize how documentation supports or refutes if the standard of physical therapy care was met.
3. Explain the meaning of "not documented, not done."
4. Recognize common legal documentation problems and pitfalls.
5. Recognize ways to mitigate legal documentation problems and pitfalls.

KEY TERMS

Medical malpractice
Medical negligence

Standards of physical therapy practice

Introduction

This chapter focuses on explaining the importance of documentation as it relates to how documentation is used legally. Accordingly, this chapter starts with an explanation of malpractice and how malpractice is determined. Next, examples of common documentation problems are examined. Lastly, suggestions for documentation that will assist you in mitigating legal exposure as it relates to your documentation are presented.

Generally speaking, you probably believe documentation is primarily used so that you can obtain reimbursement. Obviously, reimbursement for the physical therapy services you delivered is important, but, from a legal perspective, documentation explains what services you provided, when the delivery of services occurred, where the delivery of services occurred, how you implemented the delivery of these services, and why you provided the service to a patient or client. It can also explain why a treatment or intervention was not delivered, which could mitigate a patient or client or family member asserting that something should have been done that was not. Thus, documentation

explains what was assessed on the patient or client, what services and/or interventions were provided, and how the patient or client responded to the intervention.

Additionally, your documentation should identify when the service was provided, where the service was provided, and why you decided to do what was done. You likely think that these are the same reasons that are also critically important when documenting for reimbursement. You would be correct. Throughout the years, a variety of guidelines and forms have been developed and revised and now have evolved into electronic resources that aim to cue you as to what content to consider and what content to document as a result of an encounter with a patient or client. However, you must remember, no form or template, paper or electronic, can ever replace the education, knowledge, skill, and critical thinking of you, the therapist. It is appropriate to utilize a framework for your documentation content such as that indicated in TABLE 12-1; however it is paramount to realize that no process, framework, or guideline will ever replace the critical analysis that you

TABLE 12-1 Content of Legally Sound Documentation

What assessments were done on the patient or client?
What services and interventions were provided for the patient or client based on the completed assessments?
Why were the services and interventions chosen for the patient or client?
How did the patient or client respond to the delivered services and interventions?
When were the services and interventions provided to the patient or client?
Where were the services or interventions delivered to the patient or client?
Did your documentation meet the prevailing professional standard of care?

must apply to every patient or client at every encounter to produce consistently successful documentation. Each patient or client encounter must be completely documented to support, justify, and explain what you did and why you did it every time so that any question that surfaces in a legal proceeding could be answered based on the content of your documentation. It is therefore important to have an appreciation and understanding of:

○ Malpractice and how malpractice is determined
○ Common documentation problems and pitfalls
○ Suggestions that will assist you in mitigating legal exposure as it relates to your documentation

Documentation Supports or Refutes Malpractice

The primary way any litigant, usually known as a plaintiff, proves that a healthcare provider was negligent (**medical malpractice**) is through the use of documentation. Likewise, the primary way you would defend against a malpractice lawsuit is through your documentation. Specifically, your documentation will nonverbally explain how you met the prevailing professional standard of care (duty). Thus, recognizing what this means is critical to an understanding of legally sound documentation.

Medical malpractice is really the same thing as **medical negligence**. To establish a medical malpractice claim, a litigant (plaintiff) must prove:

1. You owed a duty to them and what that duty was.
2. You breached that duty.

3. The breach of the duty was the legal cause of harm, damage, and/or injury.
4. What the damages are.

The duty you owe a patient or client is established through peers, experts, research, and publications that state what a reasonably prudent physical therapist or physical therapist assistant would do under like circumstances. Then, a comparison is done between what a reasonably prudent therapist would do under like circumstances and what you did, which is supported through your documentation. When your documentation does not support that you delivered what the "standard" indicates; then the litigant may be able to prove that your failure to provide the "standard" is what harmed them.

Consider the following scenario. Part of a standard physical therapy examination is a vital signs assessment. Likewise, vital signs should be taken every visit. If a decision is made not to collect vital signs at every visit then your documentation should reflect this omission. Sometimes the patient or client's circumstances may warrant that vital signs are taken more frequently such as during and after your intervention session. The only way to really prove that you did this would be through your documentation for that patient or client. Thus, the duty owed a patient or client is that vital signs are taken at least every visit. The only true way to prove that you did this would be for your documentation to show that the vital signs were taken and recorded at every patient or client encounter.

If you were able to remember the patient or client and the specific details of a particular patient or client encounter, you might be able to testify in a legal proceeding that you remember taking the patient or client's vital signs at every visit. You might further be able to comment that since the vital signs were within a normal range you chose not to record them. While you may think you could remember the specific details of your patient or client's examination findings, it is unlikely that you or anyone else will have specific recollection of any patient or client and even more unlikely that you or anyone else will remember every visit and every piece of data collected within any particular patient or client encounter. Furthermore, it is equally unlikely that you would remember that a patient or client's vital signs were always, at every visit, within a normal range. Thus, your documentation becomes the only written evidence that can corroborate and substantiate what you did. Also realize that there is typically a large gap of time, often over a year, between a clinical instance and when legal proceedings occur. Thus, relying on your memory for specific details is likely futile. An example of how this type of inquiry or legal testimony might occur is as follows.

Q: Would you agree with me that vital signs should be taken for every patient or client's evaluation?

A: Yes.

Q: Would you agree with me that the standard of care for a physical therapist requires that vital signs be taken during every examination of a patient or client?

A: Yes.

Q: Would you agree with me that every patient or client should have their vital signs taken at least once during every visit/session?

A: Yes.

Q: Would you agree with me that the standard of care for a physical therapist requires that vital signs be taken during every visit/session with a patient or client?

A: Yes.

Q: Do you specifically remember taking Mr./Mrs. _____'s vital signs during his/her initial examination?

A: No, but I take vital signs during every initial examination.

Q: Please look at this document. Is that your initial examination of Mr./Mrs. _____?

A: Yes.

Q: Please look at your initial examination of Mr./Mrs. _____. Can you show me on your examination where you documented Mr./Mrs. _____'s vital signs?

A: There is no documentation of vital signs on this examination; however, just because I did not document vital signs does not mean I did not take them.

Q: You agree you did not document Mr./Mrs. _____'s vital signs on this initial examination document?

A: Yes, but again I take vital signs during every initial examination.

Q: When you went to physical therapy school were you taught, "Not documented, not done?"

A: Yes.

Q: What does "not documented, not done" mean?

A: If you do not document something, then it is assumed you did not do it.

You can see how the failure to document completely, especially in light of knowing that you should have documented the content in question, could lead to the presumption that you did not do something that the standard of care requires you do. Refer to **APPENDIXS 12-A** and **12-B** for the American Physical Therapy Association (APTA)'s documents of the *Standards of Practice for Physical Therapy*.[1,2] In addition to these documents, you have a professional responsibility to know the minimum **standards of physical therapy practice** in your state.

Common Legal Documentation Problems and Pitfalls

Common documentation problems and pitfalls include "parrot" documentation, technical omissions, illegible entries, undefined abbreviations, lack of substance, and lack of information that demonstrates if the standard of care (duty owed) was met. Each of these problems will be discussed in further detail below.

PARROT DOCUMENTATION

One of the most common documentation problems is what can be called "parrot" documentation. This terminology indicates that the person documenting repeats most or all of what was contained in the prior session's note. While some of the same information may be applicable to the current session with your patient or client, it is very doubtful that a patient or client is exactly the same every visit. Likewise, if the patient or client's current status, interventions, response to interventions, and plan are being *recorded* in exactly the same way at every visit, then one must ask if the delivered services are being *repeated* in exactly the same way at every encounter and if that patient or client's actually requires skilled physical therapy services. This inquiry in turn leads to the issue of the ability of your documentation to support or refute reimbursement. Consider the following daily notes from an outpatient physical therapy practice.

8-18-2014

Patient or client reports that she is slowly improving her ability to reach her right arm overhead to don her clothing and to wash her hair. She states that she continues to have difficulty due to pain (8/10) and stiffness reaching posteriorly to hook her bra and for hygienic toileting tasks.

Added motor control and coordination tasks per flow sheet to improve ability to direct overhead movements during a functional task. Adjusted home exercise program to include posterior capsule stretch for the right glenohumeral joint in rightside lying 5 × 30 second hold, three times per day, followed by active reach behind back with right upper extremity (30×).

Patient or client demonstrated the ability to perform added home exercise program with a subsequent increase in right shoulder internal rotation AROM to the L1 spinous process.

Continue to improve ability to reach overhead and posteriorly for daily hygienic tasks.

8-21-2014

Patient or client states that she continues to have difficulty due to pain (8/10) and stiffness reaching posteriorly to hook her bra and for hygienic toileting tasks.

See flow sheet for therapeutic exercise and home exercise program.

Patient or client demonstrated right shoulder internal rotation AROM to the L1 spinous process and overhead reach to 100 degrees.

Continue to improve ability to reach overhead and posteriorly for daily hygienic tasks.

Even though the two entries above are not repeated verbatim, the message of the content is the same in both entries. In other words, there is no new information revealed by the second entry and no information that indicates the patient or client's response to interventions after the prior session. Similarly, there is no support for why a similar or the same intervention as those at the previous session is warranted. Recognize that repeating interventions may be appropriate for the patient or client's condition; however it is likely that you would be able

to indicate a change in an exercise's dosage or the positioning of a patient or client during a functional task to indicate a progression or some alteration from the prior session. If you are not able to identify this sort of change for the patient or client then it is pertinent to indicate why you have elected to keep your interventions the same. Overall, it is important to include in your documentation your clinical rationale for not only changing an intervention as progress is achieved, but also for leaving an intervention unchanged from session to session. This rationale could be included for the scenario above as follows.

8-21-2014

Patient or client states that she continues to have difficulty due to pain (8/10) and stiffness reaching posteriorly to hook her bra and for hygienic toileting tasks. She notes that she was able to hook her bra after performing her home exercises with less pain (4/10) but then had increasing difficulty when getting dressed upon waking in the morning.

See flow sheet for therapeutic exercise dosing. Altered timing of the home exercise program to be performed upon waking in a.m., midday, and after the workday.

Patient or client demonstrated understanding of new home exercise program plan. Right shoulder internal rotation AROM to L1 spinous process at beginning of session indicating that gains made previously have been maintained.

Determine change in functional reach to hook bra and to reach posteriorly for daily hygienic tasks as a result of changing the timing of home exercise program performance.

TECHNICAL OMISSIONS

A technical omission is leaving detail out of your documentation that is required to process the initial examination, re-examination, or intervention as a claim for reimbursement. Sometimes the omission can lead to legal difficulties with regards to proving that the standard of care owed the patient or client from a physical therapist or physical therapist assistant was met. A technical omission could be failure to date the examination or daily note, leaving a part of the documentation blank, or coding a diagnosis or intervention incorrectly or inaccurately. Thus, a technical omission is leaving something off the documentation that was required by law to be there. Consider the following example.

> You are working with a Medicare beneficiary and are due to re-examine the patient or client at the current visit, which is the tenth visit in the plan of care. You do not realize that it is the tenth visit until ¾ of the way through the session.

If you elect to defer the re-examination until the eleventh visit you are omitting an important component of the individual's plan of care that is required by law. This omission will likely affect reimbursement for the services you delivered to this patient or client. In addition, this omission has the potential to lead to legal ramifications if the lack of a timely re-examination affected the patient or client in a negative way. It is likely that the severity of the effects of a technical omission in your documentation is unforeseen or unpredictable. Therefore, it is wise to be aware of these rules and regulations and apply them consistently to your documentation practices.

ILLEGIBLE ENTRIES

Illegible documentation entries are becoming for the most part, ancient history, with the conversion from paper-based systems to electronic health records. However, there may be times such as during power outages or times of technical difficulties with electronic health systems when you will have to document on paper. In this case, you should be cognizant that your documentation is always legible. Legally, illegible documentation will be interpreted as if the documentation was not included in the health record. Another circumstance where you would be required to document on paper is if a location within the electronic software does not exist to record the content you need to document. In this situation, you are not relieved from having to capture the documentation. Rather, you are obligated to document the information using an alternative medium, such as paper, in a legible manner. Consider the following scenario.

> You are working in an outpatient environment and your patient or client calls you to relay that she is having increased pain since her session with you earlier that day.

It is important to capture the details of the phone conversation with your patient or client especially because the conversation has the potential to impact the plan of care

that you have developed on your patient or client's behalf. Even though the communication did not occur within the context of a formal patient or client encounter, an acknowledgement of the call and the detail of how the content of the call was handled should be included in your documentation on paper and then subsequently scanned into the patient or client's health record. As technology evolves and limitations of software programs are identified by program users, issues such as the one in this scenario are more and more rare. As a result of increased electronic documentation system use, nearly every documentation software package has the ability to add comments or to provide designated areas within the record to supplement documentation. However in the event that you do not see a drop-down menu or a specific designated space in an electronic template for the content you wish to include, do not assume that one does not exist within the software in an alternative location. Furthermore, never assume that you are excused from providing that documentation.

UNDEFINED ABBREVIATIONS

Abbreviations have been shown to lead to medical errors. The use of abbreviations in physical therapy documentation can also lead to errors in examination, outcome measure and evaluation interpretation, and intervention implementation. While the American Physical Therapy Association does not endorse any specific set of abbreviations and recommends that abbreviations be used sparingly,[3] it is legally acceptable to use abbreviations in a patient or client's health record. However, it is responsible clinical practice to only use those abbreviations that have been defined as standard in your organization and practice setting and recorded in policies and procedures manuals. The Institute for Safe Medication Practices (ISMP) published a list of abbreviations that have been found to be commonly misinterpreted by healthcare providers (TABLE 12-2).[4] Additionally, there are several abbreviations that have multiple meanings within the physical therapy profession that could lead to errors in the delivery of physical therapy services and further obscure documentation interpretation (TABLE 12-3).

Communicating interpretations and definitions of commonly used abbreviations[5] can help any user of your documentation including your colleagues, referral sources, internal auditors, or third-party payers avoid errors because of a misinterpretation of your

TABLE 12-2   ISMP's List of Error-Prone Abbreviations, Symbols, and Dose Designations

Abbreviations	Intended Meaning	Misinterpretation	Correction
μg	Microgram	Mistaken as "mg"	Use "mcg"
AD, AS, AU	Right ear, left ear, each ear	Mistaken as OD, OS, OU (right eye, left eye, each eye)	Use "right ear," "left ear," or "each ear"
OD, OS, OU	Right eye, left eye, each eye	Mistaken as AD, AS, AU (right ear, left ear, each ear)	Use "right eye," "left eye," or "each eye"
BT	Bedtime	Mistaken as "BID" (twice daily)	Use "bedtime"
cc	Cubic centimeters	Mistaken as "u" (units)	Use "mL"
D/C	Discharge or discontinue	Premature discontinuation of medications if D/C (intended to mean "discharge") has been misinterpreted as "discontinued" when followed by a list of discharge medications	Use "discharge" and "discontinue"
IJ	Injection	Mistaken as "IV" or "intrajugular"	Use "injection"
IN	Intranasal	Mistaken as "IM" or "IV"	Use "intranasal" or "NAS"
HS	Half-strength	Mistaken as bedtime	Use "half-strength" or "bedtime"
hs	At bedtime, hours of sleep	Mistaken as half-strength	
IU**	International unit	Mistaken as IV (intravenous) or 10 (ten)	Use "units"
o.d. or OD	Once daily	Mistaken as "right eye" (OD-oculus dexter), leading to oral liquid medications administered in the eye	Use "daily"
OJ	Orange juice	Mistaken as OD or OS (right or left eye); drugs meant to be diluted in orange juice may be given in the eye	Use "orange juice"
Per os	By mouth, orally	The "os" can be mistaken as "left eye" (OS-oculus sinister)	Use "PO," "by mouth," or "orally"
q.d. or QD**	Every day	Mistaken as q.i.d., especially if the period after the "q" or the tail of the "q" is misunderstood as an "i"	Use "daily"
qhs	Nightly at bedtime	Mistaken as "qhr" or every hour	Use "nightly"
qn	Nightly or at bedtime	Mistaken as "qh" (every hour)	Use "nightly" or "at bedtime"
q.o.d. or QOD**	Every other day	Mistaken as "q.d." (daily) or "q.i.d. (four times daily) if the "o" is poorly written	Use "every other day"
q1d	Daily	Mistaken as q.i.d. (four times daily)	Use "daily"
q6PM, etc.	Every evening at 6 PM	Mistaken as every 6 hours	Use "daily at 6 PM" or "6 PM daily"
SC, SQ, sub q	Subcutaneous	SC mistaken as SL (sublingual); SQ mistaken as "5 every;" the "q" in "sub q" has been mistaken as "every" (e.g., a heparin dose ordered "sub q 2 hours before surgery" misunderstood as every 2 hours before surgery)	Use "subcut" or "subcutaneously"
ss	Sliding scale (insulin) or ½ (apothecary)	Mistaken as "55"	Spell out "sliding scale;" use "one-half" or "½"
SSRI	Sliding scale regular insulin	Mistaken as selective-serotonin reuptake inhibitor	Spell out "sliding scale (insulin)"
SSI	Sliding scale insulin	Mistaken as Strong Solution of Iodine (Lugol's)	
i/d	One daily	Mistaken as "tid"	Use "1 daily"
TIW or tiw	3 times a week	Mistaken as "3 times a day" or "twice in a week"	Use "3 times weekly"
U or u**	Unit	Mistaken as the number 0 or 4, causing a 10-fold overdose or greater (e.g., 4U seen as "40" or 4u seen as "44"); mistaken as "cc" so dose given in volume instead of units (e.g., 4u seen as 4cc)	Use "unit"
UD	As directed ("ut dictum")	Mistaken as unit dose (e.g., diltiazem 125 mg IV infusion "UD" misinterpreted as meaning to give the entire infusion as a unit [bolus] dose)	Use "as directed"

(Continues)

TABLE 12-2 (*Continued*)

Dose Designations and Other Information	Intended Meaning	Misinterpretation	Correction
Trailing zero after decimal point (e.g., 1.0 mg)**	1 mg	Mistaken as 10 mg if the decimal point is not seen	Do not use trailing zeros for doses expressed in whole numbers
"Naked" decimal point (e.g., .5 mg)**	0.5 mg	Mistaken as 5 mg if the decimal point is not seen	Use zero before a decimal point when the dose is less than a whole unit
Abbreviations such as mg. or mL. with a period following the abbreviation	mg mL	The period is unnecessary and could be mistaken as the number 1 if written poorly	Use mg, mL, etc. without a terminal period
Drug name and dose run together (especially problematic for drug names that end in "l" such as Inderal 40 mg; Tegretol 300 mg)	Inderal 40 mg Tegretol 300 mg	Mistaken as Inderal 140 mg Mistaken as Tegretol 1300 mg	Place adequate space between the drug name, dose, and unit of measure
Numerical dose and unit of measure run together (e.g., 10 mg, 100 mL)	10 mg 100 mL	The "m" is sometimes mistaken as a zero or two zeros, risking a 10- to 100-fold overdose	Place adequate space between the dose and unit of measure
Large doses without properly placed commas (e.g., 100000 units; 1000000 units)	100,000 units 1,000,000 units	100000 has been mistaken as 10,000 or 1,000,000; 1000000 has been mistaken as 100,000	Use commas for dosing units at or above 1,000, or use words such as 100 "thousand" or 1 "million" to improve readability

Drug Name Abbreviations	Intended Meaning	Misinterpretation	Correction
To avoid confusion, do not abbreviate drug names when communicating medical information. Examples of drug name abbreviations involved in medication errors include:			
APAP	acetaminophen	Not recognized as acetaminophen	Use complete drug name
ARA A	vidarabine	Mistaken as cytarabine (ARA C)	Use complete drug name
AZT	zidovudine (Retrovir)	Mistaken as azathioprine or aztreonam	Use complete drug name
CPZ	Compazine (prochlorperazine)	Mistaken as chlorpromazine	Use complete drug name
DPT	Demerol-Phenergan-Thorazine	Mistaken as diphtheria-pertussis-tetanus (vaccine)	Use complete drug name
DTO	Diluted tincture of opium, or deodorized tincture of opium (Paregoric)	Mistaken as tincture of opium	Use complete drug name
HCl	hydrochloric acid or hydrochloride	Mistaken as potassium chloride (The "H" is misinterpreted as "K")	Use complete drug name unless expressed as a salt of a drug
HCT	hydrocortisone	Mistaken as hydrochlorothiazide	Use complete drug name
HCTZ	hydrochlorothiazide	Mistaken as hydrocortisone (seen as HCT250 mg)	Use complete drug name
$MgSO_4$**	magnesium sulfate	Mistaken as morphine sulfate	Use complete drug name
MS, MSO_4**	morphine sulfate	Mistaken as magnesium sulfate	Use complete drug name

(*Continues*)

TABLE 12-2 *(Continued)*

Drug Name Abbreviations	Intended Meaning	Misinterpretation	Correction
MTX	methotrexate	Mistaken as mitoxantrone	Use complete drug name
PCA	procainamide	Mistaken as patient controlled analgesia	Use complete drug name
PTU	propylthiouracil	Mistaken as mercaptopurine	Use complete drug name
T3	Tylenol with codeine No. 3	Mistaken as liothyronine	Use complete drug name
TAC	triamcinolone	Mistaken as tetracaine, Adrenalin, cocaine	Use complete drug name
TNK	TNKase	Mistaken as "TPA"	Use complete drug name
ZnSO$_4$	zinc sulfate	Mistaken as morphine sulfate	Use complete drug name
Stemmed Drug Names	**Intended Meaning**	**Misinterpretation**	**Correction**
"Nitro" drip	nitroglycerin infusion	Mistaken as sodium nitroprusside infusion	Use complete drug name
"Norflox"	norfloxacin	Mistaken as Norflex	Use complete drug name
"IV Vanc"	intravenous vancomycin	Mistaken as Invanz	Use complete drug name
Symbols	**Intended Meaning**	**Misinterpretation**	**Correction**
℥	Dram	Symbol for dram mistaken as "3"	Use the metric system
♏	Minim	Symbol for minim mistaken as "mL"	
x3d	For three days	Mistaken as "3 doses"	Use "for three days"
> and <	Greater than and less than	Mistaken as opposite of intended; mistakenly use incorrect symbol; "< 10" mistaken as "40"	Use "greater than" or "less than"
/ (slash mark)	Separates two doses or indicates "per"	Mistaken as the number 1 (e.g., "25 units/10 units" misread as "25 units and 110" units)	Use "per" rather than a slash mark to separate doses
@	At	Mistaken as "2"	Use "at"
&	And	Mistaken as "2"	Use "and"
+	Plus or and	Mistaken as "4"	Use "and"
°	Hour	Mistaken as a zero (e.g., q2° seen as q 20)	Use "hr," "h," or "hour"
Φ or Ø	zero, null sign	Mistaken as numerals 4, 6, 8, and 9	Use 0 or zero, or describe intent using whole words

**These abbreviations are included on The Joint Commission's "minimum list" of dangerous abbreviations, acronyms, and symbols that must be included on an organization's "Do Not Use" list, effective January 1, 2004. Visit www.jointcommission.org for more information about this Joint Commission requirement.

documentation. Furthermore, in the event that the abbreviations used in your documentation are questioned, you can support the accepted use of those abbreviations within your clinical practice with an excerpt from a policies and procedures manual. It must be understood however that miscommunication occurring secondary to the use of abbreviations can only be mitigated by a common language published in a policies and procedures manual if that resource is actually referred to and utilized by all individuals within your clinical practice. Consider the following documentation example.

You are a per diem physical therapist or physical therapist assistant working in an inpatient rehabilitation facility. Upon reviewing a patient or client's current status you read the following.

> Pt or Ct sitting EOB with min SOB after VS A determined to be WNL.

> Pt or Ct c/o n/t BK in LLE that is worse in am and ↓ in WB.

What is your interpretation of this entry? Did you find it difficult to read? The intended meaning of the above documentation is as follows.

> Patient or client sitting at edge of bed with minimal shortness of breath after vital signs assessment determined to be within normal limits. Patient or client

TABLE 12-3   Abbreviations Used in Physical Therapy Practice with Dual or Multiple Meanings

Abbreviation	Meanings
Abd	Abdominal, abduction
AD	Assistive device, Alzheimer's dementia
BS	Breath sounds, bowel sounds
CP	Cold pack, cerebral palsy
COG	Center of gravity, cognition
CX	Cancellation, cervical spine
DC	Discharge, discontinue, direct current
ER	External rotation, emergency room
DOS	Date of surgery, date of service
FX	Fracture, function
HHA	Home health aide, hand-held assist
LF	Lateral flexion, left
LOS	Length of stay, limits of stability
mm	Muscle, millimeter
Min	Minute, minimum, minimal
Mob	Mobilization, mobility
N/T	Not tested, numbness/tingling
Post	Posterior, after
PT	Physical therapist, prothrombin time
PTA	Physical therapist assistant, prior to admission
Rx	Treatment, prescription
SB	Side bending, stability or Swiss ball
TA	Therapeutic activities, tibialis anterior, transversus abdominus
Tx	Traction, thoracic spine
Sup	Supination, superior
Sx	Surgery, symptoms
VC	Verbal cues, visual cues, vital capacity
Wk	Week, weak
#	Number, pounds
√	Flexion, check
/	Extension, per

Data from The Institute of Physical Medicine and Rehabilitation *Abbreviations Frequently used in Physical Therapy documentation*; April 2008. Physical Therapy Abbreviations, http://www.physicaltherapynotes.com/2010/11/physical-therapy-abbreviation-list.html. Accessed 6/16/2015

complains of numbness and tingling below the knee in the left lower extremity that is worse in the morning and that decreases in weight bearing.

Do you have any clearer idea of the meaning of this entry now that you know the meaning of the abbreviations? Do

you have a distinct clinical picture of what assessment was done on the patient or client at the prior session? Not only can abbreviations be difficult to read and glean meaning from, they can also generate more questions regarding the intended meaning. For example, while you may have been able to infer from the context of other components of the health record that "VS A determined to be WNF" is actually "vital sign assessment is determined to be within normal limits," it is unclear which vital signs were actually measured. Rather than indicating that vital signs are within normal limits, the vital sign with the actual numbers for the measurement should be recorded as objective data. The assessment portion of the entry would then further indicate that the actual numbers obtained are within normal limits for that patient or client. Remember, that your documentation should be clear enough that there is no need for a user of your note to contact you to clarify its contents.

LACK OF SUBSTANCE

"Lack of substance" within documentation means that the documentation does not relay to the consumer of the entry what was done, why it was done, and the effect of what was done. Therefore, when the documentation is reviewed, a clear clinical picture of the patient or client or the response to the interventions is not relayed. One common example of a lack of substance in a daily note is a response to intervention or assessment section that reads, "Patient or client tolerated treatment well." This entry is essentially meaningless since it in no way explains the patient or client's response to the interventions provided during the visit. Furthermore, you could be questioned regarding why skilled physical therapy services are warranted if a patient or client "tolerated treatment well." Therefore, the failure to document substantive information about what was done with the patient or client during the encounter, why it was done, and the response to that intervention must be avoided.

LACK OF INFORMATION TO SUPPORT IF THE STANDARD OF CARE HAS BEEN MET

As discussed previously in the context of medical malpractice, documentation is used to establish whether or not you met the prevailing professional standard of care. Again, the likelihood that you will remember the specifics of any patient or client's initial examination, re-examination, or treatment session is very small. Thus, the way to prove whether or not something was done is through documentation. Likewise, if research has established that the best evidence is to include a certain assessment tool or intervention approach and you did not, then your documentation would need to explain why you chose to do something alternative to what has been proven or accepted in the physical therapy community as best practice. While research does not mandate the delivery of physical therapy services, it does establish best practices against which you must apply your clinical reasoning skills, the characteristics of your individual patient or client, and your experience to decide if the chosen intervention is the appropriate approach for you to pursue with your patient or client. If for whatever reason it is not, then your documentation should explain why, along with your rationale for why you chose to utilize an alternative intervention. Consider the following documentation example.

> You are working in a skilled nursing facility with a frail older adult patient or client who has not been out of bed for the last 6 hours. You are concerned that she could develop pressure sores and suffer the consequences of immobility if she does not achieve some sort of movement soon. Unfortunately, she complains of severe dizziness with any movement and becomes nauseated with any attempt to raise the head of her bed or to turn her for pressure relief. When you comment that you want to transfer her to her recliner so that she can look out the window and have an opportunity to change positions, she groans and tells you that she is not going to be able to participate in therapy today. You attempt to persuade her to try to sit up but she adamantly refuses.

Documentation that would reinforce a lack of information to support if the standard of care had been met might appear as follows.

> Patient or client complains of dizziness and refuses to participate in therapy session today.

Documentation that would relay adequate information to support that the standard of care had been met might appear as follows:

> Patient or client complains of dizziness and nausea with any movement of her upper body and head.

Supine BP = 123/87 mmHg, no dizziness; BP with head of bed elevated to 30 degrees = 104/61 mmHg, reports moderate dizziness; BP with head of bed elevated to 60 degrees = 74/55 mmHg, reports severe dizziness, lightheadedness, and nausea. Symptoms diminished to minimal within 3 minutes of returning the head of bed to zero degrees of elevation; BP retaken in supine at 5 minutes = 127/85 mmHg. Nurse alerted of findings and cardiologist contacted for immediate consultation. Performed upper and lower extremity passive range of motion for pressure relief and joint movement to prevent contractures and muscular shortening. Patient or client unable to participate in active activities such as bed mobility or transfers.

Even though this patient or client refused your attempts to participate in her physical therapy session, the above entry into this patient or client's daily note indicates that attempts were made to identify the cause of her refusal to participate in physical therapy. Consider now if the assessment of the patient or client's dizziness revealed no information that could explain the etiology of her complaints. In this case, the documentation might read as follows.

> Patient or client complains of dizziness and nausea with any movement of her upper body and head. Supine BP = 123/87 mmHg, no dizziness; BP remains stable without symptoms of dizziness with varying degrees of head of bed elevation to approximately 75 degrees. Nurse alerted of patient or client's complaints and results of orthostatic BP monitoring in bed. Performed upper and lower extremity passive range of motion for pressure relief and joint movement to prevent contractures and muscular shortening. Patient or client unwilling to participate in vestibular or oculomotor testing or to sit at edge of bed or to participate in active activities such as bed mobility or transfers.

Regardless of the outcome of the scenario presented above, if there is a future occasion where the patient or client's health record is consulted, a clear indication of substantial information to support that the standard of care has been met is provided. In other words, if this patient or client ultimately developed a pressure wound, your documentation would reflect that you took action to prevent it. Alternatively, if you took measures to determine the root cause of this patient or client's dizziness but did not document your actions in the record, it will be assumed that no attempt to identify the etiology of this patient or client's symptoms was made.

Documentation Suggestions to Mitigate Legal Exposure

Often the common problems and pitfalls that occur in documentation are not intentional. However, regardless of your intentions you have a professional responsibility as a physical therapist or physical therapist assistant to create successful documentation on your patient or client's behalf so that your patient or client will continue to be able to benefit from the skilled services you provide and so that you will be reimbursed for those skilled services. Also, remember that successful documentation can be used for making programmatic decisions, to determine best practices, and for research. Consider that there are a few underlying principles that can assist you in creating documentation that can ultimately help to lessen the likelihood that your expertise will be legally challenged.

- ○ Documentation must be truthful.
- ○ Documentation should be done contemporaneously with the patient or client encounter.
- ○ Documentation should be done utilizing a method that is compliant with HIPAA laws and regulations.

DOCUMENTATION MUST BE TRUTHFUL

Any and all documentation must be truthful. Not only is it unethical, but it is illegal to document something that did not occur. Recall the scenario above of your patient or client who reported dizziness with any movement. Assume that your director expressed concern that your facility may not be reimbursed for the services you provided to this patient or client because you have been unable to document her full participation in therapy. Truthfully documenting how much time the patient or client actually participated in preventative interventions such as pressure relief and contracture management and what activities she was unable to perform is ultimately important for future decisions made regarding her health care. Even exaggerating the time spent with the patient or client on preventative interventions

or indicating an effort level that was above or below the patient or client's actual achievements is considered falsifying information in the health record. Documenting an action or activity as being done when it was not could be considered fraud. For example, consider that you forgot to re-measure the above patient or client's blood pressure at rest prior to initiating upper extremity and lower extremity passive movement as was requested by the patient or client's occupational therapist. Inaccurate documentation based on this scenario might appear as follows.

> Patient or client is supine with head of bed flat at beginning of session. No report of dizziness or nausea. Able to participate in upper and lower extremity active assisted range of motion and tolerate rolling to the right and left with moderate assistance × 1 and one upper extremity on the bed rail without complaint of dizziness. BP at rest prior to activity = 135/89 mmHg.

Although you might speculate that no one would ever know that you did not actually take this blood pressure prior to activity, your action is not compatible with the APTA's *Code of Ethics* (**APPENDIX 12-C**).[6] A truthful representation of actual events might appear as follows.

> Patient or client is supine with head of bed flat at beginning of session. No report of dizziness or nausea. Able to participate in upper and lower extremity active assisted range of motion and tolerate rolling to the right and left with moderate assistance × 1 and one upper extremity on the bed rail without complaint of dizziness. BP taken in supine 5 minutes after conclusion of therapeutic activity = 135/89 mmHg.

It is always inappropriate to document actions that you did not complete or events that did not occur, even if you do not believe that your entry into the documentation might negatively affect your patient or client's future outcomes or your credibility as a healthcare provider. Many State Practice Acts establish that it is an absolute violation to falsify documentation. Thus, your documentation should accurately and truthfully reflect all parts of your initial examination and any follow-up encounters you have with your patient or client every time.

DOCUMENT CONTEMPORANEOUSLY WITH THE PATIENT OR CLIENT ENCOUNTER

Documentation should be completed contemporaneously, at or around the same time, as the encounter with your patient or client. There are times you may be tempted to delay completing your documentation until the next day. You should not delay completing your documentation because you cannot control what may happen with your patient or client during times when you are not in direct contact with them. Furthermore, events that may occur in your own life could prevent you from being able to complete your documentation the next day. Therefore, best practice is to complete documentation contemporaneously as the physical therapy services you deliver are rendered. This practice will assist you in being as accurate and truthful as possible as well as provide you the best opportunity to document the most thorough information on your patient or client's behalf.

COMPLY WITH HIPAA LAWS AND RULES

When documenting you must ensure your compliance with the Health Insurance Portability and Accountability Act (HIPAA). This federal law, passed in 1996, dictates laws and rules that exist to impart privacy and security measures to protect a patient or client's personal health information. Essentially, anyone who is not authorized to read or be aware of your patient or client's health information should not have access to your documentation. Gaining access to health information can be as simple as leaving your written notes or electronic device available to someone who is not authorized to see that information. In practice, this means that when you are documenting, no unauthorized person should be able to see, read, and/or hear what you are documenting. Likewise, you should not be discussing your patient or client's protected health information with anyone not authorized to receive that information. The HIPAA privacy rule indicates that those who are authorized to receive an individual's personal health information without the patient or client's authorization include any healthcare provider or personnel who is directly involved in the delivery of care or any transactions associated with the delivery of that care. Therefore, taking a patient or client's health information home with you for completion of your documentation could lead to HIPAA violations. Consider the following scenario.

You are late to pick up your children from school so rather than stay later in the clinic to complete your documentation, you gather your things in your work bag, which includes your computer on which you document as well as some paper-based information such as the intake paperwork, a medication list, and MRI results from the initial examination you conducted for your new patient or client earlier that day. Your intention is to complete your documentation at home so that you are caught up by tomorrow when you return to the clinic.

As indicated above, the moment you remove from your workplace any materials that represent access to protected health information, you have surrendered express control over those materials. There is no way you could predict your involvement in a car accident, which may potentially deposit your patient or client's health information all over the road, nor can you predict if your car will be vandalized and your work computer stolen and accessed while you quickly run an errand. While there are specific requirements in the HIPAA law applied to electronic devices used for creating, transmitting, and storing protected health information such as encryption software and passwords, mistakes can occur. Hardware malfunctions and breaches in technology resulting in stolen healthcare information has occurred. Therefore, it is important for you to consider how you ensure that your patient or client's health information is kept private and secure so that you are not in violation of the HIPAA law. Remember, no one's protected health information should be visualized or verbalized unless either authorized by your patient or client or as necessary for the delivery of care to your patient or client.

Summary

Documenting your interactions with your patient or client is a necessary component of physical therapy practice. There are important considerations to ensure that you consistently create legally sound documentation regardless of the setting in which you practice or the patient or client's ability to pay for the services you deliver. Documentation should be done well to:

○ Serve as a record of the services provided to your patient or client.

○ Protect yourself and your professional license.

○ Ensure reimbursement to you and your employer for the services you deliver.

Remember that legally sound documentation should include what assessments were done on a patient or client, what services and interventions were provided, why these services were chosen, the response to the chosen services and interventions, when services and interventions were delivered, where this occurred, and if the prevailing professional standard of care was met. Your consistent regard for the quality of your documentation will translate to a consistent perception not only from the patient or client but also from any other consumer of your documentation that the care you deliver as a physical therapist or a physical therapist assistant is necessary and value-added.

BOX 12-1 The Electronic Health Record: Legal Considerations in Documentation

Electronic health systems are the vehicles you will use at some point in your healthcare career to document your physical therapy interactions with your patient or client as paper-based systems succumb to advances in technology. No matter which documentation software you use, the likelihood is high that it will not provide the optimal framework for every patient or client in every care setting. Thus, you must learn the features that exist within the system you use that will allow you to document additional comments or explanations that you need to include in your documentation. Attempting to excuse any lack of documentation because of flaws and limitations inherent in the electronic health record software will never prevail as an excuse in a court of law.

Electronic health record software utilizes templates and drop-down menus so that you might be able to navigate more quickly through your documentation process making more efficient use of your time. It is prudent however to be aware that some shortcuts implemented in an EHR may actually put you at risk for creating documentation that would not adequately support your position should the delivery of your physical therapy services be questioned in a legal proceeding. Consider for example that you are performing the initial examination on a patient or client in a facility that offers occupational and speech therapy services in addition to physical therapy services. An understanding may exist among your colleagues that the speech language pathology discipline performs initial cognitive screenings and assessments for the patient or client populations served at this institution. However, if there is a location within the physical therapy initial examination template to input this information, then you must populate the field with "not tested" or "tested by speech language pathologist." If left blank, a third party reviewing your documentation will not know if you neglected to collect the information, if you collected it and forgot to include it in your documentation, or if you collected the information at a subsequent encounter with the patient or client. Regardless of your intentions, a blank area in your documentation will be interpreted as "not documented, not done."

It is important to be cautious that some EHR systems may feature an option to carry forward to your current daily note the content of your previous daily note. This could occur automatically upon opening your daily note for that day's session or after the click of a tab that directs the software to copy previously recorded data into the current note. It is important for you to recognize this feature so that the proper areas of your current note can be updated to reflect your patient or client's actual current status, the actual services delivered in that session, your patient or client's actual response to those interventions, and the actual plan for the next encounter.

Electronic documentation systems also have the capacity to limit the use of abbreviations that are not recognized or supported. Therefore, the conversion from paper-based documentation to electronic documentation will automatically reduce this problem. Similarly, electronic systems utilize predetermined sentence structures such as "Patient or client tolerated treatment well" or "Continue plan of care." This content, which often populates automatically upon opening the note, could compromise the quality of your note as well as put you at risk for creating documentation with a lack of substance. Therefore, it is important to be aware of this feature so that you can include the appropriate detail within the note.

Using electronic documentation systems requires you to use some sort of hardware as the medium to collect, store, and retrieve your patient or client's data such as a desktop computer, a laptop computer, or a tablet. Transitioning from a paper-based system can challenge your ability to document contemporaneously, or around the same time as the actual encounter with your patient or client. Consider, however, that as you become more proficient with the features of the electronic system you use, that your ability to streamline how you capture your documentation will also improve. Be cautious during this learning process that you are not sacrificing or compromising the quality of the information you include in your patient or client's health record. It would be valuable to keep track of the variables and features of the EHR system you use that inhibit you from efficiently documenting your patient or client's encounters. This information will serve as valuable feedback to your employer as well as to the vendor who created and provides support for the system.

The use of electronic devices for documentation also poses additional threats to the privacy and security of your patient or client's health information. For example, if you step away from your electronic device and workstation to interact with a patient or client, it is necessary for you to lock your computer's screen so that health information is not displayed on the screen. If you are utilizing paper, it is appropriate to cover the material so that it is not picked up or reviewed in your absence. Lastly, consider that if you use paper to supplement your documentation style such as jotting notes for transfer to your electronic system at a later time, it is appropriate to shred the paper once you are through with it.

Discussion Questions

1. Review one of your daily notes.
   a. Have you created what could be defined as "parrot" documentation?
   b. Are there components or sections of your daily notes that are repeated or copied from the prior session's note?
   c. If so, what type of content do you tend to repeat?
   d. How could the repeated note have been written to avoid "parrot" documentation?
2. Revisit a recent daily note in your physical therapy documentation. After your review of the note, consider the following.
   a. Would your documentation support that the physical therapy services you delivered were medically necessary?
   b. Would your documentation support that you provided at least the standard of care?
   c. Can you identify content, such as "parrot" documentation, that should be changed to improve the quality of the note?
   d. Is there evidence of a "lack of substance" in the note?
   e. Repeat this process for your initial examination documentation, a re-examination note, and a conclusion of the episode of care summary.
3. Exchange initial examination documentation, daily note, or re-examination documentation with your colleague.
   a. Describe the patient or client back to your colleague.
   b. According to your colleague, was your description of the patient or client accurate?
   c. Did you identify any gaps in the content of the note?
   d. Did you identify any technical omissions?
   e. How can the documentation be improved?
4. Review your recent initial examination, daily note, re-examination, or exercise flow sheet.
   a. How many abbreviations did you use?
   b. Are the abbreviations used accepted by your employer?
   c. Exchange this note with a colleague. Does your colleague recognize the meaning of the abbreviations used in your note?
5. In what ways have you seen patient or client privacy and security enforced in your organization?

Case Study Questions

1. Consider the following documentation of a patient or client in a skilled nursing setting who had a total knee arthroplasty 8 days ago.

   9-2-2014

   Patient or client reports 8/10 pain in anterior right knee when transitioning into and out of bed.

   Neuromuscular electric stimulation applied to right medial quadriceps adjacent to surgical dressing for muscle activation for 10 minutes.

   Patient or client demonstrated ability to activate quadriceps after session without electric stimulation.

   Practice entering and exiting hospital bed from both sides next session.

   09-05-2014

   Patient or client reports that her pain has not changed in her right knee since the last session.

   Neuromuscular electric stimulation applied to right medial quadriceps adjacent to surgical dressing for muscle activation for 10 minutes.

   Patient or client able to activate quadriceps when getting in and out of bed.

   Continue with bed mobility tasks.

   a. Is there evidence of a "lack of substance" within these notes?

   b. If not, what content distinguishes the meaning of these notes from each other?

   c. If so, identify ways in which you would enhance the content of the note.

2. You are working in a busy clinic with a 10-year-old boy who has difficulty walking and communicating due to cerebral palsy. One of your other young patients or clients, a 7-year-old girl who is working on regaining her mobility after being immobilized from a tibia fracture, asks you what is wrong with the 10-year-old boy.

   a. What is your response?

   b. Do you think that this response represents a HIPAA violation?

3. Yesterday you treated a workers' compensation patient or client for your colleague who went home sick. Today your colleague informs you that a status update is due to this patient or client's case manager. Because of this, your colleague tells you that he added some objective measures and any comments regarding the patient or client's progress to date to the note from yesterday's session so that it could be sent over to the patient or client's case manager and physician.

   a. Discuss the primary therapist's actions regarding this patient or client's documentation.

   b. Do you think that he was acting in a legal manner? Why or why not?

   c. Do you think that he was acting in an ethical manner? Why or why not?

References

1. American Physical Therapy Association (APTA). *Standards of Practice For Physical Therapy.* Arlington, VA: American Physical Therapy Association; June 2013.

2. APTA *Criteria for Standards of Practice for Physical Therapy.* Arlington, VA: American Physical Therapy Association; 2014.

3. APTA. *Defensible Documentation Additional Topics.* Arlington, VA: American Physical Therapy Association; 2011.

4. Institute for Safe Medication Practices. *List of Error-Prone Abbreviations, Symbols, and Dose Designations.* Horsham, PA: Institute for Safe Medication Practices; 2013.

5. Mangusan D, Jr. *Physical Therapy Abbreviations.* Physicaltherapynotes.com; June 2010. Available at www.physicaltherapynotes.com/2010/06/physical-therapy-abbreviations-g.html. Accessed on August 26, 2014.

6. APTA. *Code of Ethics.* Arlington, VA: American Physical Therapy Association.

Appendix 12-A

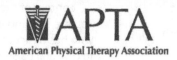

American Physical Therapy Association

Last Updated: 10/1/13
Contact: nationalgovernance@apta.org

STANDARDS OF PRACTICE FOR PHYSICAL THERAPY HOD S06-13-22-15 [Amended HOD S06-10-09-06; HOD S06-03-09-10; HOD 06-03-09-10; HOD 06-99-18-22; HOD 06-96-16-31; HOD 06-91-21-25; HOD 06-85-30-56; Initial HOD 06-80-04-04; HOD 06-80-03-03] [Standard]

Preamble

The physical therapy profession's commitment to society is to promote optimal health and functioning in individuals by pursuing excellence in practice. The American Physical Therapy Association attests to this commitment by adopting and promoting the following *Standards of Practice for Physical Therapy*. These standards are the profession's statement of conditions and performances that are essential for provision of high-quality professional service to society, and they provide a foundation for assessment of physical therapist practice.

I. Ethical/Legal Considerations

    A. Ethical Considerations

        The physical therapist practices according to the *Code of Ethics* of the American Physical Therapy Association.

        The physical therapist assistant complies with the *Standards of Ethical Conduct for the Physical Therapist Assistant* of the American Physical Therapy Association.

    B. Legal Considerations

        The physical therapist complies with all the legal requirements of jurisdictions regulating the practice of physical therapy.

        The physical therapist assistant complies with all the legal requirements of jurisdictions regulating the work of the physical therapist assistant.

II. Administration of the Physical Therapy Service

    A. Statement of Mission, Purposes, and Goals

        The physical therapy service has a statement of mission, purposes, and goals that reflects the needs and interests of the patients/clients served, the physical therapy personnel affiliated with the service, and the community.

    B. Organizational Plan

        The physical therapy service has a written organizational plan.

    C. Policies and Procedures

        The physical therapy service has written policies and procedures that reflect the operation, mission, purposes, and goals of the service, and are consistent with the association's standards, policies, positions, guidelines, and *Code of Ethics*.

    D. Administration

        A physical therapist is responsible for the direction of the physical therapy service.

    E. Fiscal Management

        The director of the physical therapy service, in consultation with physical therapy staff and appropriate administrative personnel, participates in the planning for and allocation of resources. Fiscal planning and management of the service is based on sound accounting principles.

F. Improvement of Quality of Care and Performance
The physical therapy service has a written plan for continuous improvement of quality of care and performance of services.

G. Staffing
The physical therapy personnel affiliated with the physical therapy service have demonstrated competence and are sufficient to achieve the mission, purposes, and goals of the service.

H. Staff Development
The physical therapy service has a written plan that provides for appropriate and ongoing staff development.

I. Physical Setting
The physical setting is designed to provide a safe and accessible environment that facilitates fulfillment of the mission, purposes, and goals of the physical therapy service. The equipment is safe and sufficient to achieve the purposes and goals of physical therapy.

J. Collaboration
The physical therapy service collaborates with all disciplines as appropriate.

III. Patient/Client Management

A. Physical Therapist of Record
The physical therapist of record is the therapist who assumes responsibility for patient/client management and is accountable for the coordination, continuation, and progression of the plan of care.

B. Patient/Client Collaboration
Within the patient/client management process, the physical therapist and the patient/client establish and maintain an ongoing collaborative process of decision making that exists throughout the provision of services.

C. Initial Examination/Evaluation/Diagnosis/Prognosis
The physical therapist performs an initial examination and evaluation to establish a diagnosis and prognosis prior to intervention. Wellness and prevention visits/encounters may occur without the presence of disease, illness, impairments, activity limitations, or participation restrictions.

D. Plan of Care
The physical therapist establishes a plan of care and manages the needs of the patient/client based on the examination, evaluation, diagnosis, prognosis, goals, and outcomes of the planned interventions for identified impairments, activity limitations, and participation restrictions.

The physical therapist involves the patient/client and appropriate others in the planning, anticipated goals and expected outcomes, proposed frequency and duration, and implementation of the plan of care.

E. Intervention
The physical therapist provides or directs and supervises the physical therapy intervention consistent with the results of the examination, evaluation, diagnosis, prognosis, and plan of care. The physical therapy intervention may be provided in an episode of care, or in a single visit/encounter such as for a wellness and prevention visit/encounter or a specialty consultation or for a follow-up visit/encounter after episodes of care, or may be provided intermittently over longer periods of time in cases of managing chronic conditions.

An *episode of care* is the managed care provided for a specific problem or condition during a set time period and can be given either for a short period or on a continuous basis, or it may consist of a series of intervals marked by 1 or more brief separations from care.

F. Reexamination

The physical therapist reexamines the patient/client as necessary during an episode of care, during follow-up visits/encounters after an episode of care, or periodically in the case of chronic care management, to evaluate progress or change in patient/client status. The physical therapist modifies the plan of care accordingly or concludes the episode of care.

G. Conclusion of Episode of Care

The physical therapist concludes an episode of care when the anticipated goals or expected outcomes for the patient/client have been achieved, when the patient/client is unable to continue to progress toward goals, or when the physical therapist determines that the patient/client will no longer benefit from physical therapy.

H. Communication/Coordination/Documentation

The physical therapist communicates, coordinates, and documents all aspects of patient/client management including the results of the initial examination and evaluation, diagnosis, prognosis, plan of care, intervention, responses to intervention, changes in patient/client status relative to the intervention, reexamination, and episode of care summary. The physical therapist of record is responsible for "hand off" communication.

IV. Education

The physical therapist is responsible for individual professional development. The physical therapist assistant is responsible for individual career development.

The physical therapist and the physical therapist assistant, under the direction and supervision of the physical therapist, participate in the education of students.

The physical therapist educates and provides consultation to consumers and the general public regarding the purposes and benefits of physical therapy.

The physical therapist educates and provides consultation to consumers and the general public regarding the roles of the physical therapist and the physical therapist assistant.

V. Research

The physical therapist applies research findings to practice and encourages, participates in, and promotes activities that establish the outcomes of patient/client management provided by the physical therapist.

VI. Community Responsibility

The physical therapist demonstrates community responsibility by participating in community and community agency activities, educating the public, formulating public policy, or providing pro bono physical therapy services.

(See also Board of Directors standard Criteria for Standards of Practice)

(Clinical Practice Department, ext 3176)

Explanation of Reference Numbers:
BOD P00-00-00-00 stands for Board of Directors/month/year/page/vote in the Board of Directors Minutes; the "P" indicates that it is a position (see below). For example, BOD P11-97-06-18 means that this position can be found in the November 1997 Board of Directors minutes on Page 6 and that it was Vote 18.

P: Position | S: Standard | G: Guideline | Y: Policy | R: Procedure

Appendix 12-B

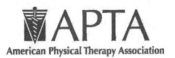

Last Updated: 04/15/14
Contact: nationalgovernance@apta.org

CRITERIA FOR STANDARDS OF PRACTICE FOR PHYSICAL THERAPY BOD S01-14-01-01 [Amended BOD S03-06-16-38; BOD S03-05-14-38; BOD 03-04-19-44; BOD 03-00-22-53; BOD 11-99-20-53; BOD 03-99-15-45; BOD 02-97-03-05; BOD 03-95-22-58; BOD 11-94-30-100; BOD 03-93-21-58; BOD 03-91-31-79; BOD 03-89-28-88; Initial BOD 11-85-13-56] [Standard]

The *Standards of Practice for Physical Therapy* (HOD S06-13-22-15) are promulgated by APTA's House of Delegates; Criteria for the Standards are promulgated by APTA's Board of Directors. Criteria are italicized beneath the Standards to which they apply.

Preamble
The physical therapy profession's commitment to society is to promote optimal health and functioning in individuals by pursuing excellence in practice. The American Physical Therapy Association attests to this commitment by adopting and promoting the following *Standards of Practice for Physical Therapy*. These standards are the profession's statement of conditions and performances that are essential for provision of high-quality professional service to society, and they provide a foundation for assessment of physical therapist practice.

I. Ethical/Legal Considerations
   A. Ethical Considerations
      The physical therapist practices according to the *Code of Ethics* of the American Physical Therapy Association.

      The physical therapist assistant complies with the *Standards of Ethical Conduct for the Physical Therapist Assistant* of the American Physical Therapy Association.

   B. Legal Considerations
      The physical therapist complies with all the legal requirements of jurisdictions regulating the practice of physical therapy.

      The physical therapist assistant complies with all the legal requirements of jurisdictions regulating the work of the physical therapist assistant.

II. Administration of the Physical Therapy Service
   A. Statement of Mission, Purposes, and Goals
      The physical therapy service has a statement of mission, purposes, and goals that reflects the needs and interests of the patients/clients served, the physical therapy personnel affiliated with the service, and the community.

      The statement of mission, purposes, and goals:
      • *Defines the scope and limitations of the physical therapy service.*
      • *Identifies the goals and objectives of the service.*
      • *Is reviewed annually.*

   B. Organizational Plan
      The physical therapy service has a written organizational plan.

      The organizational plan:
      • *Describes relationships among components within the physical therapy service and, where the service is part of a larger organization, between the service and the other components of that organization.*
      • *Ensures that the service is directed by a physical therapist.*
      • *Defines supervisory structures within the service.*
      • *Reflects current personnel functions.*

   C. Policies and Procedures
      The physical therapy service has written policies and procedures that reflect the operation, mission, purposes, and goals of the service, and are consistent with the association's standards, policies, positions, guidelines, and *Code of Ethics*.

The written policies and procedures:
- *Are reviewed regularly and revised as necessary.*
- *Meet the requirements of federal and state law and external agencies.*
- *Apply to, but are not limited to:*
  - *Care of patients/clients, including guidelines*
  - *Clinical education*
  - *Clinical research*
  - *Collaboration*
  - *Collection of patient data*
  - *Competency assessment*
  - *Criteria for access to care*
  - *Criteria for initiation and continuation of care*
  - *Criteria for referral to other appropriate healthcare providers*
  - *Criteria for termination of care*
  - *Documentation*
  - *Environmental safety*
  - *Equipment maintenance*
  - *Fiscal management*
  - *Handoff communication/therapist of record*
  - *Improvement of quality of care and performance of services*
  - *Infection control*
  - *Job/position descriptions*
  - *Medical emergencies*
  - *Personnel-related policies*
  - *Rights of patients/clients*
  - *Staff orientation*

D. Administration

A physical therapist is responsible for the direction of the physical therapy service.

The physical therapist responsible for the direction of the physical therapy service:
- *Ensures compliance with local, state, and federal requirements.*
- *Ensures compliance with current APTA documents, including* Standards of Practice for Physical Therapy and the Criteria, Guide to Physical Therapist Practice, Code of Ethics, Guide for Professional Conduct, Standards of Ethical Conduct for the Physical Therapist Assistant, *and* Guide for Conduct of the Physical Therapist Assistant.
- *Ensures that services are consistent with the mission, purposes, and goals of the physical therapy service.*
- *Ensures that services are provided in accordance with established policies and procedures.*
- *Ensures that the process for assignment and reassignment of physical therapist staff (handoff communication) supports individual physical therapist responsibility to their patients and meets the needs of the patients/clients.*
- *Reviews and updates policies and procedures.*
- *Provides for training of physical therapy support personnel that ensures continuing competence for their job description.*
- *Provides for continuous in-service training on safety issues and for periodic safety inspection of equipment by qualified individuals.*

E. Fiscal Management

The director of the physical therapy service, in consultation with physical therapy staff and appropriate administrative personnel, participates in the planning for and allocation of resources. Fiscal planning and management of the service is based on sound accounting principles.

The fiscal management plan:
- *Includes a budget that provides for optimal use of resources.*
- *Ensures accurate recording and reporting of financial information.*
- *Ensures compliance with legal requirements.*
- *Allows for cost-effective utilization of resources.*
- *Uses a fee schedule that is consistent with the cost of physical therapy services and that is within customary norms of fairness and reasonableness.*
- *Considers option of providing pro bono services.*

F. Improvement of Quality of Care and Performance
The physical therapy service has a written plan for continuous improvement of quality of care and performance of services.

> *The improvement plan:*
> - *Provides evidence of ongoing review and evaluation of the physical therapy service.*
> - *Provides a mechanism for documenting improvement in quality of care and performance.*
> - *Is consistent with requirements of external agencies, as applicable.*

G. Staffing
The physical therapy personnel affiliated with the physical therapy service have demonstrated competence and are sufficient to achieve the mission, purposes, and goals of the service.

> *The physical therapy service:*
> - *Meets all legal requirements regarding licensure and certification of appropriate personnel.*
> - *Ensures that the level of expertise within the service is appropriate to the needs of the patients/clients served.*
> - *Provides appropriate professional and support personnel to meet the needs of the patient/client population.*

H. Staff Development
The physical therapy service has a written plan that provides for appropriate and ongoing staff development.

> *The staff development plan:*
> - *Includes self-assessment, individual goal setting, and organizational needs in directing continuing education and learning activities.*
> - *Includes strategies for lifelong learning and professional and career development.*
> - *Includes mechanisms to foster mentorship activities.*
> - *Includes knowledge of clinical research methods and analysis.*

I. Physical Setting
The physical setting is designed to provide a safe and accessible environment that facilitates fulfillment of the mission, purposes, and goals of the physical therapy service. The equipment is safe and sufficient to achieve the purposes and goals of physical therapy.

> *The physical setting:*
> - *Meets all applicable legal requirements for health and safety.*
> - *Meets space needs appropriate for the number and type of patients/clients served.*
>
> *The equipment:*
> - *Meets all applicable legal requirements for health and safety.*
> - *Is inspected routinely.*

J. Collaboration
The physical therapy service collaborates with all disciplines as appropriate.

> *The collaboration when appropriate:*
> - *Uses a team approach to the care of patients/clients.*
> - *Provides instruction of patients/clients and families.*
> - *Ensures professional development and continuing education.*

III. Patient/Client Management

A. Physical Therapist of Record
The physical therapist of record is the therapist who assumes responsibility for patient/client management and is accountable for the coordination, continuation, and progression of the plan of care.

B. Patient/Client Collaboration
Within the patient/client management process, the physical therapist and the patient/client establish and maintain an ongoing collaborative process of decision making that exists throughout the provision of services.

C. Initial Examination/Evaluation/Diagnosis/Prognosis
    The physical therapist performs an initial examination and evaluation to establish a diagnosis and prognosis prior
    to intervention. Wellness and prevention visits/encounters may occur without the presence of disease, illness,
    impairments, activity limitations, or participation restrictions.

    The physical therapist examination:
    - *Is documented, dated, and appropriately authenticated by the physical therapist who performed it.*
    - *Identifies the physical therapy needs of the patient/client.*
    - *Incorporates appropriate tests and measures to facilitate outcome measurement.*
    - *Produces data that are sufficient to allow evaluation, diagnosis, prognosis, and the establishment of a
      plan of care.*
    - *May result in recommendations for additional services to meet the needs of the patient/client.*

D. Plan of Care
    The physical therapist establishes a plan of care and manages the needs of the patient/client based on the
    examination, evaluation, diagnosis, prognosis, goals, and outcomes of the planned interventions for identified
    impairments, activity limitations, and participation restrictions.

    The physical therapist involves the patient/client and appropriate others in the planning, anticipated goals and
    expected outcomes, proposed frequency and duration, and implementation of the plan of care.

    The plan of care:
    - *Is based on the examination, evaluation, diagnosis, and prognosis.*
    - *Identifies goals and outcomes.*
    - *Describes the proposed intervention, including frequency and duration.*
    - *Includes documentation that is dated and appropriately authenticated by the physical therapist who
      established the plan of care.*

E. Intervention
    The physical therapist provides or directs and supervises the physical therapy intervention consistent with the
    results of the examination, evaluation, diagnosis, prognosis, and plan of care. The physical therapy intervention
    may be provided in an episode of care, or in a single visit/encounter such as for a wellness and prevention
    visit/encounter or a specialty consultation or for a follow-up visit/encounter after episodes of care, or may be
    provided intermittently over longer periods of time in cases of managing chronic conditions.

    An *episode of care* is the managed care provided for a specific problem or condition during a set time period and
    can be given either for a short period or on a continuous basis, or it may consist of a series of intervals marked by
    1 or more brief separations from care.

    The intervention:
    - *Is based on the examination, evaluation, diagnosis, prognosis, and plan of care.*
    - *Is provided under the ongoing direction and supervision of the physical therapist.*
    - *Is provided in such a way that directed and supervised responsibilities are commensurate with the
      qualifications and the legal limitations of the physical therapist assistant.*
    - *Is altered in accordance with changes in response or status.*
    - *Is provided at a level that is consistent with current physical therapy practice.*
    - *Is interdisciplinary when necessary to meet the needs of the patient/client.*
    - *Documentation of the intervention is consistent with the <u>Guidelines: Physical Therapy Documentation of
      Patient/Client Management</u>.*
    - *Is dated and appropriately authenticated by the physical therapist or, when permissible by law, by the
      physical therapist assistant.*

F. Reexamination
    The physical therapist reexamines the patient/client as necessary during an episode of care, during follow-up
    visits/encounters after an episode of care, or periodically in the case of chronic care management, to evaluate
    progress or change in patient/client status. The physical therapist modifies the plan of care accordingly or
    concludes the episode of care.

    The physical therapist reexamination:
    - *Is documented, dated, and appropriately authenticated by the physical therapist who performs it.*
    - *Includes modifications to the plan of care.*

G. Conclusion of Episode of Care
    The physical therapist concludes an episode of care when the anticipated goals or expected outcomes for the patient/client have been achieved, when the patient/client is unable to continue to progress toward goals, or when the physical therapist determines that the patient/client will no longer benefit from physical therapy.

    Conclusion of care documentation:
    - *Includes the status of the patient/client at the conclusion of care and the goals and outcomes attained.*
    - *Is dated and appropriately authenticated by the physical therapist who concluded the episode of care.*
    - *Includes, when a patient/client is discharged prior to attainment of goals and outcomes, the status of the patient/client and the rationale for discontinuation.*

H. Communication/Coordination/Documentation
    The physical therapist communicates, coordinates, and documents all aspects of patient/client management including the results of the initial examination and evaluation, diagnosis, prognosis, plan of care, intervention, responses to intervention, changes in patient/client status relative to the intervention, reexamination, and episode of care summary. The physical therapist of record is responsible for "hand off" communication.

    Physical therapist documentation:
    - *Is dated and appropriately authenticated by the physical therapist who performed the examination and established the plan of care.*
    - *Is dated and appropriately authenticated by the physical therapist who performed the intervention or, when allowable by law or regulations, by the physical therapist assistant who performed specific components of the intervention as selected by the supervising physical therapist.*
    - *Is dated and appropriately authenticated by the physical therapist who performed the reexamination, and includes modifications to the plan of care.*
    - *Is dated and appropriately authenticated by the physical therapist who performed the episode of care summary and includes the status of the patient/client and the goals and outcomes achieved.*
    - *Includes, when a patient's/client's care is concluded prior to achievement of goals and outcomes, the status of the patient/client and the rationale for conclusion of care.*
    - *As appropriate, records patient data using a method that allows collective analysis.*

IV. Education
     The physical therapist is responsible for individual professional development. The physical therapist assistant is responsible for individual career development.

     The physical therapist and the physical therapist assistant, under the direction and supervision of the physical therapist, participate in the education of students.

     The physical therapist educates and provides consultation to consumers and the general public regarding the purposes and benefits of physical therapy.

     The physical therapist educates and provides consultation to consumers and the general public regarding the roles of the physical therapist and the physical therapist assistant.

     The physical therapist:
     - *Educates and provides consultation to consumers and the general public regarding the roles of the physical therapist, the physical therapist assistant, and other support personnel.*

V. Research
    The physical therapist applies research findings to practice and encourages, participates in, and promotes activities that establish the outcomes of patient/client management provided by the physical therapist.

    The physical therapist:
    - *Ensures that their knowledge of research literature related to practice is current.*
    - *Ensures that the rights of research subjects are protected, and the integrity of research is maintained.*
    - *Participates in the research process as appropriate to individual education, experience, and expertise.*
    - *Educates physical therapists, physical therapist assistants, students, other health professionals, and the general public about the outcomes of physical therapist practice.*

VI. Community Responsibility
The physical therapist demonstrates community responsibility by participating in community and community agency activities, educating the public, formulating public policy, or providing pro bono physical therapy services.

The physical therapist:
- *Participates in community and community agency activities.*
- *Educates the public, including prevention, education, and health promotion.*
- *Helps formulate public policy.*
- *Provides pro bono physical therapy services.*

(See also Board of Directors standard <u>Criteria for Standards of Practice</u>)

(Clinical Practice Department, ext 3176)

Explanation of Reference Numbers:
<u>BOD P00-00-00-00</u> stands for Board of Directors/month/year/page/vote in the Board of Directors Minutes; the "P" indicates that it is a position (see below). For example, BOD P11-97-06-18 means that this position can be found in the November 1997 Board of Directors minutes on Page 6 and that it was Vote 18.

P: Position | S: Standard | G: Guideline | Y: Policy | R: Procedure

Reprinted from Criteria for Standards of Practice for Physical Therapy, with permission of the American Physical Therapy Association. Available at http://www.apta.org/uploadedFiles/APTAorg/About_Us/Policies/BOD/Practice/CriteriaforStandardsofPractice.pdf. © 2012 American Physical Therapy Association.

Code of Ethics for the Physical Therapist

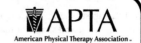

HOD S06-09-07-12 [Amended HOD S06-00-12-23; HOD 06-91-05-05;HOD 06-87-11-17; HOD 06-81-06-18; HOD 06-78-06-08; HOD 06-78-06-07; HOD 06-77-18-30; HOD 06-77-17-27; Initial HOD 06-73-13-24] [Standard]

Preamble

The Code of Ethics for the Physical Therapist (Code of Ethics) delineates the ethical obligations of all physical therapists as determined by the House of Delegates of the American Physical Therapy Association (APTA). The purposes of this Code of Ethics are to:

1. Define the ethical principles that form the foundation of physical therapist practice in patient/client management, consultation, education, research, and administration.

2. Provide standards of behavior and performance that form the basis of professional accountability to the public.

3. Provide guidance for physical therapists facing ethical challenges, regardless of their professional roles and responsibilities.

4. Educate physical therapists, students, other health care professionals, regulators, and the public regarding the core values, ethical principles, and standards that guide the professional conduct of the physical therapist.

5. Establish the standards by which the American Physical Therapy Association can determine if a physical therapist has engaged in unethical conduct.

No code of ethics is exhaustive nor can it address every situation. Physical therapists are encouraged to seek additional advice or consultation in instances where the guidance of the Code of Ethics may not be definitive.

This Code of Ethics is built upon the five roles of the physical therapist (management of patients/clients, consultation, education, research, and administration), the core values of the profession, and the multiple realms of ethical action (individual, organizational, and societal). Physical therapist practice is guided by a set of seven core values: accountability, altruism, compassion/caring, excellence, integrity, professional duty, and social responsibility. Throughout the document the primary core values that support specific principles are indicated in parentheses. Unless a specific role is indicated in the principle, the duties and obligations being delineated pertain to the five roles of the physical therapist. Fundamental to the Code of Ethics is the special obligation of physical therapists to empower, educate, and enable those with impairments, activity limitations, participation restrictions, and disabilities to facilitate greater independence, health, wellness, and enhanced quality of life.

Principles

Principle #1: Physical therapists shall respect the inherent dignity and rights of all individuals.
(Core Values: Compassion, Integrity)

1A. Physical therapists shall act in a respectful manner toward each person regardless of age, gender, race, nationality, religion, ethnicity, social or economic status, sexual orientation, health condition, or disability.

1B. Physical therapists shall recognize their personal biases and shall not discriminate against others in physical therapist practice, consultation, education, research, and administration.

Principle #2: Physical therapists shall be trustworthy and compassionate in addressing the rights and needs of patients/clients.
(Core Values: Altruism, Compassion, Professional Duty)

2A. Physical therapists shall adhere to the core values of the profession and shall act in the best interests of patients/clients over the interests of the physical therapist.

2B. Physical therapists shall provide physical therapy services with compassionate and caring behaviors that incorporate the individual and cultural differences of patients/clients.

2C. Physical therapists shall provide the information necessary to allow patients or their surrogates to make informed decisions about physical therapy care or participation in clinical research.

2D. Physical therapists shall collaborate with patients/clients to empower them in decisions about their health care.

2E. Physical therapists shall protect confidential patient/client information and may disclose confidential information to appropriate authorities only when allowed or as required by law.

Principle #3: Physical therapists shall be accountable for making sound professional judgments.
(Core Values: Excellence, Integrity)

3A. Physical therapists shall demonstrate independent and objective professional judgment in the patient's/client's best interest in all practice settings.

3B. Physical therapists shall demonstrate professional judgment informed by professional standards, evidence (including current literature and established best practice), practitioner experience, and patient/client values.

3C. Physical therapists shall make judgments within their scope of practice and level of expertise and shall communicate with, collaborate with, or refer to peers or other health care professionals when necessary.

3D. Physical therapists shall not engage in conflicts of interest that interfere with professional judgment.

3E. Physical therapists shall provide appropriate direction of and communication with physical therapist assistants and support personnel.

Principle #4: Physical therapists shall demonstrate integrity in their relationships with patients/clients, families, colleagues, students, research participants, other health care providers, employers, payers, and the public.
(Core Value: Integrity)

4A. Physical therapists shall provide truthful, accurate, and relevant information and shall not make misleading representations.

4B. Physical therapists shall not exploit persons over whom they have supervisory, evaluative or other authority (eg, patients/clients, students, supervisees, research participants, or employees).

4C. Physical therapists shall discourage misconduct by health care professionals and report illegal or unethical acts to the relevant authority, when appropriate.

4D. Physical therapists shall report suspected cases of abuse involving children or vulnerable adults to the appropriate authority, subject to law.

4E. Physical therapists shall not engage in any sexual relationship with any of their patients/clients, supervisees, or students.

4F. Physical therapists shall not harass anyone verbally, physically, emotionally, or sexually.

Principle #5: Physical therapists shall fulfill their legal and professional obligations.
(Core Values: Professional Duty, Accountability)

5A. Physical therapists shall comply with applicable local, state, and federal laws and regulations.

5B. Physical therapists shall have primary responsibility for supervision of physical therapist assistants and support personnel.

5C. Physical therapists involved in research shall abide by accepted standards governing protection of research participants.

5D. Physical therapists shall encourage colleagues with physical, psychological, or substance-related impairments that may adversely impact their professional responsibilities to seek assistance or counsel.

5E. Physical therapists who have knowledge that a colleague is unable to perform their professional responsibilities with reasonable skill and safety shall report this information to the appropriate authority.

5F. Physical therapists shall provide notice and information about alternatives for obtaining care in the event the physical therapist terminates the provider relationship while the patient/client continues to need physical therapy services.

Principle #6: Physical therapists shall enhance their expertise through the lifelong acquisition and refinement of knowledge, skills, abilities, and professional behaviors.
(Core Value: Excellence)

6A. Physical therapists shall achieve and maintain professional competence.

6B. Physical therapists shall take responsibility for their professional development based on critical self-assessment and reflection on changes in physical therapist practice, education, health care delivery, and technology.

6C. Physical therapists shall evaluate the strength of evidence and applicability of content presented during professional development activities before integrating the content or techniques into practice.

6D. Physical therapists shall cultivate practice environments that support professional development, lifelong learning, and excellence.

Principle #7: Physical therapists shall promote organizational behaviors and business practices that benefit patients/clients and society.
(Core Values: Integrity, Accountability)

7A. Physical therapists shall promote practice environments that support autonomous and accountable professional judgments.

7B. Physical therapists shall seek remuneration as is deserved and reasonable for physical therapist services.

7C. Physical therapists shall not accept gifts or other considerations that influence or give an appearance of influencing their professional judgment.

7D. Physical therapists shall fully disclose any financial interest they have in products or services that they recommend to patients/clients.

7E. Physical therapists shall be aware of charges and shall ensure that documentation and coding for physical therapy services accurately reflect the nature and extent of the services provided.

7F. Physical therapists shall refrain from employment arrangements, or other arrangements, that prevent physical therapists from fulfilling professional obligations to patients/clients.

Principle #8: Physical therapists shall participate in efforts to meet the health needs of people locally, nationally, or globally.
(Core Value: Social Responsibility)

8A. Physical therapists shall provide pro bono physical therapy services or support organizations that meet the health needs of people who are economically disadvantaged, uninsured, and underinsured.

8B. Physical therapists shall advocate to reduce health disparities and health care inequities, improve access to health care services, and address the health, wellness, and preventive health care needs of people.

8C. Physical therapists shall be responsible stewards of health care resources and shall avoid overutilization or underutilization of physical therapy services.

8D. Physical therapists shall educate members of the public about the benefits of physical therapy and the unique role of the physical therapist.

Glossary

Accountable care organization (ACO) Network of healthcare providers who are financially incentivized to provide high-value quality care to Medicare beneficiaries.

Activity Execution of a task or action by an individual.

Activity limitations A component of the ICF model that defines the difficulties an individual may have in executing tasks or actions.

Advanced Beneficiary Notice (ABN) Indicates that the Medicare beneficiary will agree to pay out of pocket or via a secondary insurance provider for therapy services received in the event that Medicare does not cover the services provided.

Affordable Care Act (ACA) A federal law passed in 2010, developed to initiate comprehensive healthcare reform over a period of years to implement new consumer protections, improve quality, lower costs, and increase access to affordable health care.

Algorithm A process or set of rules to be followed in an episode of care.

Anticipated goals Statements that are patient- or client-centered, objective, measurable, functional, and include a time element for meeting the goal.

Biopsychosocial Indicates that one's level of disability is an accumulation of the characteristics of a pathologic process or medical condition, of personal qualities inherent to an individual, and of the social and physical aspects of one's environment.

Body functions Physiological functions of body systems (including psychological functions).

Body structures Anatomical parts of the body such as organs, limbs, and their components.

Clinical decision making A dynamic process used by clinicians to synthesize data collected from an encounter with a patient or client.

Clinical decision support A feature of an electronic documentation system that assists the system's user to make clinical decisions (computerized reminders, information regarding medication side effects, or contraindications to care).

Clinical impression The synthesis of all of the data collected via the history, systems review, tests and measures, and outcome measures into a narrative that relays why the patient or client requires skilled physical therapy services.

Clinical reasoning The framework that supports why clinical decisions are made.

Clinical reasoning flow sheet A component of the daily note that has an inherent structure from which decisions can be made regarding interventions for each patient or client clinical encounter.

Clinical reflection The process of allowing a future behavior to be guided by a systematic and critical analysis of past actions and their consequences.

Conclusion of the episode of care summary A component of the documentation that indicates that a single episode of care has ended when the anticipated goals and expected outcomes have been met.

Contemporaneous documentation Also referred to as *point-of-service documentation* or *real-time documentation*; documentation that is completed at or around the same time as the encounter with the patient or client.

Consolidated billing A billing practice used by Medicare-certified home health agencies and skilled nursing facilities that bundles most of the expenses that a Medicare beneficiary receives while in that setting with the exception of physician's professional services fees and room and board costs.

Contextual factors A component of the ICF model that defines the physical, social, and attitudinal environment in which people live and conduct their lives.

Co-treatments Also known as "team therapy"; physical therapists or physical therapist assistants working together as a team to treat one or more patients or clients at the same time.

Current Procedural Terminology (CPT) codes Codes created by the American Medical Association in 1996 and used by the physical therapy profession that are required in order to receive payment from the payer source for skilled services provided.

Diagnosis The patient or client's health condition and reason for seeking physical therapy services.

Direct access A state mandate that allows a physical therapist to be the practitioner of choice as a patient or client's entry point into the healthcare system.

Disability 1) Nagi: a limitation in the performance of socially defined roles and tasks within a sociocultural and physical environment; 2) ICF: the boundaries of functioning; decrements in impairments in body functions and structures, limitations in activities, and restrictions in participation of life events.

Disablement A term intended to portray that there is an "impact of chronic and acute conditions on the functioning of specific body systems and on people's abilities to act in necessary, usual, expected, and personally desired ways in their society."

Documenting by exception A documentation strategy that utilizes an examination and intervention protocol that includes predetermined assessment tools, goals, outcomes, and frequency and duration of the episode of care that is not tailored to the unique needs of a patient or client.

Duration of the episode of care The amount of time the episode of care will cover (4 weeks, 8 weeks, 6 months).

Electronic communication Transmission of information using methods such as e-mail.

Electronic health record A digital collection of a patient's health information.

Enablement A term intended to portray that disability is not the fundamental consequence of impairments and functional limitations.

8-Minute Rule A guideline for billing each unit of timed CPT codes created by the Centers for Medicare & Medicaid Services.

Episode of care summary Part of the physical therapy plan of care indicating that a single episode of care has ended.

Examination A process of collecting, synthesizing, analyzing, and interpreting data with your patient or client to determine the need for skilled physical therapy services; includes a history, systems review, test and measures and outcome measures, evaluation, prognosis, anticipated goals and expected outcomes, the frequency and duration of the episode of care, and the intervention plan.

Expected outcomes The functional status you expect your patient or client to achieve by the conclusion of the episode of care.

Evaluation A part of the initial examination that includes the synopsis of the patient or client's response to tests and measures and outcome measures that includes the integration of this information with information collected during the history and systems review to develop the diagnosis and clinical impression.

Feedback process Action that uses the details of a response to make further decisions.

Feedforward process Action that requires prior knowledge of an intended outcome or consequence to make further decisions.

Flow sheet A component of the daily note used to relay intervention details for each patient or client clinical encounter.

Frequency of the episode of care How often physical therapy services are provided to the patient or client (two times per day, three times per week, daily).

Functional limitation reporting (FLR) The use of nonpayable G-codes that are submitted with a patient or client's billing claim by healthcare professionals to capture information about a Medicare Part B beneficiary's activity limitations and participation restrictions.

Functional limitations A component of the Nagi model that defines limitations in performance at the level of the whole person.

Functioning The body functions and structures that permit an individual to experience activities and participate in life situations.

G-codes Codes with a descriptor, a severity modifier, and a therapy modifier used for functional limitation reporting to the Centers for Medicare & Medicaid Services for Medicare Part B beneficiaries.

G-code descriptor A categorical term used to classify a Medicare beneficiary's activity limitations or participation restrictions for functional limitation reporting.

G-code severity modifier An estimate assigned to a Medicare beneficiary's degree or level of functional limitation expressed as a percentage based on the data collected at an initial examination as well as a therapist's clinical expertise.

G-code therapy modifier A code that signifies which therapy discipline—physical, occupational or speech language pathology—submits G-codes for functional limitation reporting.

Goal achievement status A patient or client's progress toward the goals established at the initial examination as well as any additional goals that were added.

Group therapy 1) Outpatient setting: therapy provided simultaneously to at least two patients or clients who have similar or differing therapy needs as long as the therapist providing the group therapy gives constant attendance and provides skilled medically necessary services; 2) Long-term care setting: therapy provided simultaneously to no more and no less than four patients or clients who are performing the same or similar activities.

Health condition A component of the ICF model that defines the disease, disorder, or injury as analogous to the medical diagnosis.

Health Information Technology for Economic and Clinical Health (HITECH) Act A federal law passed in 2009 designed to promote the adoption and meaningful use of health information technology.

Health Insurance Portability and Accountability Act (HIPAA) A federal law passed in 1996 that dictates laws and rules that exist to impart privacy and security measures to protect a patient or client's personal health information.

Healthcare Common Procedure Coding System (HCPCS) A coding scheme developed by the Centers for Medicare & Medicaid Services that incorporated the fourth edition of CPT codes developed by the American Medical Association in 1983; used by physical therapists and physical therapist assistants to report the skilled services provide during an encounter with a patient or client.

History A part of the initial examination that includes a systematic gathering of data related to why a patient or client is seeking physical therapy services.

Home exercise program A unique and tailored intervention program issued to a patient or client and/or caregiver intended to be completed outside the context of the physical therapy encounter; has the following characteristics: effective, efficient, salient, individualized, brief, and explicit.

Impairment 1) Nagi: anatomical, physiological, mental, or emotional abnormalities or loss; 2) ICF: problems in body functions or structures such as a significant deviation or loss.

Initial examination The first evaluation of a patient or client's health status to determine a therapeutic course of action.

Inpatient Quality Reporting (IQR) Program Reporting on the care of and mortality of those admitted to acute care facilities with myocardial infarction, heart failure, pneumonia, or stroke, patient or client satisfaction, safety, hospital-associated infections, hospital-acquired conditions, immunization measures, emergency department throughput, and cost efficiency.

International Classification of Diseases (ICD) A diagnostic coding schema created by the World Health Organization to organize and code health information used for epidemiology, national mortality and morbidity statistics, resource allocation, research, primary care, prevention, healthcare management, and reimbursement.

International Classification of Functioning, Disability, and Health (ICF) Model A conceptual framework rooted in biopsychosocial concepts that assists a clinician in describing a patient or client's level of functioning and ability in life.

Intervention plan A conclusion or summary statement in the episode of care that relays the framework for the actual intervention approaches and techniques implemented during patient or client encounters.

KX modifier A modifier attached to billing codes to signify that a Medicare beneficiary requires medically necessary outpatient care that exceeds the therapy cap; part of the automatic exceptions process to the therapy cap.

Lack of substance When documentation does not relay to the consumer of the entry what was done, why it was done, and the effect of what was done.

Letter of medical necessity A written communication documenting that activities are reasonable, necessary, and/or appropriate, according to evidence-based clinical standards of care.

Level I Healthcare Common Procedural Coding System (HCPCS) codes Five-digit codes referred to as the "97000 series" and labeled as "Physical Medical and Rehabilitation" codes that are used by physical therapists and physical therapist assistants to define skilled services provided to a patient or client.

Level II Healthcare Common Procedural Coding System (HCPCS) codes Four-digit codes preceded by a letter for services that do not have a corresponding Level I HCPCS/CPT code such as durable medical equipment, medical supplies, prosthetics, and orthotics.

Maintenance therapy Physical therapy interventions that address needs for a patient or client that could not be addressed safely and effectively through the use of nonskilled personnel.

Manual medical review A level of the exceptions process that requires a review of therapy documentation that is implemented when a Medicare beneficiary exceeds a predetermined annual amount for outpatient therapy services received.

Medical malpractice Also referred to as medical negligence; the primary way any litigant, usually known as a plaintiff, proves that a healthcare provider was negligent.

Medical negligence Action or lack of action (error of omission) during a medical procedure that can lead to illness, disability, or death.

Minimal clinically important difference (MCID) The smallest amount of change in the results of a test or measure that would be perceived by a patient or client as a meaningful change in the attribute being assessed; a measure of clinical relevance.

Minimal detectable change (MDC) A statistical value based on the standard error of measurement that represents the smallest difference between the test values from initial exam to follow-up that is necessary to be confident that a true change has actually occurred; a measure of statistical significance.

Minimum Data Set (MDS) The process required by the Centers for Medicare & Medicaid Services to report and document the use of quality measures in Medicare-certified skilled nursing facilities.

Modified procedure Process where some change has been made to the standard procedure of performing a test or measure, which may or may not have been tested for reliability or validity in the literature.

Nagi disablement model A disablement model that emphasizes that a pathology leads to impairments and abnormalities at the body systems level that in turn defines one's functional limitations and level of disability.

Nonverbal communication Communication through gestures, facial expressions, and body positions rather than spoken language.

Outcome Assessment and Information Set (OASIS) The process required by the Centers for Medicare & Medicaid Services to report and document the use of quality measures in Medicare-certified home health agencies.

Outcome measure A tool that has established validity and can be used to determine the efficacy of an intervention by measuring change over time.

Paper-based documentation Method of recording patient health information using paper.

Parrot documentation When the person documenting repeats most or all of what was contained in the prior session's note.

Participation Involvement in a life situation.

Participation restrictions A component of the ICF model that defines the problems an individual may experience in involvement in life situations.

Pathology A component of the Nagi model that defines the interruption or interference with normal processes and the efforts of a person to regain a normal state.

Patient- or client-centered care Providing care that is respectful of and responsive to individual patient or client preferences, needs, and values and ensuring that these values guide all clinical decisions.

Patient-Specific Functional Scale (PSFS) A self-report outcome measure found to represent the activity component of the ICF model used to gather information during the initial examination to identify a patient or client's perception of his or her functioning and disability.

Physical Therapy Classification and Payment System (PTCPS) A healthcare payment reform initiative proposed by the American Physical Therapy Association in 2013 to transition from a payment system where services are reimbursed based on the procedures delivered over a certain period of time to a per-session payment system.

Physician Quality Reporting System (PQRS) A pay-for-performance (P4P) program created by the Centers for Medicare & Medicaid Services that penalizes eligible healthcare providers, including physical therapists, for not reporting the actual use of quality measures in the documentation of outpatient services furnished under Medicare Part B.

Point-of-service documentation Also referred to as *real-time documentation* or *contemporaneous documentation*; a patient or client's documentation is completed during the encounter with that patient or client.

Prevention Actions directed to avoiding illness and promoting health.

Prognosis An explicit statement regarding interpretation of the level of improvement or outcome a patient or client can achieve; and judgment of the time frame it may take to achieve this improvement.

Progress note Also known as *progress report* or *progress summary*; similar to a daily note but includes more detailed information regarding the patient or client's current status as compared to a previous time frame such as at the initial examination or the last re-examination.

Real-time documentation Also referred to as *point-of-service documentation* or *contemporaneous documentation*; a patient or client's documentation is completed during the encounter with that patient or client.

Reassessment The ongoing process of determining the patient or client's status before, during, and after every session.

Re-examination The process of performing selected tests and measures and outcome measures after the initial examination to evaluate progress and to modify or redirect interventions; includes a thorough reassessment of all of the components of the plan of care.

Reflection Systematic and critical analysis of past actions and their consequences in order to guide future behavior.

Reimbursement Payment by a third party such as an insurance company to a hospital, physician, or other healthcare provider for services rendered to an insured person.

Reliability A characteristic of a measurement that describes how confident a clinician can be that the values obtained from the measurement are free from error and would be the same if tested multiple times.

Responsiveness A characteristic of a measurement that describes the amount of change in value necessary to be confident that a change has truly occurred.

Self-reflection The ability to self-direct the process of clinical reflection.

SIRP A decision-driven documentation format intended to apply the context of a clinical encounter into a daily note using a clinical reasoning process; **S**tatus, **I**nterventions, **R**esponse, **P**lan.

SOAP A data-driven documentation format used to create the contents of a daily note; **S**ubjective, **O**bjective, **A**ssessment, **P**lan.

Standard error of measurement (SEM) The degree of variability expected in the values obtained from a given test assuming the testing procedures remains constant.

Standard of practice Established through peers, experts, research, and publications that state what a reasonably prudent physical therapist or physical therapist assistant would do under like circumstances.

Standard procedure One that has been previously described and tested in the literature and has been accepted as the usual method for performing a test or measure.

Successful documentation Documentation that contains the information that multiple consumers need to make sound decisions.

Systems review A part of the initial examination that includes a short assessment of four biological systems in the human body—cardiopulmonary, integumentary, musculoskeletal, and neuromuscular system—and information regarding a patient or client's communication and language abilities, cognitive and mental status, and learning style.

Technical omission Leaving detail out of your documentation that is required to process the initial examination, re-examination, or intervention as a claim for reimbursement.

Tests and measures A part of the initial examination used to gather data regarding some characteristic of your patient or client.

Therapy cap A predetermined monetary cap for an annual basis that when reached, terminates payment for outpatient physical, occupational, and speech therapy services to a Medicare beneficiary.

Third-party payer The entity who reimburses healthcare providers for the services delivered to beneficiaries enrolled in the provider's healthcare insurance plans.

Validity A characteristic of a measurement that describes the clinician's confidence that the measurement is truly measuring what it is intended to measure.

Value-based purchasing (VBP) program A program that rewards hospital systems with higher performance on clinical process and patient or client experience measures with higher payments than those paid to lower performing hospitals.

Verbal communication The use of words to express oneself.

Workers' compensation A form of insurance providing wage replacement and medical benefits to an employee injured in the course of employment in exchange for mandatory relinquishment of the employee's right to sue the employer for negligence.

Index

Note: Page numbers followed by *b*, *f*, and *t* indicate material in boxes, figures, and tables respectively.